(The Evening V

Amelia Moore

To my dearest friend
She She

love from
amelia Moore
xxx

J2 Press

J2 Press

An imprint of J2 Press
Brooklands, Nash, Buckinghamshire
MK17 0EN

www.j2press.co.uk

This paperback edition 2012 (1)

A catalogue record for this book is available from
The British Library
ISBN 978-0-9571136-5-7

This book is dedicated to our sister

Anna Göldi

May God forgive them for what they did to you

Christmas Day 1864

Yorkshire

England

Chapter 1

"They is t' Devil's footmarks, ah say," the woman shouted. The people standing in the small group outside the church stared at her. "'E wor 'ere last evenin' all right," she insisted. The group of people remained silent, fidgeting nervously, each trying hard not to draw the woman's attention to them. "An' tis plain t' see whose 'ome 'e paid visit to an' all," the woman shouted again, determined not to be ignored. "Tis t' Devil. 'E came 'ere to take care o' one of 'is own."

It was Christmas morning and as cold a day as it had been all winter. The snows had come early that December and the temperature had not risen much above freezing for some weeks. The gathering of people who came to worship that holy morning did so with something of a heavy heart. Christmas Eve it had snowed again which, although making their walk to church more difficult, was not the reason for their uneasiness. No, it was the tracks that could be seen entering their village in the night, then circling one of the cottages before leaving again, which was the source of their anxiety.

The people in the small village of Elmsley had woken up Christmas morning to find that they had been visited by what they believed to be an 'unnatural being'. Unnatural, because it left strange footprints in the snow. Unexplainable footprints. The gentle snowfall of Christmas Eve night gave witness to a visitor, whose large, deep, clear tracks showed it was an upright-walking creature with two legs, a creature however, with horny covering of foot. In other words, it had cloven hooves.

"We must not allow old superstitions to get the better of us," the pastor told his flock during the Christmas day sermon. "Those tracks could have been made by any number of different kinds of animal." Pastor Bell was doing his best to give guidance to the good people of Elmsley sitting before him in the cold, candle-lit church. But who amongst them would believe the man?

Joseph Locke, the baker, had informed the pastor very early that Christmas morning of the strange footprints left behind the night before. Knowing of the deeply irrational fears and beliefs that some Elmsley folk still held on to, Joseph thought the pastor should know of the event, so that he could talk to them about the tracks before their imaginations and fright overtook common sense.

But few amongst his flock believed the man.

After the sermon, a number of men in the congregation decided to walk around the village, following the route of the footmarks left by the visitor. Whilst not completely believing the tracks were made by the Devil, they were not so sure as to not believe it either, and therefore wanted to look at the prints more intensely. They were also interested to see whose dwelling the creature 'called' upon.

"Thomas," one of the men called out to him, seeing Thomas ahead, hurriedly making his way through the village. "Ya wor not at church today?"

"Nay," Thomas called back, "Mi wife's about ti birth. Ah have ti fetch her mam and Anna." It was now time for Thomas to bring help for Mary, his wife, as she had been in labour since the early hours of the morning. Thomas's step was fast, as he needed to return home as quickly as possible; Dru, his small son, had been left to sit with Mary.

Whilst Thomas was on his urgent errand, the group of men continued to follow the visitor's tracks and found they led them to his cottage. The footmarks in the snow showed it had circled Thomas's home and, in one place in particular, below a bedroom window, where the tracks were very deep and wide, it seemed to have stood for a time; its weight widening the print and melting the snow about its hooves.

"It stayed fer some while 'ere, judging by them marks," one of the men stated as he bent down to examine the tracks more closely.

"Aye," the others agreed in mumbled voices. Thomas arrived back at his home with Mary's mother, Elisa and her sister Anna. The three of them looked at the group of men hovering outside the cottage.

"What's 'appenin' 'ere then?" Thomas asked them, puzzled by the gathering. The two women said nothing and went straight inside to Mary.

"Tis these footmarks Tom," one man told him, pointing to the prints in the snow.

"Aye. What about 'em?" Thomas asked, still mystified.

"Do ya not find 'em strange?" another member of the group asked him.

"What are ya talkin' about man?" Thomas replied. He was becoming angry with his uninvited guests. "Mary's about ti give birth an' ah don't have time fer all this." He turned to go into his home.

"We think ya wor visited by t' Devil 'imself last night," a voice spoke up. "Look, there's 'is footmarks around yar home Tom, an' yar wife gettin' ready ti birth last night an' all. Tis a puzzle Tom, a right puzzle," the man managed to blurt out, despite the attempts of his group members to prevent him from doing so. Thomas stared at the men in shock and disgust.

"Ah'll not 'ave this," he shouted. "Now get yarselves away from mi door an' leave us alone. Do ya hear me?"

"All right Tom, all right, calm down," one of the older men in the group said, stepping forward to appease him.

"Don't all right me, Fred Furrows!" Thomas shouted back, and stood up hard against the man in a threatening manner. "Just get yarselves away from my home. Now!" he yelled aggressively. Thomas then turned his back on the group and went into his cottage, rage and anguish churning over his stomach. Once inside, he stood by the closed door to regain his composure and control. His wife was hard in labour and she needed him to be calm.

"Don't push yet Mary, take some rest," he could hear Elisa telling her daughter from their bedroom upstairs. Mary had been in labour for many hours and was near exhaustion. This was her second birth, but she had carried the baby differently from her first born. Elisa said that was because her second grandchild was certainly to be a girl.

"Thomas, take Dru fer a walk," Elisa ordered him. "Tis Mary's time." Thomas wrapped his son against the freezing cold day and took him from the cottage. Before he left however, he checked outside. The group of men had left his frontage and Thomas could see them walking towards the outskirts of the village.

"We'll go ti church an' ask t' pastor to light a candle," he told Dru, "fer our new babby." Thomas swept his son up into his arms and carried him, shoulder-high to the church, to wait for Mary's

9

birthing to be completed. Elisa returned to her daughter.

"Now my sweet, ya have ti push," she told Mary gently. Mary responded by bearing down as hard as her strength would allow.

"Good lass," Elisa said. "Ah can see t' baby's head. One more push. Come on, try now."

"Ah can't push any more mam, Ah can't," Mary complained.

"Ah know ya tired love, but ya must push as hard as ya can," Elisa lovingly stroked her daughter's head. "Take a deep breath an' push. One more, come on...that's it, the baby's head's out. Now its shoulders...push. It's coming...there," Elisa held her granddaughter's head, then her tiny wet frame, as she finally gushed from Mary's body.

"Oh mam," Mary cried as she looked upon the baby lying between her legs. "Ya wor right. Tis a girl." She rested for some moments, mesmerised by the sight of the new life she had just born. Elisa and Anna smiled at one another, Elisa holding back tears of happiness.

"Ya have ti make one more push now Mary," she told her daughter calmly. "One more ti get rid of t' afterbirth, then ya can rest." Elisa gently put her hand on her daughter's lower stomach and massaged it. "Good...there now, tis done."

Mary laid still and silent, soaked and drained with

the effort of birthing, as her mother cut the umbilical cord. Anna picked up the baby and slowly rubbed her tiny body clean, then her arms and legs, and then wrapped her in a swaddling cloth.

Elisa and Anna were present at many of the births in their village, but this was a precious moment, especially for Elisa. To bring into the world her own flesh and blood, as her mother had done for her birth and the women in her family had done so for as far back as could be remembered. This is the way it had always been. Mary reached out for her newborn.

"Mam, her mouth, is it well?" Mary asked urgently.

"Aye," Elisa replied quickly. "Sh's perfect. Her mouth is perfect. Look," she showed Mary the baby's face before settling her into her arms. Mary, relieved, kissed the little girl's head as she cradled the small bundle and delicately touched her tiny lips. She then opened the swaddling cloth to inspect the rest of her baby to make sure that everything else was also as it should be.

"Ah'm goin' to call the baby Eve, mam," Mary smiled wearily at her mother. "What do ya think of that?" She knew Elisa would be happy that she had decided to call her little girl Eve; it was Elisa's own mother's middle name and she was content that her new granddaughter was to honour her in that way.

"That's wonderful my sweet," Elisa said as she

lovingly washed Mary down. "Ya Nanna would be proud."

"Aye, ah can just see t' smile on 'er face," Anna contributed. She had grown up with Elisa. Elisa's mother had taken Anna in as a child when she was orphaned at the age of three years of age during an epidemic of influenza in the village. Anna had lost both parents and two siblings to the virus and had it not been for Elisa's family adopting her, she would have been condemned to the work house. Anna was eight years younger than Elisa, who spoilt her. Anna, in turn, idolised her 'big sister'. The pair was inseparable as children and had stayed together all through their adult lives; neither woman marrying.

"Aye, ah can just see 'er lookin' down right now an' smilin' at ya Mary," Anna told her. "Sh' loved ya so much. Never hear said a bad word against ya sh' wouldn't, even when ya wor naughty, sh' wouldn't hear of it."

Mary rested her head back into the soft pillow and smiled weakly. She remembered her grandmother so clearly, even though it had been six years since she passed; only days before Dru, her first child, was born. Mary still felt sad that her Nanna Maria had not seen her grandson come into the world.

"Sh's wi' us," Elisa had reassured her daughter at the birth of baby Dru. "Never ya worry, Nanna's 'ere looking down at her first-born grandchild."

"Ah hope sh's here now," Mary reflected. "An' ah hope sh's happy that ah give this little girl her name."

"Aye, sh' is," Elisa told her. "Now then lass, we need to get ya cleaned up proper before ya man an' little Dru come home." Once Mary had been washed and changed, Anna went to fetch Thomas and Dru from the church.

Chapter 2

"Oh Mary," Thomas said as he kissed his wife and then the baby's head gently. "Sh's beautiful, just like 'er mammy." Mary smiled. She was happy and relieved. Happy, because the birth had gone better than she had feared, after what had been a difficult pregnancy. She had fallen with child twice since the birth of her son six years ago, but had lost the babies after only a few months. So, going full-term and delivering this child safely was a great joy. It was not unusual to lose babies during pregnancy in Mary's village; it was an accepted part of life. Nor was it uncommon to have a still-born baby and for women to die in childbirth.

Although there was a doctor in the local market town, Elisa was the only kind of midwife in the community, and, with the help of Anna, they did most of the birthing amongst the poor of the parish, doing their best for those in their care. However, it was largely the strength of the mothers and babies that determined life or death. As well as the midwife, Elisa acted as something of a medicine woman, using ancient knowledge passed down through her family, of wild flowers and herbs and plants, to benefit her neighbours when they were sick.

Mary was also relieved that her precious baby girl was born perfect; she had not inherited her own cleft

14

lip.

"Sh's well Thomas," Mary told him. "Our little girl's mouth is well."

"Aye," Thomas replied, kissing Mary again. "Ah told ya the baby would be well. Dru was, wasn't he? Ah told ya not to worry."

"Ah know, but ah couldn't bear thinkin' of my child livin' wi' the same disfigurement as me," Mary said.

"That's maybe," Thomas replied caringly. "But it never stopped me choosin' you fer my wife, did it?"

"Nay, it didn't," Mary smiled. "'Tis because ya're a good man Thomas Dru Jennus, a good man."

"He is that," Elisa said, as she brought a bowl of hot rabbit broth into the bedroom for Mary. "Mary needs warmin'," Elisa told Thomas and ordered him to put more wood on the fire in the corner of the room. "Sh' needs somethin' inside her as well, to get her strength back. There's a bowl of broth fer you and Dru on t'able."

"Thank ya mam," Thomas replied. "Ah'll take my broth then look in at the smithy." He kissed Mary again.

"Now get that down ya, daughter," Elisa ordered, taking the baby from her so she could sip at the hot bowl. "When ya've finished, ah'll put baby on yar breast." Before Mary began to feed little Eve, Dru was allowed to come up and meet his new sister.

"Mammy, mammy," he shouted as he burst into

the bedroom and ran to his mother's bedside. "Where's t' babby mammy, t' babby?" he screamed out in his excitement.

"Shush Dru, shush little man," Mary calmed him. "Ya'll waken babby, an' look, sh's sleepin'. This is yar new sister. Her name is Eve," she told her son, and opened the swaddling cloth for him to get a good look at his new sibling. Dru's face changed from excitement to puzzlement, then to wonder, and then back to excitement, all in the space of a few moments.

"Can ah touch it mammy, can ah?" he asked his mother.

"Of course ya can. Be gentle now though," Mary told him and directed the boy's hand to the top of the baby's head, controlling it as he gently stroked Eve's soft brown hair.

Dru had been born with the same thick, brown mane of hair, which was hard to believe now, looking at his long golden locks. As Mary watched her little boy's fingers caressing his baby sister's head, the memories of his birth came back in her mind. Although Eve looked like Dru in many ways, Mary was becoming aware of the differences, seeing their faces side by side. From the moment Dru was born, she thought he looked like a boy and now, watching Eve, Mary could see she was clearly a little girl. The baby began to stir and make sucking noises with her mouth, her tiny lips pursing for a nipple. It was time for Eve to suckle her mother's milk.

Elisa would stay with Thomas and Mary to look after her daughter for a few days whilst she recovered from the birth, doing and caring for all the family. The delivery had taken all of Mary's strength, and Elisa would not leave until she was sure that her daughter was strong enough to manage without her.

It was only when she left their cottage and returned to her own home that she heard about the visitor to the village on Christmas Eve. Thomas had not told her anything of what the group of men had said to him outside on Christmas morning, and Elisa had not asked. A cold chill ran through her body whilst Anna was relaying the story to her, in spite of the heat rising from the large open fire by which she was sitting.

"There's been talk o' t' creature's footmarks goin' around our Mary's cottage," Anna said. "An' they reckon that it stood fer some while outside 'er bedroom window, 'cos o' t' deep prints it made int' snow just there."

"Well, they wor bound to see tracks near me or mine, weren't they?" Elisa remarked sarcastically. "Ah reckon they didn't look too hard fer 'em anywhere else, either. An' they 'onestly believe that those marks wor made by t' Devil?" she asked, laughing aloud as she said it and shaking her head in disbelief. However, behind the laughter there was some concern.

"They is sayin' that t' creature walked on two legs, 'cos there wor only two tracks set down at a time, not four, like cattle," Anna said. "They is sayin' t' creature walked upright, like a man, only it had cloven hooves, like t' Devil."

"An' how would them ignorant so-an'-sos know that then?" Elisa asked. "How would they know it only walked on two legs? There's nothin' walks on two legs an' has hooves, nothin'!" Elisa said angrily as she stared into the fire.

"That's why they is sayin' tis t' Devil," Anna replied anxiously. Her face looked frightened in the light from the fire. "Ah just hope it ain't all startin' again," she said, looking nervously across to Elisa for reassurance. "Ah just hope we don't get all that trouble startin' again," she repeated quietly.

"Aye," Elisa said simply. She continued to study the fire, thoughts crowding her mind. Anna had become more and more stressful as she told the story, but Elisa needed to be quiet and think on what she had heard.

"Stop frettin'," Elisa told Anna.

"But they won't stop talkin' about it." Anna blurted out. "They is still goin' on about how t' creature stopped outside our Mary's cottage, an' 'er birthin' that night as well. They is askin' why 'e wor interested in Mary's babby, sh' bein' born on Christmas day an' all," Anna continued. She was afraid, and beginning to babble. "Ah'm tellin' ya Eli, ah'm not happy about what they is sayin'."

"They'll have ti talk!" Elisa responded sharply. "Ah can't stop that, but if they bother my daughter, it won't just be Thomas who'll be dealin' with them. It'll be me as well."

Although dismissive, Elisa was worried about the rumours that Anna had reported to her and knew of their implications for Mary and her children, especially for baby Eve, if they did not abate. However, much to her relief, as the weeks and months passed and the bitterly cold days and nights of winter turned into spring, the visitor to Elmsley on Christmas Eve was talked of less and less. The story faded slightly into a tale that was occasionally brought up at the Bull, the local inn, and argued over; between those who believed that the Devil had visited the village that night and those that did not. Whenever it was discussed however, somebody would mention how it, the creature, stood outside the Jennus cottage, and then questions would be raised as to why it, the creature, should do such a thing. Why did it single out the Jennus home, that very night of all nights, when baby Eve was about to be born?

No one ever brought up the tale of the visitor in front of Elisa however, although she occasionally heard whisperings going about as she entered the local shops. Nor was the visitor now ever mentioned in front of Thomas. Nobody dared. He once overheard someone make a comment at the wood yard about this very thing. The man, who did not realise that Thomas was standing close by, mentioned Mary and baby Eve and how much interest the Devil seemed to have shown them. Thomas pinned the man to the side of a barn, almost chocking him to death, and it had taken three other men there to make Thomas release his grip on him. News of this confrontation soon spread around Elmsley and at least acted as something of a deterrent for others to guard their careless and derogatory remarks. It did not stop the mumbled gossiping that penetrated every crack and corner of the village however. The story would simply be added to those tales of strange happenings that surrounded the females from the Shetcliffe family lineage, Shetcliffe being Elisa's surname and Marys', before she married Thomas Jennus. And what stories they were!

However, with the coming of summer, little Eve blossomed. Mary, although slight in stature, recovered well from the birth and was able to give her baby daughter the good nourishment she needed and Eve got on very well. Although life was hard for everyone at that time, the country was at peace with the world and Mary and Thomas, along with their neighbours in the village and the local tenant farmers, were managing to sustain themselves fairly well. The previous two winters, although cold for long periods, were not as harsh as they had been known to be and with two good summers behind them, many of the farmers had built up larger herds of livestock and felt somewhat prosperous because of it.

This made a difference to the work coming into Thomas's smithy, which resided in the heart of the village, and he and Mary were living quite comfortably because of it. Thomas had been left the smithy and a small forge that stood next to it, by his father, Thomas Jennus Senior, Master Blacksmith and Master Gunsmith, who had passed away some four years earlier. Young Thomas had completed his apprenticeship with him and more than earned the right to call himself a Master Blacksmith and Gunsmith also. As well as the smithy and forge, his father had left him a cottage with a small holding of two acres at the back. It was rare for a mere tradesman to own property or land at this time, but old Tom Jennus had done a lot of good work for King James, making superior weapons for his army, and as a reward, was given the right to buy his livelihood and home. The land owner, the local Squire, whose large estate included much of Elmsley, was 'obliged', by Royal Command, to settle all the deeds on him.

On half of their land, Mary and Thomas kept chickens and geese for poultry and eggs, a few cows and a goat for milk, and fattened up pigs for slaughter. Thomas sold the surplus meat and poultry at the local market town. The rest of their land was used for grazing, growing animal feed and a small amount of produce. Life was quiet and normal for the Jennus family and, over the last few years they appeared to have achieved some respectability in the community, although Elisa knew this was largely due to Thomas. He was a mountain of a man and a physical match for any male in the village. When he took Mary as his wife, Thomas accepted the role of her protector and guardian against the prejudice that she had suffered all of her young life. Being born with a cleft lip, although slight, compared to others with the same disfigurement, had been hard for her to bear in a small, closed community. Living with any facial deformity was difficult for a woman and it marred what would have otherwise been a very pretty face. But Mary had a captivating personality and was always full of joy. She laughed at herself and refused to hide her face away, mostly due to the strength of character that her mother, Elisa, helped instil in her daughter from a child, to enable her to cope with the abnormality. When Thomas came courting her, Mary did not allow herself to feel undeserving of his love. She knew she would make him a good, loving wife and that is exactly what she had done.

Chapter 3

Elisa was a wise woman and understood how fragile existence can be. She had seen many changes of fortune in her own life and of those around her. She worried for her daughter and believed that Mary's sweet nature and oft-time poor health, made her too gentle and delicate for the harshness of the world. Elisa was also concerned that with a young child, and now a baby, Mary had to rely heavily on the strength and protection of her husband, as did all the women in the village. For Mary though, Elisa had added worries. Ever since her early childhood, Mary had been singled out. One reason for this was that she was illegitimate. Elisa had given birth to her daughter out of wedlock. Having never named the father, it was left to the speculation of the villagers as to who he was, and some of the suggestions were obscene, ludicrous and at times, dangerous for her. However, Elisa would not divulge who the father was. For whatever reasons she had, Elisa kept the identity of Mary's father a secret; one that she swore she would take to her grave.

So, when Mary was born with an obviously deformed lip, it was there for the entire world to see...God's punishment for her mother's wicked ways! Mary was shunned, humiliated and scorned as a child and as a young woman, stigmatised and isolated by the other young people in the village and local market town. Mary was also not robust. A childhood illness, one that could have taken her life, left her weak at times and vulnerable, especially during the cold winter months. Her breathing often became laboured and Elisa had to take extra care of her daughter when the damp mists of autumn came in.

When Thomas Jennus began to call on the young Mary, most of the community were shocked. He was not only a handsome and bright young man, but a Master tradesman who owned property and land. He was well-placed in the whole area, not just Elmsley, and deemed to be a very good catch for any lass. To choose therefore an 'undeserving', 'deformed' and 'sickly' creature like Mary, coming from a family of ill repute, actually caused frenzy. When Thomas announced his betrothal to her, both she and Elisa had to endure a storm of disbelief and anger from their neighbours and fight all of the old accusations and prejudices that came flooding back again.

Thomas stood fast however, and he and Mary were married in Saint Guthlac Church, much to the disgust of many in the village. Mary had not been baptised into the faith and therefore had to agree to 'become' a Christian before being allowed a church wedding. Even so, only a small number of well-wishers came to support the couple. But the day was a happy one for everyone who attended, especially for Elisa, who was relieved that a good, strong and true man had chosen her precious daughter for his wife.

Five years passed relatively calmly in Elmsley. Elisa and Anna went about giving their usual midwifery help to the women of the village who asked for it and Elisa supplied her old remedies, medicines and curing pastes to those in need. Thomas was steadily building up more custom for his smithy and forge, and was now being called upon to do work for farmers and tradesmen much further afield than Elmsley. His reputation for good work was spreading far and wide. Dru had just left the local village school to join his father in the smithy and learn Thomas's trade. Eve was also growing up fast and Mary thought it might benefit her daughter to send her to school, as most of the village children of that age were now attending, even if it was only for half a day. For the other half day, many of the youngsters over the age of ten were going to work at the local cotton and wool mills that were springing up near Ashton, the nearby market town.

Although school started well for little Eve, who was as bright as a button and excited to be so grown-up, some older children at the school decided to make her life difficult. Eve began to take home stories of her treatment at their hands. Being only just five years of age, she did not understand the taunting and jibing that was directed at her by these children, who had obviously inherited their parent's bigotry towards Mary, her mother, and her grandmother, Elisa. The bullying escalated and culminated in Eve having pebbles from the playground flicked into her face during one break in lessons. In spite of Mary's complaints to the teacher about this behaviour of some of the children however, little was done to reprimand the culprits. After a further attack on her daughter, which left Eve with cuts to her face and neck, Mary withdrew her from the school altogether. The village elders made some fuss over this at first, as the children were required to go to school, but even they conceded that there was a real threat to Eve's well-being and were contented, and probably relieved, to be reassured that she would be taught at home. The school was linked to Saint Guthlac, which had the patronage of the village elders, and the truth was, they mostly cared little for any child descending from the Shetcliffe line.

It was only after these incidents with her daughter that Mary found out her son, Dru, had also been bullied whilst attending the school, but he had never told neither her, his father nor his grandmother. Mary took this news very badly, as did Elisa. She had always suspected that Dru was being bullied, but these latest reports of her other grandchild suffering in this way upset Elisa a great deal. She had hoped that her neighbours had gotten over her past by now. But as she thought about this, she knew that was never going to be the case. Much of what she had done in her life had always been used as a weapon against her family, as she herself had suffered for her own mother's actions. She was therefore not surprised that Eve, as Mary before her, was being singled out and bullied.

The community had always sought the Shetcliffe's help in times of need, but despite that help given freely and kindly, some Elmsley folk remained uneasy and slightly fearful of the family. Others in the village were just openly hostile towards any Shetcliffe and did not miss an opportunity to dispraise them. Only a small number of villagers respected the family for their kindness and goodness and were prepared to speak up for them.

And so Mary withdrew Eve from school. She wanted to confront some of the parents of those children who had bullied her daughter, but Thomas thought it best to put the incidents behind them as soon as possible. There was really no more to be done. Although he was unafraid of anyone in the village, he did not court trouble either. Thomas was very aware of how quickly the goodwill of neighbours can turn against someone. He particularly remembered old Alfred Sacker, an agricultural servant to one of the big local farmers in the area. He was set on by the whole community. The unfortunate man was probably no more than losing his mental faculties, as he was almost eighty years-of-age. Alfred became very obstinate about things and shouted profanities a lot in public. The final straw was him blaspheming in the middle of Elmsley one day and refusing to go to church because he said that the Devil had moved in there. The community put pressure on the farmer, who Alfred had served well and under whose roof he had lived for many years, to throw him out. Alfred turned to the villagers for their charity, but the poor soul was physically driven out of Elmsley. Nobody knew what became of him, but being sick and elderly, with no home, work, or means by which to feed himself, death would have been a certainty. With the treatment of the unfortunate Alfred Sacker in his mind, Thomas wanted this whole episode to quietly settle down. He was content to see his daughter now at home with her mother.

Mary would teach Eve to read and write and have numbers herself as she had been taught by her own mother. Although Dru had attended the local school, he received far more education from Mary than he had done from there anyway. Dru was always encouraged by Thomas to learn, even though he was following him into a trade. Learning was important to the Jennus family as it had been to the Shetcliffes, going back generations. And, long before the school had been established in the village, the children of this lineage were always given an education. When Elisa was a child, there were no such schools in Elmsley. Some teaching was given to the poor of the parish at Sunday school, but generally not much learning apart from religious instruction. Some of the newly founded local factories provided their employee's children with a very basic education, but for those youngsters whose parents remained working on the land, they, for the most part, were illiterate. Elisa was one of the few children from a farm-labouring father, who could read and write at that time, which set her apart from her neighbours and their children, many of whom disliked or were envious of the fact that someone from the same labouring class should have learning.

Elisa was now comforted that her granddaughter would be safer away from the school and be protected from being bullied. It was another reminder to her that Mary must for ever be vigilant for herself and the children. Elisa, in calm moments would discuss this with her daughter, again and again, now that there was some urgency. What she would like to have told her daughter over many years, Elisa had to try to now impart to her in a short time. She would also have to pass the care of

Mary and her grandchildren entirely into the hands of Thomas. Elisa had been ill for some months and knew that she would not recover; she had an incurable disease. Over the years, Elisa had nursed others with the same illness and understood that she was dying and did not have long to live. She would have to hand over the future of the Shetcliffe line to her daughter and she hoped that Mary would be strong enough to cope with what that responsibility would bring.

The following six months were very hard for Mary. Words could not describe her anguish and desperation at the thought of losing her mother. As the days and weeks passed and Elisa became weaker and weaker, had it not been for the care of Anna and the support of Thomas, Mary would not have coped with seeing her mother slowly drift towards her end. The evening Elisa finally passed peacefully away, Mary sat holding her mother's hand until she gave up her last words and her final breath to her, the proud daughter of Elisa Maria Shetcliffe, granddaughter of Maria Eve Shetcliffe, great granddaughter of Elyse Mary Shetcliffe, and descendent of Esabel Eve Shetcliffe.

She and Anna cried all night long by Elisa's body until the morning light forced its way into the darkened room. Mary then came to the knowing that she must let her mother go from the world, if not from her heart and soul. After the fourth day of mourning was over, Elisa's body was taken from her cottage to the far north corner of the Saint Guthlac churchyard and buried, at the mercy of Pastor Bell, without ceremony, as was her wish. Elisa was laid to rest next to her mother and generations of grandmothers, who were only allowed to be buried on the north side of the church because they were not deemed to be 'good' Christian people. This mare's nest did not worry Elisa in any way; she just wanted to lay with her kinfolk for eternity.

Mary was heartbroken at her mother's funeral. She stood sobbing, her arms surrounding Eve and Dru, watching her mother's coffin slowly and quietly being lowered into the ground. Death was no stranger to any family in Elmsley, but Mary was not just losing her beloved mother, but her protector and dearest friend, and she knew that life without Elisa was going to be harder and less safe. She was now also the next in line to continue the destiny of the female line of her family and she was a little afraid and anxious for what that obligation would bring.

Summers turned into autumns and then winters, and back into springs and summers. Mary had taken her mother's place with Anna as midwife to the community, with the knowledge learnt at Elisa's side for some years. She would soon begin to pass that on to her own daughter, as Anna was getting on in years and kept talking of retiring. Mary had also been administering healing mixtures and remedies and curing pastes, as her mother had done, to any of those in the village who wanted and needed them. From a very early age, Eve had also been taught by her grandmother and mother about the ancient ways. Like all of her female ancestors before her, Eve became an apprentice to this role in readiness for when her turn would come to continue on with these duties. She became used to collecting the wild flowers, berries, fungi, plants and herbs from the local meadows, hedgerows and woodlands for her mother, and helping Mary to mix the tinctures and curing pastes for the remedies. She even ran the preparations to the homes of those in the village wanting them. Eve grew up knowing everyone in Elmsley and, apart from the occasional confrontation with some of the local children, did not feel particularly different from anyone else in any way. She was loved and cared for by wonderful parents and an older brother, who adored her, and Granny Anna, as she fondly named her.

Eve had now turned twelve and was at the crossroads between still being a child in mind but showing clear signs of womanhood with a changing shape and budding breasts. Her dark brown hair had never lightened, as Dru's had done, but remained very dark, like Mary's. Eve inherited her father's steel blue eyes however, not her mother's, which were deep brown. Dru had those, 'like deer's eyes', Elisa used to say. No, Eve's eyes were cool blue and sharp, and as her face started to take on a woman's contours, the promise of beauty began to appear. Her skin was pale and white, too pale for a peasant girl, but no amount of sun turned the milkyness of her skin dark. Her lips were becoming full and red and tempting. It was also clear that Eve was not going to be as slight in body as her mother. She was physically strong and, along with her brother Dru, she had taken some of Thomas's powerful frame. Eve was going to be a stunning woman to look at, and when her father noticed that his little girl was growing up so quickly, he knew she would have many a young lad chasing after her. She was going to break a few hearts.

Chapter 4

It had been a perfect summer that year. The rains had been gentle but steady all through the season and the local farmers' crops promised to be abundant at harvest. Mary was busy baking bread that morning and Eve was playing at the front of the cottage with her Raggy Polly, as she called the doll that her father and mother had made for her; the head, feet and hands carved out of wood by Thomas, and the soft-stuffed cloth body and arms and legs sewn together by Mary. Dru, a young man by now, was working alongside his father at the smithy as usual. He was a quick learner and a good worker, and had just completed his seven years of apprenticeship. Under Thomas's supervision, Dru was now doing some of his own small jobs; his father slowly giving him increased responsibility in the workshop. It was, by all accounts, a normal day.

As Mary pulled the tray of cooked loaves from the bread oven at the side of the large inglenook which housed it, she paused. In the pit of her stomach, she knew something was wrong. Mary looked over towards the open front door, as if expecting a dark cloud to enter the cottage and fill the room. She stared out at the bright sunlight for a few moments, listening and waiting, but there were no sounds other than the chatter-boxing of her daughter Eve to

Raggy Polly, telling her off for being naughty. But Mary strained to listen to other sounds. And then they came. At first it was a faint cry, then a louder call and then a hysterical shouting, which suddenly entered her home, followed quickly by Dru, black-faced and sweating from the heat and smoke of the smithy workshop.

"Tis father, come quick mam, tis father," he screamed at Mary. She dropped the tray of bread and ran to the door.

"Eve, stay there," she ordered her daughter then she followed Dru quickly the hundred yards or so down the lane to the smithy. There, on the floor, just inside the entrance, was Thomas. He was laying face down, his arm twisted awkwardly beneath his torso.

"Thomas!" Mary shouted as she fell on her knees and leaned forward to see to her husband. "Dru, help me," she told him. He was stood there, shocked, and looking on in a daze. Responding to his mother's plea, he bent down to his father and helped her slowly turn him over.

"Oh Thomas," Mary cried, looking at his forehead and nose, both bloodied from the fall. "What happened?" she asked Dru.

"Ah don't know mam, ah don't know," he replied. "Ah wor bringin' in some pieces of iron from out back an' when ah got here father wor on't ground."

"Did ya not see what happened to him?" Mary

asked again, but Dru just kept shaking his head and mumbling that he did not know. "Go fetch some men," she ordered her son. "Quickly. Fetch some help," Mary shouted again and Dru ran from the smithy. She very carefully rested Thomas's head on her lap and put her hand close to his nose and mouth to feel for breathing. He was alive, but clearly unconscious. As he lay cradled on her, Mary looked over her husband's body, arms and legs, but could see no obvious injuries.

"What's wrong my love?" she asked him. "What happened to ya Thomas?" she said, tears rolling down her face. She was desperately trying not to become hysterical. As she began to wipe the blood from Thomas's face with her apron, three men ran into the smithy.

"What 'appened?" one asked.

"We don't know," Mary sobbed. "Please help me get him up," she begged.

"Move back lass," another man told her and taking the weight of Thomas's head from her lap, ushered Mary away, so that the three of them and Dru could lift Thomas onto his bench, which Dru had just cleared of tools. They carefully laid him out, Mary placing a roll of cloth beneath her husband's head to cushion it from the hard wood of the bench.

"He don't seem to be injured any," one of the men said. He was Joseph from the bakery, a good friend

37

of Thomas. "Maybe he's just fainted or sommit," he continued, trying to keep Mary calm. He could see she was turning very pale and her whole body was trembling with fear. "'Tis a hot day Mary, an' there's not much air in here," he told her, searching for reasons why Thomas should have fainted.

"Aye, maybe he did faint," Mary replied, but she instinctively knew this was far more serious. "Oh, Thomas," she cried, burying her face in her hands. She then thought of her daughter.

"Go to Eve," she ordered Dru, "an' wait there fer us." Mary turned to the men. "Can ya get Thomas back to my cottage?" she asked them. They looked at one another and nodded a yes. Thomas's cart was brought around to the front of the smithy to take him home. He was a large man and it was thought best to carefully convey him back, not knowing the cause of his collapse.

Four days later, Thomas passed away without opening his eyes again. He had, according to Doctor Selby, who practised mostly in Ashton, apoplexy; the symptoms known to accompany the suffering of a stroke. Selby had been brought to Elmsley to look at Thomas by Joseph, but after his first visit, at which Mary refused to allow him to perform bloodletting on her husband, the doctor angrily withdrew his services, leaving Mary to nurse the stricken Thomas.

"Ah'll not have that man near Thomas again," she

stated to Anna, who had come to help with caring for her husband and to look after Eve. "Ah'll not have him bloodletting my Thomas," she added. "Ah've seen the results of him doin' that too many times. It does nay good. My mammy always told me never to let any doctor do it an' ah trust that, allus." Anna had heard Elisa complaining about that particular medical practice numerous times herself, but was concerned for Mary all the same. Anna had been a witness to many an argument that Elisa had with the very same doctor over bloodletting and now Mary was setting herself against the man as well. She feared that no good would come of it, and she was right.

Within days of Thomas's death, rumours, no doubt started by Doctor Selby, were spreading around the village that Mary refused to let Thomas have the medical treatment he needed to survive. Although not accusing her of actual murder, because that would have been ridiculous, the implication was that she showed little care for her husband and thus contributed to his untimely demise. Thomas had no family still living, so at least Mary was spared having to face them with such a dreadful allegation. Apart from suffering the indignity of having his authority questioned and diminished by Mary in her refusal to allow the bloodletting, the doctor was also denied what he thought was his by professional right. He wanted to carry out a post mortem on Thomas's body, but Mary would not let him do this either. Doctor Selby was furious, but as he had been witnessed in the Bull Inn by a number of villagers saying he categorically knew Thomas died of apoplexy, he could not force the issue with the village elders; the reason for death was already given, and by him.

Thomas was buried in a quiet and respectful way with just a handful of friends present. Mary, Dru and young Eve were supported by Anna and Joseph, he having made most of the arrangements. Mary was not coping at all well and had hardly spoken a word since Thomas had died. Anna was very worried about her. Mary had never been robust and was truly suffering with her loss, both physically and mentally.

She went back to work making up remedies far too soon, and whilst delivering some of them in Elmsley, Mary came face to face with the viciousness of those in the village who believed the gossip being spread around by Selby. When she heard the things they were saying about her, Mary fell into a black depression. Dru did his best to help his mother ignore this malicious gossip, but Mary's life had been shattered and she could not cope with her overwhelming grief at the loss of Thomas, and the ill feelings of some of her neighbours, from whom she needed sympathy, help and support, not cruelty. Anna eventually took Eve home to look after her whilst Mary went through her grieving and hopefully make a recovery from it. But instead of improving, she got worse over the following weeks. Mary then became a recluse. She would not leave her cottage or see anyone, other than Anna and her children. She then refused all food and just lay in a dark room day and night in a state of total distress. Anna, no matter how hard she tried, could not get through to her, nor could Dru. Eve, who was suffering herself at the sudden loss of her father, desperately needed her mother at this time, but Mary could not pull herself from the dark, despairing place she had fallen into.

"Something has to be done about Mary Jennus," Doctor Selby reported to the village elders. "She's got mania," he told them dispassionately.

"She's suffering, the poor woman," Pastor Bell remarked sympathetically. "She has just lost her husband."

"That's maybe, but she's gone into madness and should be put in to the asylum at Paddow," the doctor replied coldly.

"I do not agree," the pastor argued. "Mrs Jennus has melancholia. She's grieving for her husband." He and Doctor Selby rarely saw things the same way, but the pastor was still shocked at the extreme opinion given by him on Mary Jennus.

"Ah've seen it before," Selby told him loudly. "She'll not recover from this unless she gets proper treatment. Sommit has to be done."

"What do ya propose we do?" the other man present at the meeting asked. He was Jonathan Barlow, who was a local businessman. Barlow owned a large wool mill near Ashton where a number of Elmsley residents now worked. He had taken a modest inheritance left to him by his father and with it built himself a thriving business in the woollen industry, an industry that was just beginning to boom in that part of Yorkshire. Barlow was one of the first entrepreneurs to embrace a new mechanistic age, moving the woollen cloth-making trade from being a cottage industry into an expanding and lucrative enterprise. Because of his growing wealth and importance in the area, he had some influence and sway over the local judiciary also, but he was not the area's Justice of the Peace. That role was taken by one higher up the social scale, the elderly Squire Edmond Addington. Barlow did a lot of the work in the community that Addington should have done however, had he been bothered to, so felt he could make decisions on behalf of the J.P. in his absence.

"Ah propose she be taken to Paddow Asylum," Doctor Selby replied. "They can take care of her there."

"I really must protest doctor, this is...," the pastor tried to say something, but Barlow interrupted him.

"Ah think Doctor Selby knows best Pastor Bell," he told him. "You take care of the souls of Elmsley folk an' let the good doctor here look after their bodies an' minds." The pastor was silenced. He relied on the goodwill of the Squire for his very living, and a bad report back to him from his lap-dog, Jonathan Barlow, and he would be in trouble. He was outnumbered. As well as the doctor, Barlow also disliked the Shetcliffe family and hated their influence in the community. He was a fiercely God-fearing and devout man and could not understand why a Christian community such as Elmsley tolerated the likes of them. If he had his way, the Shetcliffes would have been driven from the village years ago. There was some bad history between his family and theirs, although nobody in the community would speak of it.

It was no surprise therefore that when he heard his eldest son James had been mixing with Eve, a child from this family, Barlow was mortified and very angry. Eve was also the daughter of a tradesman, and on her mother's side, came from peasant stock, hardly the type that he wanted his son to associate with. As his eldest boy, Barlow had very high aspirations for James.

"Mary Jennus is the mother of that wild bairn, Eve,

isn't she?" he asked the doctor.

"Yes, the child Eve is her only daughter," Selby replied.

"Aye, Ah caught her on my land encitin' James to get up to mischief," Barlow said. "She's like the rest of them Shetcliffes, she's nay good. Ah soon put a stop to her mixin' wi' my son though. Ah skelped her," he boasted.

"You beat her?" the pastor asked incredulously.

"Aye," Barlow replied. "Ah saw her talkin' to James an' ah beat her. She'll not be goin' near my boy again." He stated triumphantly, puffing out his chest as he put his hands into the small pockets either side of his garish waistcoat. The pastor was sickened upon hearing this.

"But she's just a child," Bell said.

"She might be a child, pastor, but she's still a bad-un. All the Shetcliffes are," Selby joined in. Pastor Bell felt very uneasy in the company of his colleagues. He was basically a good man, but unfortunately, a weak one. Frightened for his own interests, he knew he could not show too much concern for any member of the Shetcliffe family, even for the young Eve; it would not serve him well. Pastor Bell was not a native of Elmsley, or even from that part of Yorkshire. He had moved to the region with a young wife and two children only three years earlier from Liverpool. When he first joined the community, he had found the beliefs and attitudes of some of his flock difficult to deal with and decided that it would be his pastoral duty to curb the more extreme religious views that some of the zealous members of his parish held. A fate of fire and brimstone and being dammed to Hell for so-called unchristian behaviour lurked around every corner of Elmsley, according to some villagers who were avid believers in the Devil and his doings. The Shetcliffe family were unfortunately deemed to belong to the unchristian members of the community.

"When did you beat her?" he asked Barlow.

"Two days ago," he bragged. "Anyway, enough about the bairn. Tis the mother needs seein' to. Do what ya have to do doctor," Barlow told Selby. "Ah'll bring the whole business before Squire Addington myself, but ah'm sure he'll agree wi' our decision. If ya say the Jennus woman should be in Paddow Asylum then it must be done."

By the end of that week, Doctor Selby had called upon the staff at Paddow Lunatic Asylum to collect Mary Jennus from her cottage and take her back there. They came for her in the afternoon of Friday. Neither Dru, who was working his father's smithy by himself, nor Anna, knew what was about to be done. It was a sympathetic neighbour of Mary's who ran to the smithy and then to Anna's cottage to tell them what was happening. Dru rushed to his home, as did Anna, Eve chasing behind her. The men from the asylum had already broken down the door to Mary's cottage by the time Dru reached there. Anticipating any resistance from her son, Doctor Selby had enlisted the help of three men from the village to hold him back should he try to prevent the Paddow staff from taking his mother. He also had Elmsley's police officer, Samuel Jowett, present at the Jennus home to show that the action was enforced by the law. Dru ran as fast as he could; the screams he heard from his mother as he neared the cottage, piercing his brain. By the time he reached it Mary was being carried out by two men, having already been physically restrained in a jacket and now gagged around her mouth. As the realisation of what was happening sunk in, Dru became aggressive and tried to pull one of the men off of his mother. The other men from the village 'hired' by the doctor stepped forward and tussled him to the ground, the largest pinning the youngster to the floor. Meanwhile, Doctor Selby stood in front of the cottage watching the procedure with cold indifference. He stonily glanced at Mary as she was carried past him.

"Leave mi mam alone," Dru screamed and struggled hopelessly beneath the weight of the man. "Leave her," he yelled again, but the Paddow men continued with their job and carried Mary into an awaiting carriage, locking the barred doors behind them.

Anna had been standing outside the cottage, shocked, terrified and helpless as she watched Mary being removed from her home in such a dreadful way. She covered Eve's eyes, pulling her face into her, shielding them from the spectacle of watching her mother from being forcibly taken away. But Eve understood enough to know that something dreadful was happening and screamed uncontrollably into Anna's arms. She was still traumatised and hurting from the attack upon her person by Jonathan Barlow only days earlier; an attack that Anna made Eve promise she would tell nobody about, especially Dru. Anna knew that if he heard how she was attacked, he would have gone after Barlow and paid a terrible price for doing so. Barlow was too powerful in the community to be crossed and as Eve was not seriously hurt, she would have to accept the beating and remain silent about it. To Dru, she would say that she had fallen over, cutting herself as she fell. As he would not see the marks from the lashing to her body, just those on her hands, where she had covered her face from the whip as Barlow brought it down, he would accept that story. Dru would not have imagined that any grown man could inflict such cruelty on to a young girl, so Eve's explanation of her injuries would be believed.

When the Paddow Asylum carriage with Mary in

had left the village and travelled a considerable distance, the men holding Dru to the floor released him. He stood up, distraught at what had just ensued.

"Ah'll not forget this," he shouted at the men as they began leaving. "Ah'll nay forget what ya did to mi mam," he continued.

"Tis fer 'er own good," one of the men retaliated loudly.

"Doctor told us it wor for Mary's own sake son," another added.

"Ya let 'em take mi mam to that place," Dru cried. "Ya let them take her." The men looked sheepish as they left the cottage, unable to look Anna in the eye as they passed her. Eve, who had stopped screaming by now, looked up at the men as they filed past. She was not going to forget them either.

Chapter 5

Paddow Lunatic Asylum was an old deserted manor house that had been pressed into use a few years earlier as a place to incarcerate those suffering with mental disorders from the communities that surrounded it. It was one of the 'newer' establishments created to take in the growing numbers of mentally ill. Before Paddow Asylum was founded, the sick in the area were simply sent to the work houses, or worst still, local jails, where they mixed with killers and violent criminals and lived in appalling conditions, often being treated worse than animals. Very few came out of those places alive.

The Paddow Asylum stood in its own grounds some thirty miles from Elmsley, just outside the small market town of the same name, Paddow. It was largely the mentally ill from the poor and lower middle classes who ended up in there however; the wealthy tended to keep their own deranged family members locked up at home. Fortunately for Mary, the dreadful treatment given to the mentally sick in earlier times had improved dramatically during the previous few decades, and she was therefore not as unsafe as she could have been. Paddow Asylum was still a daunting place to end up in however. Its patients lived their lives at the mercy of unqualified staff, usually hired from the labouring classes, they being chosen for their physical size and aggression, and the other patients, who included those capable of extreme violence. With a slight change of attitude towards the mentally ill in recent years, lunatic asylums were hailed as being more humane places for the patients in them, which was some consolation to Anna and Dru. However, the truth was that many of the old practices and treatments still persisted in these 'new' mental asylums, including chaining the inmates up for hours and giving beatings to quieten them.

Anna had known of people over the years that had been taken into Paddow 'House', as it became known locally, but she had never heard of anyone coming out of it. This was the dreadful fear that hung over Dru and Anna like a thick, dense fog. Following Mary's taking, they had spent weeks trying to see her, endlessly making the journey to Paddow. This was difficult for the ageing Anna in particular, as she had to rely on the kindness of Joseph, the baker to take her by horse and cart, because she and Dru took it in turns to go to the asylum. Eve was not allowed to go there and had to be looked after, as she was too traumatised to be left alone and would not stay with anyone else in the village other than her brother or Anna. However, every time either Dru or Anna tried to see Mary, they were refused entry; the man guarding the gate turning them away without grace. Paddow Asylum did not welcome visitors.

"Ah'm lookin' after Mary Jennus myself," Doctor Selby told Dru. He was coming out of the main entrance on one of the days when Dru was attempting to get into the place.

"Ah want ti see mi mam," Dru insisted loudly to the doctor.

"All in good time Mr Jennus," Selby replied. "Your mother is being well cared for."

"Cared for?" Dru questioned loudly. "Sh's no place bein' in there."

"You should be grateful young man that your mother's here, being looked after," Selby snapped back at him. "She would have died if left at home. So just think yourself lucky."

"Lucky?" Dru rounded on the doctor again angrily. "Ya wouldn't have dared to do this to mi mam if mi dad wor still alive. Ya had nay right puttin' her in there. May God have mercy on yar soul fer what ya're doin' to mi mam."

"Do not worry about my soul Dru Jennus," Selby shouted at him. "And coming from the family you come from, you have no right to bring God into this either."

"Ah want to see mi mam," Dru yelled in Selby's face; he had no intention of backing down. The doctor ignored him and quickly began walking towards his carriage, Dru following behind, loudly repeating the sentence again and again. He was fighting the urge to get hold of the doctor and dash him to the ground, murderous thoughts tearing through his mind. Sensing the intense anger emanating from Dru, Selby hurriedly climbed up onto his carriage.

"If you do not stop Jennus, ah'll have you arrested," he turned and shouted down to Dru. "Ah've said you can see your mother soon. Let that be an end to this now."

"There'll be nay end ti this until mi mam is out of that place Selby," Dru screamed back. "An' if owt happens to mi mam in there, it'll be you ah'll be comin' to see," he warned the doctor. Selby whipped his horse and tore away from the asylum, Dru having picked up a handful of gravel from the pathway and thrown it at him as he moved off.

"There'll be nay end to this Selby," Dru repeated to himself, "not till mi mam is home."

More weeks went by and summer turned to late autumn. Still Dru had not been allowed into the asylum to see his mother. In desperation, he went to Squire Addington at the big house to beg him for his help. Anna had told Dru to go and speak with the Squire and present his mother's case to him. He was to particularly mention to the Squire that his grandfather was Jabez Dru Bowlin. Jabez had worked for Squire Addington's father as an out labourer on his estate's farm for many years and there had been some kind of respectful alliance between the two men, despite their very different stations in life. Rumour had it in the village that Jabez had saved the Squire's life on one occasion when he fell from his horse. For this act, the Squire had settled the deeds of his tied cottage on him, which meant that neither he nor his family would ever have to leave their home when he was too old or sick to work any longer. Jabez was always thankful for this gift and when he and Maria both passed on, the cottage was left to Elisa and Anna. As neither woman had ever married, they were at least secure in their home.

But getting to even see the Squire was difficult. It had taken Dru three attempts to be granted a hearing. However, he persistently called at Addington House until he was standing in front of the Squire in the Great Hall, his cap-in-hand.

"I do not see what it is you expect me to do," the Squire said to Dru after he told him the whole story. Squire Addington had just returned from his morning ride and, still dressed in his riding clothes, reluctantly agreed to give Dru a few minutes of his time. "I leave these sorts of matters to Mr Barlow," the Squire said. "Barlow did speak to me about your mother, I seem to remember. Doctor Selby said she had suffered some kind of mental breakdown; that she had gone mad, and needed treatment or she might die."

"That is not true Sir," Dru argued. "Mi mam wor grievin' fer mi father. Sh's not mad. Please Sir, ah need ya to help us," he pleaded.

"I am sorry Jennus," the Squire told him dismissively. "I really cannot interfere with such medical matters. Doctor Selby is my own personal physician and a very good one at that. If he said that your mother is mad, then she is, and therefore she is in the best place she can be. Surely you can see that?" he put forcefully to Dru. "Doctor Selby is just doing his job and there is no more to say." He stood up and motioned to Dru that his time to speak was over. Dru was mortified and panicked.

"Please Sir," he begged again. "Please. They won't even let mi see mi mam. Ah've got to see mi mam, to make sure sh's alright. Mi mam's not a strong woman, an' ah'm worried about her Sir."

"Jennus," the Squire said angrily. "I have said all that I am going to say on this. I am sorry about your mother, but I simply cannot help you. Now go home young man." Dru left the big house devastated. He had waited three weeks to be given an audience with the Squire, only to be allowed less than five minutes to put his mother's case before him. He made his way home in a state of total hopelessness; there was no one else left to turn to. He and Anna had put all of their faith in the Squire having some care, but he did not.

"What 'appened?" Anna asked Dru expectantly on his return. "What did t' Squire say? Is 'e goin' ti 'elp our Mary?"

"Is he 'eck!" Dru spat out. "He's nay better than the rest of 'em. He said he could not interfere wi' what Selby had done. He said mi mam wor in the best place fer her." Anna was very surprised to hear this. She had always thought that Squire Addington, whatever else he may or may not have been, was a decent and merciful man.

"Did ya tell 'im who yar grandfather wor?" she asked Dru.

"Aye. Ah told him," Dru replied.

"What did 'e say when ya told 'im that?" she said.

"He said nowt. He just looked at me, blank like, but he never said owt," Dru told her.

"Oh," was all Anna could think of saying.

"Ah'll tell ya sommit though," Dru said. "It wor Barlow that spoke to the Squire. He told him that Selby said mi mam wor mad. They is all against us Anna. None of them care what happens to her. An' what did mi mam ever do to any of them? Sh's never hurt anyone in her whole life." Dru sat holding his head in his hands. He felt defeated, angry, disappointed and exhausted. "Ah don't know what else to do," he said.

"Ah know lad," Anna replied sadly. "Yar mam is a sweet thing and sh' don't deserve this. But ya have ti be strong. We all 'as ti stay strong, fer Mary's sake. We can't just go givin' up, not now."

It was Anna's turn to go to the asylum the following day and what occurred there was something of a miracle. At least that was what she told Dru it was. To her astonishment, soon after her arrival outside of the gates, Anna was unexpectedly taken inside the asylum to see Mary. As she stood at the entrance, preparing herself to beg to be allowed in, Doctor Selby had seen her from a window and sent a message to the man on the gate to unlock it for her. She was then unceremoniously ushered in and guided along a wide hall, either side of which were people sitting, walking and generally moving around. Anna did not linger or stare at the folk she passed; it was clear from their demeanour that they were residents. Then, in a corner at the end of the hall, Mary sat staring at the floor. Anna was shocked at the sight of her and for a few moments needed to confirm in her mind that it was actually Mary to whom the staff member had taken her.

"Mary, oh Mary," she cried and bent down to touch her face. "Tis you Mary," she said. Mary slowly looked up, studying Anna's face as if she were trying to recognise her.

"Mary, tis me," Anna told her, "tis yar Anna, mi sweet," she said, unable to prevent herself from sobbing loudly.

"Umm," Mary barely mumbled, slightly gesturing with her head a 'yes'. Anna wanted to hold her tightly and kiss her, but Mary looked so frail, she dare not for fear of hurting her. Mary had always been petite, but now she was painfully thin; her beautiful long, dark brown hair badly cut to her shoulders and matted and unkempt. Mary was always so proud of her hair, 'yar crowning glory', Thomas used to tell her. She was dressed in a dull, loose-fitting garment, her thin legs hanging carelessly from it. On her feet were overly-large shoes that exaggerated her bony feet swimming in them. She was hunched forward, her hands limply settled in her lap. The shock of seeing Mary's poor physical condition was made worse when Anna looked at the bandages tied up along her bruised arms, some appearing to seep small traces of blood. She realised immediately that the good Doctor Selby had been bloodletting her. Anna was mortified and felt sick to her stomach. Her first thought was how Dru would bear the sight of his mother, especially her tortured arms.

"Ya can take 'er 'ome," the member of staff told Anna brightly. "Doctor Selby said there's nowt much more we can do fer this one now. Sh's quiet enough an' 'e said that as sh's beginnin' to eat, sh' can go 'ome."

"Can ah take 'er wi' mi now?" Anna asked, afraid to walk away from Mary and leave her one more hour even, just in case they changed their minds.

"Ah don't see why ya can't," the man said, "as long as ya can manage 'er." Anna would. She had been taken to the asylum that day by Joseph Locke, whose kindness towards her, Dru and Eve had been unwavering. He took some time out of his day, having baked early that morning, to use his delivery cart to take Anna to Paddow. She fetched him to help her with Mary. Between them, they wrapped her in a blanket and walked her slowly out of the asylum, Joseph helping her up into his cart. Anna sat holding Mary, gently supporting her as they made their way back to Elmsley.

It was almost dark by the time they reached Mary's home, the autumn nights now drawing in fast. The oil lamps had been lit, and Mary, who had not spoken a word all the way back, looked up at the light coming from her cottage as they approached it.

"Thomas," she mumbled. "Thomas," she repeated and reached out her hand.

"Thomas is passed Mary," Anna whispered to her kindly, and she went silent again. Joseph called to Dru to come and help him with getting Mary down from his cart and into her cottage. As he came out of the door and took the first sight of his mother, Dru gasped in both horror and delight.

"Mam," he shouted, "Mam." Dru ran to Mary and carried her in his arms from the cart indoors, crying as he did so. Thankfully, Eve was sound asleep and did not see her poor mother's frail body being brought home. Dru took his mother to her bed and gently laid her on it. He covered her with another blanket against the cold night, kissing her and stroking her hair as he did so. Eve, who was asleep in her bed in the corner of her mother's room, woke up with the sound of voices. Although drowsy, she quickly understood what was happening and rushed over to her mother's side.

"Mammy, mammy," she screamed and threw herself on to her.

"Careful Eve," Dru said, lifting her away from Mary. "Ya have to be careful, mammy isn't well. Ya must be careful sweet." But Mary opened her arms out for her daughter and Eve gently rested her head on her mother's breast as Mary's arms surrounded her. Mary then gestured to Dru, and he too knelt next to his mother. They all held one another and cried, Anna standing at the doorway weeping uncontrollably.

"Anna," Mary whispered to her. "Anna," she repeated.

"Aye, mi precious one," Anna replied.

"Thank you," Mary whispered. "Thank ya fer bringin' me home."

"Oh, Mary," she sobbed. "Ah just can't say 'ow 'appy we are ti 'ave ya back wi' us. Ah just can't say." Mary managed to smile faintly. She was clearly exhausted and Dru thought it prudent to usher Eve away to her bed, so that their poor mother could rest. He built a fire in the room to give extra warmth to Mary, while Anna went off to get her some hot milk and honey. Mary would take two spoonfuls of the nectar before falling into a deep and relieved sleep. Dru closed the door to his mother's bedroom and he and Anna crept downstairs.

"Ah'm goin' to kill him," Dru told Anna. She did not need to ask him who he meant. "Ah'm goin' to make him suffer fer what he did to mi mam. He's goin' to pay fer it."

"Dru, Dru. Listen ti me, please," Anna begged. "Yar poor, wretched mam an' little Eve, they need ya. Ah do as well. If ya take revenge on t' doctor, 'e'll get ya sent away. Ya know 'e will. Please promise me ya won't do fer 'im. An' if ya kill 'im, it'll mean t' gallows. Promise me ya won't touch 'im?" But Dru's mind was elsewhere, fixed on the sight of his mother, particularly her thin, damaged arms, and he was beyond being angry; he wanted total revenge.

"He did that to mi mam," he seethed. "That man, that cunte, he hurt mi mam like that."

"Oh Dru, ah know 'ow ya must be feelin'" Anna said.

"Nay Anna," he told her. "Ya don't know how ah feel. Ah couldn't stop 'em takin' mi mam, an' look what they did to her. They'is nearly killed her, an' tis my fault."

"That's not true," Anna replied. "Ya couldn't stop 'em takin' our Mary, nobody could've done. Now listen to me," she said very firmly. "Ah'm just old Anna. Ah'm not clever like yar Nanna Eli wor, but ah know what sh'd be sayin' to ya right now Dru Jennus, if sh' wor 'ere. Sh'd be tellin' ya to get those thoughts of murder from yar mind. Ya'll be nay good to those who need ya otherwise. Do ya hear mi Dru?" Dru did not answer; he just lowered his head and sobbed. He was such a grown lad now, but he cried as if he were a little boy. Dru cried for his mother and what she must have gone through, for the loss of his dear father and his beloved grandmother. He also cried for little Eve, because he had watched his sister suffering for all those months that Mary was taken from her, just when she needed her mother. He had lain in his bed listening to Eve crying herself to sleep, night after night.

"Ah know what ya're tellin' mi," Dru finally told Anna, when he had composed himself. "Ah know ya're right. But as God is my witness, if that man ever comes near mi mam or Eve, or you Anna, ah'll not be responsible fer what ah'll do to him. So pray to God that he keeps away."

Chapter 6

The days of autumn passed, and as the season headed into winter, Mary grew a little stronger, nursed by Anna and Eve, who did not leave her mother's side, day or night. Anna bathed Mary's body and Eve made the pastes that she spread over the wounds on her mother's arms, and they slowly began to heal. The scars of bloodletting would remain however, both physically and mentally. Mary would not speak of this episode to her children or Anna, not yet anyway. She began to eat a little so her weight improved and her lovely face acquired some colour, instead of the sickly paleness she had when she first came out of the asylum. Mary was not ever to be left alone; somebody would always be close by to protect her. Although Doctor Selby had not ventured near to the cottage, he had been seen in Elmsley and Dru could not trust that he would not try to take his mother again. Such was the tension in the Jennus home. Those few people in the village, who knew they owed debts of gratitude to Mary and her mother for their help when sickness had struck their families, now looked out for Mary. No visitor called at her home without Dru being alerted immediately.

This last year had seen the lad grow into a tall, strong man, in mind as well as body; he was beginning to look just like his father. The smithy work built his boyish frame into that of a man. Like Thomas before him, Dru was now a physical match for any male in the village and he made sure everyone knew that he would fiercely protect his mother, sister and also Anna.

A small number of Elmsley folk visited during this time, bringing in gifts of food for Mary and her family. Joseph had been helping Dru and Eve with the livestock since Thomas's death, but little had been grown or harvested that summer on their small holding, so the fruit, oatmeal and porridge brought from friendly neighbours was a Godsend. Joseph also helped Dru to sell their extra poultry and pigs in Ashton, so at least the family would not go hungry that winter. Joseph had been a good friend of Thomas's. Although nine years his junior, the two men were very close. Thomas had helped Joseph through the tragic loss of his dear wife two years earlier and had always made himself available to him whenever he needed to talk. Joseph had often been invited to their home by Mary for supper, and Eve and Dru had grown very fond of him. When Thomas died, Joseph was deeply upset and promised his friend, as he was being laid to rest, that he would look out for Mary and the children. He was devastated therefore to have been away from Elmsley, buying flour in the local town, the day that

Mary was taken to Paddow Asylum. When he heard of this outrage, Joseph was beside himself, and had thereafter done all he could to help Dru and Eve cope without their mother.

It was on one of the visits into Ashton market, when Eve saw James Barlow again. Anna was looking after Mary that day, so that Eve could join her brother to sell their produce at the monthly market. James was sitting in his father's carriage outside a shop, on the other side of the road. Eve had just helped Dru unload the crates of poultry onto the siding for him to take them into the market place, when she noticed the lad. He sat quite still and upright, dressed smartly, from what Eve could see, wearing a small hat and high collared shirt and jacket. She stared at his profile.

James was the eldest son of Jonathan and Florence Barlow and at fifteen years of age was two years older than Eve. He was tall, with fair hair that curled around his face and neck. Eve teased him about this, but she was secretly envious. She had always wanted curls, instead of her own straight locks. James however, liked Eve's hair and told her so, which caused her to girlishly blush. He had blue eyes, much paler than hers, but he had long blond eye lashes, which fascinated Eve. She marvelled at the length of them. James's facial features were fine and delicate, which gave him a sensitive appearance.

Eve found looking at him quite pleasurable.

Although from completely different worlds, the two children instantly made friends. They had met when Eve was delivering one of her mother's curing pastes to Abel Fenley, to spread on his daughter's blisters. The child had gone down with a painful rash and Mr Fenley was at a loss as to know what to do for her. Mary had been visited and an appeal was made for one of her pastes. James was on a rare visit home to his parent's house. He had been sent away to boarding school from a very young age to acquire a good education, the best that his father could buy, and only came home occasionally during some of his holidays. Free to roam the fields around his father's estate for a few carefree weeks, James had decided to go out walking on the day he crossed paths with Eve.

"Hello," he said to her, as they found themselves walking towards one another along the same lane.

"Hello," she replied, "who are you?"

"Ah'm James, James Barlow," he told her.

"Where are ya from?" Eve asked him.

"Ah'm from Stockley House, over there," James said, pointing back in the direction from which he had just come.

"Don't know much of it," Eve said. "Do ya live there?"

"Yes," he replied.

"How comes ah've not seen ya before?" Eve asked.

"Ah'm not home very often. Ah go to Briddlington Boys School. It's a long way from here," James told her. "But ah've seen you before. Ah've seen you in town." He had seen Eve on several occasions, from his father's carriage, as he was never allowed to walk around in Ashton. Eve always went with Dru and her father to town once a month on market day. It was a treat for her when she was allowed to go into the sweet shop there and choose some sweets from out of the row of jars lined up along its shelves. The sweet shop in Ashton was her most favourite place in the world. James had first noticed Eve on one of those days. She was playing along the side of the road with her hoop and stick whilst Dru and Thomas sold their produce. James watched her as he waited for his father to finish business with one of the town's shopkeepers.

"Ah've seen you a few times," he told her. "Where do you live?"

"Ah live in Elmsley," she answered. "'Ave ya ever been there?"

"No, ah'm not allowed to go to the village," James said.

"Why not?" Eve asked him.

"Ah'm not sure, but ah think my father does not want me to mix with people from there," James replied. "He wants me to be gentlemanly and educated so I can follow him into his business."

"What do ya mean by 'his business'?" Eve asked.

"My father owns a wool factory up at Stockley Hill. When ah've finished school, ah'm to go and work with him there," James explained.

"Oh," Eve remarked. She did not really understand much of what James was telling her, but she was content to listen to him. Eve found his tone of voice and friendliness appealing. "Well, ah've got to go," she told him.

"Will you come back here tomorrow?" he asked her.

"Don't know, why?" Eve said.

"'Cause ah'll come here if you do," James told her.

"All right," Eve replied simply. "Ah have to do my chores first though, so it'll have to be late in the day."

"Can you tell the time?" James asked her.

"Of course ah can," she replied indignantly. "Ah'm not stupid."

"No, no, ah did not mean you were. Ah just wanted to make sure we did not miss each other," he said apologetically. "Can you come at three o'clock?"

"Aye," Eve replied. "Ah'll be here at three o'clock. Mind ya do as well," she added.

"Ah promise. Do you?" James said.

"Aye," Eve replied. The following day at three o'clock the two of them met on the same lane going out of Elmsley at the wooden fence leading into

Britchit Lane. From there they walked and ran across fields and climbed over stone walls as they talked and laughed with one another, each telling their secrets. Over the following few weeks, James and Eve met whenever they were both free to do so. James's father was busy at the factory and was not studying what his son was doing during the day, and Eve combined her meetings with collecting the wild produce for her mother to make the remedies and pastes from. She even taught James some of what to pick for a particular ailment and where to find it.

Then Eve came one day to tell James of her father's death. He was kind and caring towards her and sat under a tree with Eve as she cried for hours. They promised always to be friends and arranged to meet up some weeks later to say goodbye. James would be busy until then, preparing to return to his boarding school. It was as they met by the wooden gate to Britchit Lane that day, when Jonathan Barlow rode up to them on his horse. He yelled at his son to go home as he dismounted. Turning on Eve angrily, he shouted, asking her what she thought she was doing with his son. Barlow forbade her to ever speak with James again. She, being Eve, was not fazed by the man, and stood up to him, saying that they were only meeting to say goodbye. This seemed to anger him further and it was then that he lashed out. Seeing him lurching towards her with a raised whip,

Eve covered her face with her arms and hands as Barlow struck her about the head and body at least five times. She screamed in pain at the first blow, but this did not stop the man. He left Eve on the ground, sobbing. James had witnessed this attack and he was devastated for his new friend, but the fear of his father made him keep walking towards home. He had been on the receiving end of his dreadful temper many times and was now afraid that he too would be beaten. His father rode past him without stopping when he had finished with Eve and shouted that he would deal with him back at home. The prospects for the lad were not good.

As she watched James sitting in the carriage, the pain that his father, Jonathan Barlow inflicted on her that day flooded back into her mind. She had not seen James since then and she missed him. Eve had made very few friends in her short life and she and the Barlow lad seemed to have got along so well. She knew however, that should she go anywhere near him, she risked the wrath of his father, and Eve remained very much afraid of the man. At this point, James looked across the road in her direction and for a fleeting moment smiled in recognition, quickly turning away again as he heard his father's voice coming out of the shop. Within minutes, father and son had ridden off in their carriage, out of Ashton. Eve would not see James again for some years.

"Who wor that?" Dru asked Eve. He had noticed his sister looking over at the lad and wondered what her interest in him was.

"James Barlow," she replied. "Ah met him once on the way to Mr Fenley's farm."

"Ya do know who his father is don't ya?" Dru asked.

"His father?" Eve said innocently.

"Aye, his father," he replied. "He's Jonathan Barlow, one of the village elders. It were him an' that Pastor Bell, who must have agreed wi' Doctor Selby to send our mam to Paddow House. Selby could never of done it on his own. They all had sommit to do wi' it. All of them." Eve was shocked. She did not know much about those in charge of the village. She only understood that Squire Addington lived in the big house and made the law. If you got into trouble, he sent the police to arrest you and you got put in jail. She thought that it was only Doctor Selby who took her mother away; she did not know that Barlow and Pastor Bell were also to blame. Perhaps it was because she had played with James that Barlow sent her mother to Paddow Asylum, she began to think. Perhaps it was all her fault?

"Why would they do that to our mam?" she asked Dru. "Ah like Pastor Bell. He asked if our mam wor gettin' better the other day. Why would he send our mam to Paddow House?"

"Because of who we are," he told her.

"Who are we?" Eve asked him. She did not understand.

"We're descended from Esobel Shetcliffe," he replied, but that still made no sense to her. She knew that was the name of a great grandmother, but her mother had always told her she must be proud of that fact.

"Ah don't know what ya're sayin' Dru," Eve told him.

"Ya'd be better to talk to our mam about this sweet. Sh's the one to tell ya," Dru said. "Sh's the one to tell ya." When Eve got back home, she went straight to her mother with some questions. Mary knew that this day would come, when Eve would ask her about her family and why the community had problems with them. Mary, now stronger, was able to sit with Eve and tell her all she needed and wanted to know. Her daughter would soon be a young woman and there were family secrets she must now know. Dru knew what these were, and although the eldest, he was a male child and the old knowledge was only handed down through the female line. His job was to protect his mother and sister, as best he could, so they could fulfil their destiny and carry out their duty.

Chapter 7

Another Christmas descended on Elmsley and the Jennus family quietly celebrated Eve's thirteenth birthday. She was now a woman as far as Mary was concerned, and therefore given more responsibility for running the home and helping make the remedies and curing pastes. Mary needed that help. She remained weak from her ordeal and could not stand up for very long and sometimes slept for much of the day. Some days she seemed quite well, but that would be followed by three or four where she was weak and out of salts. Some days she smiled a lot and even laughed, but that would be followed by days where she hardly spoke a word and seemed to be unable to raise her face to the day. Mary's body seemed to be healing, albeit slowly, but what of her mind and soul? Many nights Eve could hear her mother weeping softly, trying not to let her daughter hear her torment. Occasionally she was woken up by Mary's faint cries of help that she made in a half-sleep state. Eve would leave her bed and go to her mother and whisper that she loved her and kiss her cheek. Sometimes she would cover Mary up when she had been thrashing around and lay cold without cover against the night.

Eve also overheard Anna and Dru talking downstairs about her mother on a number of occasions. She was not supposed to have heard the conversations, as they were all held in hushed tones, but she did understand some of their content. Dru would ask Anna if she thought his mother would ever fully recover from being in Paddow House with what they might have done to her in there. Anna said that she did not know if Mary would ever be the same as she was before she was taken, and that only time would tell. She told Dru that, with God's mercy, his mother would one day be well and stronger, like she used to be. Then Dru would ask her if he should take his mother and sister from this place, where nobody had ever heard of Esobel Shetcliffe. Perhaps his mother would be safer in this supposed 'other place', he pondered. Anna said that it would be very hard to start their lives in another village or town. Where would they live, what would they live on? And why should they be driven from their cottage and land? It had belonged to his father and his father before him. In spite of what had happened to poor Mary, Anna told Dru that he must remember how lucky they were. They had a home. The smithy and forge belonged to him by right and he must honour his father, who had worked so hard to maintain his reputation. He was now the man of the family and must provide for them all. No, Anna argued. Both his mother and his father's roots were in Elmsley, for good or for bad, and that is where they belonged and should stay.

It was also because of what happened on one occasion soon after hearing this conversation that Eve finally understood why she had not been allowed to bathe her mother, or be in the room when she was bathing. Eve had long found this to be puzzling, because before she went into Paddow House, she always bathed with her mother. Anna was putting some remedy on Mary's back one evening when Eve unexpectedly walked into the bedroom. She was shocked to see that over the whole of her mother's back, there were long scars.

"Mam," Eve said. "What are those marks on yar back?"

"They is nothin'," Mary replied, quickly trying to cover her body up.

"What are they Anna?" Eve turned and asked her.

"Yar mother had an accident when sh' wor in t' asylum," she calmly replied.

"They look like ya wor thrashed mam," Eve shouted. She began to cry. "Someone thrashed ya mam, didn't they?"

"Eve, Eve, come here to me," Mary told her. "Come to me." Eve sat beside her mother and Mary put her arm around her daughter. "Ah wor thrashed, but ah'm fine now," she told her. "But ya must promise never to tell Dru. Do ya hear what ah'm sayin'?"

"Who did it? Wor it Doctor Selby?" Eve questioned

her mother.

"Nay, nay sweet," Mary said. "It wor a patient in there. He wor wavin' a stick around and ah got in the way, that's all. Ya promise to say nowt to Dru, don't you?"

"Ah know," Eve said sarcastically. "Ah mustn't tell Dru. Dru mustn't be told owt must he?"

"What do ya mean?" Mary asked her. "What does sh' mean by answering me like that?" she repeated, looking at Anna.

"Nothin'," Eve replied sullenly.

"Is there somethin' ah should know?" she questioned the pair of them. Anna and Eve looked at one another.

"If ah should know somethin', then ya'd better tell me," Mary quizzed them again.

"Tis better ya don't know," Anna told her. "It won't do ya any good."

"Well, ah want ya to tell me all the same," Mary replied. Between them, Anna and Eve told her about the beating that Jonathan Barlow had given Eve. When they had finished, Mary asked her daughter to show her where she had been whipped. She wanted to see if it had left any marks.

"Tis fine," Eve told her. "There's nothin' to see. Everythin' healed up. Ah'm fine." Mary was very, very angry and had to fight hard to control her tears.

"Has he ever come near ya again?" she asked her

daughter calmly.

"Nay," Eve answered simply. "Ah've not seen him since that day."

"An' Dru doesn't know?" Mary asked.

"Nay," Anna spoke up. "Ah didn't know what ti say ti Eve when sh' came 'ome after that beatin'," she said guiltily. "Ah thought that if Dru knew what Barlow 'ad done ti Eve, 'e would 'ave gone after 'im, an' ah wor afraid o' what would've 'appened ti im fer doin' it. Ah'm sorry Mary. Did ah do wrong?"

"Nay Anna, ya did right. Ya did right by our family, just as ya always have," Mary told her. "Thank ya fer lookin' after my children when ah wor in the asylum. Tis not yar fault. Tis Barlow who should be sorry. One day he'll pay fer what he did to our Eve." Mary sat holding her daughter for some time, crushed with the thought of her being beaten by the man Barlow, knowing that she dare not say anything about it, especially to Dru. Mary also knew full well that Barlow, and even Pastor Bell would have had to agree with Doctor Selby for her to be taken into Paddow House. Mary understood that Pastor Bell was not a strong man and she could see how easily he might have been intimidated into agreeing to her being committed. Barlow however, was another story. Squire Addington had given him far too much authority over the villagers of Elmsley.

Ever since the Squire lost his only son to the

cancer, he had paid little interest in the day to day lives of his wards. It was as much as he could do to attend the court, but as Justice of the Peace, he had little choice. Barlow, who had delusions of grandeur way above his station, stepped in and began to take control of things he should have had no rights over, and the Squire simply allowed him to do it. But how to stop the man? After some discussion, it was agreed between Anna, Mary and Eve that Dru, for his own safety, was never to be told about either Eve's beating at the hands of Barlow or the injuries sustained by Mary at Paddow House. Dru would have wanted to take terrible revenge for both awful events.

Eve was now helping Anna with birthing in the village. Mary could not physically cope with doing it, she tired too easily, and Eve, as young as she was, took to it quite naturally. Everything about child birth fascinated her and her happiest moment was when she held the newly born babies in her arms.

"Ah want to have loads of babbies," she would tell Anna after each birth they attended. "Ah want lots of bairns."

"Ah'd wait till ya 'ad one if ah wor you," Anna would always reply, "then make up yar mind about 'ow many ya want." Whilst walking home from attending one birth, Eve turned to Anna.

"Why did ya never have any bairns yarself Granny

Anna?" she asked her.

"'Cause ah never got miself an 'usband," she replied.

"Nanna Eli never had a husband, but she birthed my mam," Eve replied cheekily.

"That's maybe," Anna said, "but sh' did 'ave a man that loved 'er, an' ah 'aven't 'ad that." Eve was suddenly intrigued.

"Did ya know who he wor?" she asked. "Did you know who my granddad wor?" Eve knew that her grandmother never told her mother, Mary, who her father was. But she now thought that she might find out; that Anna might know and tell her.

"Nay," Anna quickly answered. She was not about to tell Eve anything of it. "It wor yar Nanna Eli's secret and we should respect that," she told her sharply. "An' you lass, ya shouldn't be talkin' about 'avin' babbies at yar age. Ya've got plenty o' time ti be thinkin' on that. Ya ain't even seein' yet are ya?"

"Seein' what?" Eve teased Anna.

"Ya know what ah'm speakin' about," Anna replied. Eve laughed. She really enjoyed playing with Anna when she was in her mischievous mood.

"Nay, Anna, ah'm not seein' yet," Eve said. "Mi mam said ah should be soon though, bein' as my breasts is gettin' bigger."

"Aye," Anna said. "Don't be in too much of 'an 'urry lass. Ya'll 'ave 'em fer plenty o' years an' you'll be sick o' them by time ya've finished."

Eve always told her mother about the births when she got home and Mary listened attentively, posing questions for Eve to think about. These were designed to help her learn. Mary wanted Eve to become more and more used to seeing the process of child birth and thus experience the problems that would invariably occur. Eve then had to write in her book anything unusual that had happened during the deliveries. Anna would not be there for ever and when Eve completely took Mary's place in the community, she must know all there was to know about birthing, pregnancy and how babies got to be made in the first place. This meant telling her daughter all about sexual intercourse, and the diseases that came about because of it. She was also exposed to stories of bad treatment of some woman at the hands of their husbands; not that unusual at this time and about the act of rape and its consequences and how to treat it.

Over the following months, Eve had to grow up very quickly. She took on more of Mary's work and became a common site going about her birthing and medical duties in Elmsley. She was content to do this for her mother, but she was also beginning to have a yearning in her being, and missed the company of lasses her own age. Few youngsters in the village spoke to her and none made a friend.

Some of the lads were beginning to notice her however and she occasionally had to run the gauntlet of a group of them in the village as they shouted and called out various names to her as she passed them by. Of course, Eve made a show of ignoring them, but some of the names they called her hurt emotionally. She had the first stirrings of womanhood and what the local lads thought of her mattered. It made no difference how much Mary, or Anna or even Dru told her that these lads were stupid and cruel and that it was probably because she was attractive that they spoke to her in that way, she still got upset. But that was how Eve's life was and would remain for the next year.

It was the following summer, on her way back from visiting Joseph at his bakery, when the incident happened; a very dangerous incident for Eve. A group of young lads saw her walking home through Elmsley and decided to abuse her. They began by heckling from the other side of the main road, shouting out unkind remarks about her looks. This did not produce the reaction they wanted from Eve so they came to her side of the road and proceeded to follow directly behind her, mimicking the way she walked as they called her awful names. Eve ignored this also, so the boys began throwing things at her. To begin with, these were little bits of twigs and flotsam and jetsam, but then a larger object hit the back of her head, almost causing her to fall. It hurt Eve so badly, she turned on the lads, screaming at them and demanding to know who had thrown it. One of the boys, a William Morley, stepped forward and cockily claimed he had thrown the stone, laughing in her face as he did so. The others smirked and giggled like silly little children. Eve was furious and in a fit of pain and rage yelled at Morley that he was going to have a dreadful accident and die horribly under the wheels of a cart. She added that it would certainly all come to pass, as she had powers and could see it happening. The lad reeled from this outburst and visibly shuddered. The others stood in shocked silence, staring first at Eve, then at Morley. She then turned her back and walked away, immediately knowing she should not have said what she did. Eve could not help feeling a sense of victory however, in silencing the group. By the time she reached home though, she wished she had not opened her mouth. Eve dare not tell her mother or brother what had happened and just hoped it would all quietly go away.

Later that evening, Constable Samuel Jowett, Elmsley's only policeman, called at the Jennus home. He requested to speak to Eve. Dru stood like a wall at the door and demanded loudly to know what the constable's business was with his sister.

"Miss Eve has been accused of performin' a wicked

act," Jowett told him.

"What wicked act?" Dru asked.

"Sh' threatened young William Morley and told him his future; a grisly one by all accounts," Jowett replied. "There's been a complaint made against her by William's mother, Sarah Morley. Ah'm to take Miss Eve wi' me to the police house." Dru was speechless, and turned to see his sister clutching their mother in a corner of the room, frightened and pale. He said nothing to her, but turned back to the constable.

"Ya're not takin' mi sister anywhere," he told him.

"Now then Dru," Jowett said, but Dru interrupted him.

"Now then nothin'," he replied. ""Ah'll find out the truth of this an' ah'll bring Eve down to the police house miself later, once ah've spoken to her."

"Well, as long as ya do or ah'll have to come back. Don't make me have to come back now Dru will ya?" Jowett told him and left.

"What happened Eve?" Dru asked her loudly. "Tell me what happened." Mary brought Eve to the table and ushered her into a chair. Eve then told her mother and Dru the story from beginning to end. She did not leave anything out.

"Have ya not learnt owt Eve?" he shouted at her. Dru was furious with Eve but more afraid for her. "Have ah not told ya, time an' time again how careful we have to be? Did ya not hear me sayin' this all the time?" Eve sat with her head bowed. She knew what she had done and did not know what to say to her brother.

"What made ya say that to the Morley lad?" her mother asked Eve. "Of all things, ya said that!" Mary put her hands to her heart as if in pain.

"Ah don't know mam," Eve began to sob. "Ah just got so angry. He hurt my head an' ah just said what ah said. Ah saw William dead under a cart an' ah told him that."

"Oh Eve!" Mary cried. "What ya did was bad. Don't ya know what can happen to ya fer speakin' like that to someone? Don't ya realise?"

"Tis fine mam," Dru told his mother. He could see she was becoming distraught so he helped her into a chair. "Don't worry mam, it'll be fine," he said, realising he must remain calm for his mother's sake. Mary was panicking and finding it hard to take a breath. "Ah'll fetch Anna to sit wi' ya an' ah'll go an' sort this out wi' Jowett. Ah'll have to take Eve wi' mi mam, but ah'll sort it out."

"Nay, nay," Mary cried, "they'll not let her come home again Dru. Don't make her go, please," she begged him, holding on to her son's shirt front.

"Mam," he stressed. "Ah won't let owt happen to Eve. Ah promise." Dru went to Anna and brought her back to sit with Mary. He also called on Joseph as well; he needed his support at the police house. With Mary looked after, Dru, Joseph and Eve made their way to speak with Jowett. Eve sat and calmly told the constable what had happened and showed him the lump that by now had come up on the back of her head.

"Sh' wor defendin' herself Jowett. Those lads attacked her fer nay good reason an' sh' defended herself," Dru told the officer. "Look at mi sister's head. That stone cut it open an' could've hurt her right bad."

"Ah can see that," Jowett agreed, examining Eve's head, "but sh' shouldn't have put a curse on the Morley lad. That's the problem here. Eve shouldn't have said what sh' said."

"Ah never cursed him," Eve told the officer defensibly.

"Then why did ya say what ya said to him then?" Jowett asked her.

"Ah don't know, ah just said it," she replied. Joseph spoke up.

"Sh's just a young lass. Ya know what they are like at this age, they say anythin' that comes to mind. Sh' didn't mean any harm to t' lad. Can't ya get Sarah Morley to stop this now? Tell her that Eve's sorry."

"Tis out of my hands Joseph," Jowett replied. "Sarah Morley took this to Jonathan Barlow. It's him who's callin' fer Eve to go before the Squire, not me. Ya know ah would've done all ah could to stop this. Ya know ah would've done that. Ah think it's all utter nonsense. Look...," Jowett paused and scratched his head. "Ah'll let Eve go home now," he told a relieved Dru, "but sh's still goin' to have to stand before the Justice of the Peace. Morley said sh' put a curse on him an' told 'is fortune. Barlow is sayin' Eve's broken the law. Ya know that it's against the law Eve to tell fortunes, don't ya?" Jowett turned and asked her. Eve nodded.

"Barlow!" Dru mumbled as they made their way home. "Barlow again."

Chapter 8

A week later, Eve was called to stand before Squire Addington in the court house in Ashton. Mary, in spite of being unwell, had insisted on going to speak for her daughter. Anna and Joseph were in the public seating area to support the family, and Joseph, if need be, would talk on behalf of Eve. He held a lot of respect in the village and the hope was that his voice might be heard, even if Mary's was not. As Dru entered the courtroom with his mother they were surprised to see the large number of people sitting in the public area.

"Look at 'em," Dru said to her. "Like a pack of dogs waitin' to be fed." Mary did not reply, she just nervously looked across the crowd and then sat down. Dozens of people from Elmsley had made their way to town to listen to the case. Many of them stared at Mary, seemingly shocked at the sight of her. Most had not seen her for some time and had not realised how frail she now was. When Eve entered the room by the side of Officer Jowett, the crowd became noisy, some even booed her. A man's voice shouted 'witch', followed by a round of gasps and mumbles, and then a woman shouted 'devil's choice'. Eve flinched at these insults and moved closer to Jowett, who steadily looked over the crowd in disgust. Dru stood up and glared at the crowd defiantly to defend his sister, but was urged to sit back down by Mary.

"It doesn't matter what they think," she told him quietly, "it only matters what the Squire thinks."

"All stand for Squire Addington," a loud voice boomed across the courtroom, and the crowd stood whilst he walked in and took his place on the bench. Eve was directed to stand and face him. She looked so young and terrified, standing alone in the high dock.

The first person to take the witness stand was William Morley. He acted as if he would rather be somewhere else entirely and stood sheepishly, avoiding any eye contact with Eve. He was made to swear on the bible by an officer of the court, who then asked him to tell his account of what happened. Morley mumbled his way through his story, the part where he threw the large stone at Eve's head was almost inaudible to the room.

"Speak up," the Squire ordered him. Morley spoke a little louder, especially when he described the way that Eve screamed at him, with her eyes fiery and wild. Her stare penetrated his very being, he recalled. Then he recounted how she cursed him to hell and told him she was going to make him die beneath the wheels of a cart. The crowd hissed and groaned at hearing this, and looked over at Eve, who sat with her head bowed. She showed no reaction to this fanciful story. Then the other boys who had been with William on the day spoke one by one, each virtually telling the same story, word for word.

"Eve Jennus. What do you say to the accusations that have been made against you?" the Squire asked her, after needing to call three times for the public to be quiet. "What do you say to the charge of laying a curse on William Morley and telling him he that was going to die?"

"Ah did not put a curse on him Sir, but I did tell him he were goin' to die. I did not tell William that ah was goin' to kill him though," Eve answered quietly. "Ah'm sorry ah said any of it Sir," she added.

"This is a serious offence young woman," the Squire said sternly. "You could be sent to jail."

"Ah know Sir," Eve replied sheepishly. "But ah didn't mean owt by it Sir."

"Even if you did not put a curse on William Morley, you do know that it is against the law to tell fortunes?" the Squire questioned her.

"Aye Sir," Eve answered. "Ah didn't mean any harm to come to William."

"Well you did harm him, did you not?" the Squire said haughtily. "You frightened him!"

"Aye Sir," Eve whispered.

"Please Sir," Mary stood up. "Ah would like to speak fer my daughter."

"Very well Mrs Jennus," the Squire told her. "Take

the stand." She moved slowly across to the witness box.

"Please Sir," Mary said shakily. She was barely able to stand up with the stress of the day and was supporting her body against the rail.

"Somebody get Mrs Jennus a stool please," the Squire barked. A chair was quickly brought and Mary sat down.

"Thank ya Sir," she told the Squire humbly. When she gained her composure Mary began to speak, but very quietly. A hush spread over the room as everyone strained to hear her voice. "Eve's just a silly girl Sir. Sh' didn't mean any harm by what sh' said to the Morley lad," Mary pleaded. "Sh's a good girl really Sir. William Morley, he threw a large stone at Eve an' hurt her Sir. Sh' just said the first thing that came to her mind. Sh' didn't mean any harm to the lad. Sh's very sorry an' won't do nowt like it again."

The Squire sat pensively for some moments, seemingly deep in thought. He looked over the people crowding out his courtroom. He then looked across at Mary. His face seemed to soften, somewhere around the eyes, just for a second or two. The Squire then took in a deep breath and straightened up, his cool, detached demeanour returning.

"Thank you Mrs Jennus," he said to Mary. "You can leave the stand." Mary looked over to her daughter as she stepped out of the witness box and gave her a reassuring look that belied the stomach-wrenching pain from fear she was feeling for her. Constable Jowett was next called and he described to the Squire the condition of Eve's head when he saw her on the day of the incident. He also said that he had never had cause to speak to Eve before, as she was a good, law-abiding citizen. The Squire listened to Jowett's testimony and then turned to Eve.

"Eve Jennus," he said. "I am going to fine you for your outburst, by way of compensation to William Morley. His mother and father will decide the amercement. On this occasion, I shall not send you to jail. But if I ever see you before me again in my courtroom for either cursing someone or telling them their fortune, then I will send you to jail. Do you understand that?" Eve nodded a 'yes', as the noise in the courtroom grew louder and some people began to grumble that the Squire was being too lenient on Eve. The Squire ignored them.

"Speak up girl," he told Eve.

"Yes Sir," she replied loudly.

"And," Squire Addington added. "From this day forth, you will attend church every Sunday. Pastor Bell informs me that you do not go to church. You will go in the future. Perhaps we can make a good Christian out of you, young lady?" This was greeted with more mumbles and grumbles of disbelief from the public. "This case is dismissed," the Squire said. "And," he turned to the crowd before him. "I will not ever tolerate this kind of behaviour in my courtroom again," he levelled at them loudly, which produced instant silence in the room. He then prepared himself to leave, and a voice called for everyone in the room to stand. They stood and waited for the Squire to exit before they too left. Eve ran from the dock to her mother and Dru. Anna and Joseph met them outside the court house.

"Let's get home," Dru told everyone. He helped his mother and Eve into his cart and Joseph took Anna with him. The journey back to Elmsley was silent, but the family had plenty to talk about once they got home. Eve had to be secured and made to understand how near disaster she had just been. Dru and Mary needed to ensure that Eve did not tell anyone else anything of what she 'sees'. They were aware of her ability, which was becoming more powerful as she grew older. Now they had to protect her from the consequences of using it.

"Ah'm not sure ah agree on what ya did wi' Eve Jennus, Squire," Barlow told Squire Addington later that day at a meeting of the elders back at Elmsley.

"Really?" the Squire replied indifferently.

"Aye Sir. Sh' should have been sent to jail fer what sh' did to the Morley lad," Barlow said.

"William Morley attacked the Jennus girl and hurt her," the Squire stated strongly. "He deserved what he got as far as I am concerned."

"Aye Sir," Barlow continued, "but Eve Jennus cursed him an' then sh' broke the law when she told him his .fortune. Sh' should be punished fer what sh' did. There wor plenty of people in the courtroom today who would agree wi' me Sir."

"Barlow, I have heard as much as I want to about this case," the Squire told him. He was finding the man tedious. "I think the Jennus family have been through enough over the past couple of years and sending the girl to jail would have simply been unchristian. Would you not agree Pastor Bell?" The Squire turned to the pastor.

"Yes Sir, I absolutely agree," he said, feeling rather brave with the Squire there. Doctor Selby had not commented up until this point.

"What do you say doctor?" the Squire asked him.

"Ah leave all legal judgements to you Sir," he said smartly. Doctor Selby never disagreed with Squire Addington; he paid him too well for his services. "Ah don't think we have seen the last of Eve Jennus and her doings mind," he added. "But maybe this'll teach her a lesson." Selby said that, but hoped it would not, because, like Barlow, he would rather have seen Eve in jail; anything to silence that family.

"Well, she is under your care now pastor," the

Squire told him. "I would like to see you teach the Jennus girl to be a good Christian. I trust you can do that?"

"I will certainly try Sir," Pastor Bell replied.

"That is the end of the matter then," the Squire said with authority, much to the intense rankling of Barlow. He was unhappy that his plan to inflict damage on the Jennus family had not worked.

And so, Eve was to be turned into a devout and obedient Christian. Dru paid the Morley family compensation for the injury that Eve caused William Morley, and everyone hoped that would be the end of the affair and they could return to a normal life, or at least, as normal a life as possible.

"Ah'm not goin' to church," Eve protested early the following Sunday morning.

"Ya have nay choice," Dru told her. "If ya don't do what the Squire ordered, then ya'll be in fer it," he pressed on her. "Ya've brought enough trouble down on us heads."

"That's not fair Dru," Mary rounded on her son. "Sh's just a lass. Sh' doesn't understand the wicked ways of folk, especially not thems around here." Mary could see that Eve was upset by what Dru had just levelled at her, which was unusual for him. It was not like Dru to be so unkind to his younger sister.

"Ah'm sorry sweet," he told Eve. "Ah know ya didn't

mean any harm by what ya did. Ah'm just tired. Tis really hard fer mi sometimes to do everythin'. Tis hard enough workin' in the smithy all day, let alone worryin' about mi family." He walked over to Eve and kissed her forehead.

"Tis fine," she told him. "Ah just don't want to go to church."

"Look...ah'm comin' wi' ya," Mary said, smiling. "Let's get us best clothes on an' go to church together. Let's show 'em, shall we?"

The unusual sight of Mary and Eve at church that next Sunday caused something of a commotion to those attending, but Pastor Bell was very welcoming towards them. Mother and daughter sat in a pew towards the back of the church; the only people joining them there were Anna, and then Joseph, both of whom often attended. Mary and Eve sang the hymns enthusiastically and listened to the sermon with interest. It was all about love and forgiveness and Mary could not help but think that it was written by the good pastor for their benefit. Squire Addington sat in his seat at the front of the church along with his granddaughter, Jayne Addington and his grandson, Frederick Addington. It was Jayne and Frederick's father who was the son and heir that the Squire lost to the cancer. He died when Jane was seven and Frederick was ten. The Squire took charge of the children's future, especially that of the boy, given that he was to inherit his title and fortune. Frederick, now twenty years of age was a troubling young man however, proving very difficult for his aging grandfather to control. He had been over-indulged as a lad and the Squire was now paying the price for spoiling him. Behind Squire Addington and his grandchildren sat the Barlow family. James was not with them of course, he was away at school. Jonathan Barlow was disgusted to have to endure the presence of Mary and Eve Jennus in his church. Doctor Selby attended another church, thankfully for Mary.

The weeks went by and Eve continued to attend Sunday worship, as she had been commanded to do. Barlow made no secret of his disdain at her presence there however, and expressed his outrage at every opportunity. He would spend many evenings at the Bull Inn, after having downed a significant amount of alcohol, complaining about the unholy people now being allowed to worship in St Guthlac. His disgust was made all the more frustrating because Eve Jennus was there due to the Squire himself having ordered it. Barlow could therefore do absolutely nothing about that.

It was some six months later, after one of his drunken nights at the inn that Jonathan Barlow disappeared. He had ridden into Elmsley on his horse, which was not unusual. He was an excellent horseman and boasted ownership of some valuable pure-blooded stock. His pretentions towards being a gentleman had urged him into setting up a magnificent stables and buying quality horses to fill it. Barlow had left the Bull Inn at around midnight. The landlord said that he had drank rather excessively the whole evening and was very loud and, as usual, the conversation had turned to his foul-mouthing some Elmsley villagers, the Jennus family amongst them. Over the other side of the inn, in a quiet corner, Dru and Joseph sat talking over a glass of cider. Barlow's voice grew louder with every pint of ale he drank and his remarks became so offensive that Dru and Joseph left before Dru became angry and took the man to task over what he was saying. Joseph had persuaded Dru to leave, knowing the consequences if they stayed.

Barlow did not arrive home later that night however, even though at least six people saw him leave the inn and mount his horse outside. His wife, the following morning, sent a message to Elmsley that her husband had not returned from the village, but his horse had. It strolled into the stable yard, without its rider, in the early hours of the morning, according to Jacob, their stable lad. Constable Jowett was called upon and a search party went out to look for Barlow.

He was found, lying stone-cold dead, some miles

from home. The route his body lay beside was the road from Elmsley to Ashton, Barlow's estate being some three miles off of this main route. His neck was broken, as the autopsy carried out by Doctor Selby confirmed. It was determined at the public inquest into the death of Jonathan James Barlow that was held in Ashton some weeks later, that he died of the injuries he sustained from a fall from his horse. The fact that he was extremely drunk that night was played down by Selby, so as not to damage Barlow's reputation, him being an elder of the village and a pillar of the society. The Squire was satisfied that Barlow's death was purely accidental and the case was closed. Officially, that was the verdict, but people being people, some had come to their own conclusions and theories as to how Jonathan Barlow had met his end. A few pointed out that Dru had long hated the man and that if anyone wanted him dead, he did. Given the size and strength of the now fully grown Dru, he could easily have snapped Barlow's neck 'like a twig', it was surmised. However, as Dru had been in the company of Joseph all evening and they had both returned to Mary's cottage directly after leaving the Bull Inn that night, the blame could not have reasonably been put on to him, although Jowett, due to accusations flying around the village, had duly looked into this possibility. The other more ludicrous theory was that

Mary Jennus had used her 'powers', those inherited from her Shetcliffe lineage, to take revenge on the man who helped put her into Paddow Asylum.

With his father dead, James Barlow was called back from boarding school within the month. At the young age of eighteen, he was to take over the running of his father's business. Fortunately, Jonathan Barlow had previously installed two good managers at his factory, so James would not have to do the job without experienced help. Eve heard in the village that James Barlow had returned to Stockely House, and she was fleetingly interested in the news, but not having seen or spoken to him for over three years, the lad was now virtually a stranger to her. At least that is what she thought, until she saw him some weeks later. When she watched James enter the church that first time, with his mother and younger brothers, and find his family seating near the front of the church, James Barlow was no stranger to Eve. He was taller than she remembered him being, but he walked the same way she noted, head down and quickly. Other than that glance at him when he entered the church, she did not really get much more of a look at James.

St Guthlac was divided into two parts, the one area where those high in the social ranking sat, such as the Addingtons and Barlows, and the other part, where the poor sat. Eve was at the back of the second part, therefore sitting quite some way away from James and his family. When they occasionally happened to be outside the church at the same time, he was very careful not to look in Eve's direction. Even when she stared across at him, he would not glance back at her. However, she knew, that he knew, she was looking at him, and it amused her.

Chapter 9

For the next two years, Eve attended church most Sundays, as was instructed by Squire Addington. The silence remained between her and James Barlow and their earlier friendship faded into memory and was almost as if it had never been. Eve did as she had been ordered and did not curse anyone or tell them of a horrible fate awaiting them in their future. Whilst she kept her own counsel and did what she could not to draw attention to herself, she was left alone by her would-be abusers. Any 'curse' or 'vision' coming from a female descended from the Shetcliffe line was taken seriously by some Elmsley folk however, and William Morley, being one of them, was taking great care around horses and carts after his encounter with Eve that day. If ever they passed in the village, William would divert his eyes from her for fear of further retribution. Since the incident with Morley however, Eve had paid a heavy price. She was further ostracised by the other youngsters in the village, but seemed to have accepted this as being inevitable, resigning herself to a lonely existence.

She was not idle though. Eve took on much of the heavy work on their family small holding behind the cottage; Dru was busy in the smithy and forge, and she also more or less ran the home. Mary had not gained her former strength; that which she had before she was put in Paddow House, but thankfully, seemed much happier. Her nights were not full of so many terrors and frights. Mary and her daughter settled into tending the family's graves every week without trauma and Eve felt some peace in her life. It was quiet, and at times very solitary, but she looked after her mother and brother's needs in the home and spent much of her time caring for Mary and also Anna, who was beginning to feel her age.

Doctor George Selby died that year at the age of sixty-three, with hardly a raised eyebrow or comment from the community. He went down with some kind of infection and was taken within a week. It was a horrible death, according to the gossip that a neighbour brought into the Jennus home one morning. Not that anyone there was saddened to hear of his demise; his name had not been spoken by Mary, Eve, Dru or Anna for a very long time and he, in turn, had avoided coming anywhere near their homes. In the year leading up to Selby's death, his visits to Elmsley had already become fewer by the month. Apparently, there was a new, young doctor who had also taken up a practice in Ashton, and, according to the gossip, he had become more popular in the area than the crusty old Doctor Selby.

"'Ave ya seen t' new doctor?" Margaret, the gossipy neighbour asked Eve.

"Nay," she replied.

"Well, 'e's quite a looker," Margaret told her with a glint in her eye. "'E's almost worth gettin' sick fer," she joked. "My Ethel is right stuck on' 'im. 'E's got the blackest hair ya've ever seen an' eyes ti match. They reckon he came up here from down south."

"Eve's not interested in nay doctor," Mary said abruptly.

"Ah reckon sh'd be interested in this 'un," Margaret quipped. "Ya'd have ti be blind not ti look kindly at this man." Eve smiled. She liked Margaret. She always had a good story to tell when she visited.

"What's his name?" Eve asked.

"'Is name's Doctor Lawson. They reckon he lives in a big 'ouse in Ashton an' he's not got a wife," Margaret told her, raising her eyebrows sassily. Eve smiled again and nodded. She had to admit to being slightly pleased with the man's description.

"Anyways, ah'd best be off," Margaret said and left.

"Ya make sure ya don't have owt to say to this new doctor if ever ya see him," Mary told Eve, who was surprised at the sharpness of her mother's order.

"Why should ah not speak to him?" she asked.

"Because ah said," Mary replied. "Ah don't want ya to ever speak to the man." Eve was even more surprised at her mother's continued insistence.

"Ah don't understand what ya're sayin' this to me for," Eve said. "Ah wasn't goin' to speak to Doctor...whatever his name is, anyway. But why are

103

ya so against me doin that?"

"Ah'm not arguin' wi' ya Eve," Mary shouted. It was so unlike her to even raise her voice and Eve did not know how to respond.

"All right mam," she told her mother. "Ah'll not ever speak to the doctor. Does that please ya now?"

"Don't cheek me," Mary said. "Ah'll not have ya cheekin' me."

"Ah'm sorry mam," Eve told her. "Ah didn't mean to cheek ya." Mary did not reply, just carried on rolling out the dough on the table top. Eve could not understand why her mother was talking to her in such a way, but as she was clearly getting upset, Eve changed the conversation to something lighter.

"Ah want to go to town tomorrow an' buy some claht," she told Mary. "Ah want to make myself a new dress. Will ya come wi' me to choose it?"

"Ah don't think so," Mary replied. "Ah'm not feelin' too good."

"Why, what's wrong?" Eve asked. Mary always loved going to the shops, so she knew her mother must have felt very unwell to turn down the trip.

"Ah'm just tired ah think," Mary told her. "You go. P'raps Dru'll take ya in?"

"Tis fine. Joseph said he were goin' to get some flour, so ah'll go wi' him," Eve told her. "But ah don't like leavin' ya if ya're not feelin' well mam."

"Ah'll go an' sit wi' Anna," Mary replied, "so ya

don't have to worry about me." The following morning Eve went to Ashton with Joseph. Whilst he went off in his cart to collect flour from the miller, she found the store selling dress material. Eve picked the fabric she wanted and then made her way across the road to the haberdashery. As she came out of the shop, carrying the parcel of cloth and a bag of cottons and buttons, Eve walked straight into James Barlow. Both stood for some moments in silence, not knowing what to say or do, each looking uncomfortable at the unexpected meeting.

"Miss Jennus," James eventually said, lifting his hat politely.

"James," Eve replied. She smiled nervously. Another few moments of silence passed.

"How are you?" James enquired.

"Ah'm well, thank ya fer askin'," Eve answered. "Ah've never seen ya walkin' about in town before," she added.

"No," James replied. They looked at one another, each inspecting the other's face, eyes, lips, cheeks and hair. They had not been this close since just before James's father had attacked Eve, over five years earlier. Each thought the other had barely changed, and yet thought they had completely changed. Eve recognised James's soft curls and long, blond eyelashes, and he, her thick, shiny dark brown hair and stunning blue eyes. The years melted away for just a few seconds as they stood, almost mesmerised, exploring each other.

"James?" a shrill voice broke the spell. "I am ready," the voice continued. Eve turned to face a small blond-headed female with a pink and white face that she recognised as belonging to the Squire's granddaughter, Jayne Addington. She was dressed superbly in a light blue satin, bustled dress, which was trimmed around the neck line and cuffs in delicate white lace that matched her gloves. She wore a magnificent blue hat that was adorned with a large white feather. Eve had never seen such a spectacle in her life. She could do nothing more than stare at the woman in astonishment.

"Who is she?" Jayne asked James.

"Oh...er, this is Miss Jennus," he fumbled to say.

"Who?" Jayne asked him again abruptly.

"Eve Jennus. She is an old acquaintance of mine," James said almost apologetically.

"Oh," Jayne replied. She looked at James disapprovingly. "Well, we have to go. Nice to meet you Miss Jenny," she said insincerely, turning to Eve.

"Aye," was all Eve could say in return. She looked blankly at James as she gaped after them until they disappeared into a shop at the end of the parade. At that moment, Joseph's cart came along side of her.

"Are ya finished lass?" he asked Eve. She was still

staring up the road after the couple.

"Aye," she eventually responded.

"Are ya all right Eve?" Joseph asked her. Her mind seemed to be somewhere else.

"Aye, ah'm fine," she replied. But she was not, not really. It was as if a light had been switched on inside her brain. The vision of the Squire's granddaughter in the blue shiny dress completely swamped and occupied every miniscule part of her mind and remained there for the entire journey home.

"Did ya get what ya wanted in Ashton?" Mary asked Eve on her return.

"Aye," Eve replied.

"Show me what ya got then," Mary told her enthusiastically. Eve unwrapped the parcel of cloth she had purchased and laid it out on the table. "That's really pretty," Mary said. Eve looked down at the roll of material she had just bought. Two hours ago it was the loveliest, most colourful cloth she had ever seen, and she was very excited at the dress she was going to make for herself. Now, it looked like an old piece of rag and the dress she was going to make seemed ordinary and dull. In fact, she would look awful in it, and she was not going to make the dress now anyway. Nothing, absolutely nothing, compared to the blue shiny dress she had just seen. Not only that, she would never own such a magnificent hat as the one Jayne Addington wore, with or without a feather in it. Then she looked at what she had gone to town in. It was her best outfit, the one she and her mother had spent hours making. Eve suddenly hated it, hated herself and hated her life. Within minutes she was laying on her bed sobbing. An astonished Mary was left standing by the table, staring at the material, and looking for the reason as to why her daughter was upstairs crying her eyes out. Eventually, Mary went to see what was troubling her.

"What's wrong Eve?" she asked her calmly.

"Nowt," Eve replied abruptly.

"There must be somethin' wrong," she argued. But Eve just lay on her bed, head buried in her pillow, crying. Mary was at a loss as to what to say.

"Can't ya tell me what's wrong lass? Did somethin' happen to ya in town?" Mary asked.

"Ah want to be on my own," Eve snapped at her mother in between her sobs. "Just leave me alone." Mary was surprised. Eve had very few such outbursts, so few in fact, that Mary could remember what they were over even, and she had not had one since she was a young child.

"Ah'll let ya cry it out," she told her daughter. "If ya're not goin' to tell me, then ah can't help ya."

"Ya can't help me anyway, nobody can," Eve blurted out.

"Well…if ya tell me what's troublin' ya then maybe ah can," Mary said. "At least give me the chance to try." Eve controlled her crying for some moments and sat up. She wanted to talk to her mother, but was not really able to express what she was feeling. Eve did not even know what was wrong herself, except that she knew her life had just gone through some kind of major change and she could not cope with it.

"Ah saw him today in Ashton," she mumbled, sniffing and wiping her eyes.

"Who?" Mary asked.

"James Barlow," Eve said. "Ah saw him there an' he wor with the Squire's granddaughter, Jayne Addington. Sh' were all dressed up, beautiful like. Sh's right pretty an' sh' wor with James. They were walkin' out together in town." She paused for thought. "He never goes to town," she said angrily, "but he wor there today wi'er." Eve then began to sob again.

"Oh," Mary said simply. She now knew what was wrong with her daughter and put her hand on Eve's shoulder. "Don't cry my sweet," she told her gently. "Did the lad say anythin' to ya? Did he speak to ya?"

"Aye," Eve replied. "Ah can't remember the exact words, but he did say hello and told Jayne that ah wor an old acquaintance."

"So, he wasn't unkind to ya then?" Mary said

109

softly. "Sounds as if he wor polite?"

"Aye," Eve answered, "he wor polite." Mary kissed her daughter and left her to be quiet and collect her thoughts.

"When ya calm down we'll talk all about James Barlow if ya want to," she told her. Mary understood exactly what was troubling Eve, but knew there would be little she could do about it. This was something that she would have to find her own way through. Later that evening, Eve, having finally stopped crying, sat staring out of the bedroom window, re-living every second of the meeting she had with James earlier that day, trying to recall what he said to her, what she said back to him, how his voice sounded, was he pleased to see her, how did he look at her? She then went over and over in her mind what Jayne Addington was like. Eve had never seen her so close up before. She pieced together every inch of her face, her dress, and that hat. Then she looked at herself through James's eyes. What must he have thought of her, standing there in her simple dress and walking boots? She did not even have her bonnet on. Her hair was loose around her shoulders, and not even showing a colourful ribbon. How plain and ugly she must have seemed to him. Eve wished she had not gone to Ashton today, then she would not have seen James or the Squire's granddaughter, who he was obviously now walking out with. Was he engaged to her, she asked herself? Did he love her?

Seconds later, Eve changed her mind. She was glad she went to Ashton, glad she saw James, glad she saw Jayne Addington. Now she would force him from her mind, never think of him again, never speak to him again. Then she felt even more distraught; the thought overtaking her that she was in love. She loved James Barlow and he did not love her. He loved Jayne Addington, the rich and pretty Squire's granddaughter. The dark cloud came out again and the tears returned, this time silently and more painful than before.

Some hours passed then Eve made her way downstairs. Mary was sitting by the range, with supper cooking in two large pots. Dru was working on something at the table and looked up at Eve as she came down the last step. He noticed her puffy face and red eyes.

"What's the matter sweet?" he asked.

"Nowt," Eve replied.

"Sh's not feelin' well," Mary said quickly.

"Oh," Dru murmured and returned to his job. Mary studied her daughter's face for some moments.

"Do ya feel any better?" she asked her.

"Aye," Eve replied sullenly. She did not feel better at all, but she needed to get out of the room she had been hiding in for the past three hours.

"Ah'm goin' fer a walk," she told her mother and brother. Mary was concerned.

"Tis gettin' late Eve," she said. "Ah don't want ya out int' dark."

"Ah'll not be long mam," Eve replied, taking down her shawl from the hook by the front door and putting it around her shoulders. "Ah'll not be gone fer too long." She just wanted to go out and get some fresh air. She left the cottage and walked a little way. It was a warm night, with darkness just descending. But the sky was clear with a full moon, which gave some light to her way. Eve had not planned to walk far, but she started walking and just kept on going, out of Elmsley and on to the road towards Ashton. It was now getting quite dark, but this did not bother her any; she could have walked that route blindfold. When she got to the road leading off to Stockley House, she turned and walked towards it. She was not heading for the house however, but to a nearby field where she looked for the gate leading to Brickets Lane. She just wanted to sit on it and think. It had been five years since she had spoken with James there, and although she had seen him almost every week at church over the last two years, they had not spoken during the whole of that time, save when meeting in town today. In all those years, he had barely come to her mind. Why was she suddenly so bothered about the man and who he was with, she asked herself? Why was she so suddenly and utterly sick with love for James Barlow? The night air suddenly turned much cooler and Eve knew she should go home. Dru and her mother would be getting concerned and it would take her at least an hour to walk back.

"Where've ya been?" Dru questioned Eve as she came into view. He was standing at the door of the cottage, watching out for her return.

"Ah just went fer a walk," she snapped back at him.

"Well, ya've been gone a long time an' we wor worried fer ya," he replied angrily.

"Ah'm sorry," Eve relented. "Ah didn't mean to be gone so long, ah just walked." She was sorry, especially after seeing the relief on her mother's face as she walked in. "Ah'm sorry mam," Eve told her, and kissed Mary. Mary knew what the kiss was for. She had an idea where Eve had gone, but did not say anything to Dru, that was clear. If Dru had thought for one second that Eve was liking or forming any kind of attachment to James Barlow, they would both be in trouble. Dru hated the very name of Barlow, and although Jonathan Barlow was dead and buried, and his son had nothing to do with committing his mother to Paddow House, James carried his blood, and that would be considered by Dru to be reason enough for his sister to keep away from him.

"Where did ya go?" Dru asked Eve.

"Ah just went fer a walk," she told him again. "Ah can go fer a walk can't ah?"

"On yar own?" he questioned firmly.

"Of course ah went on my own," she replied, irritated by the question. Dru was becoming more and more suffocating to her in recent months and wanted to know her every movement.

"Ya'd better not be lyin' to me," he told his sister loudly.

"Dru!" Mary stepped in. "What are ya sayin' to Eve? Sh' told ya sh' were out walkin'. Ya've nay right to be layin' into her like this."

"Ah just don't want her to be gettin' our family more of a bad name, any more than it's already got, anyhow," he told his mother in a loud voice. Mary was astonished. Dru had never spoken to her like that before. What with Eve's emotional outburst earlier and now Dru's angry behaviour, she felt quite upset and sat down, dejectedly, in her chair. Eve was furious with her brother.

"What are ya shoutin' at mammy fer?" she rounded on him. "There's no call to speak to her in that way. An' as fer what ah do...tis nowt to do wi' you either." Dru stood in silence, contemplating what had just happened.

"Ah'm sorry ah shouted at ya mam, but ah'm not

havin' her spoilin' my life," he blurted out. "Ah know sh's yar favourite, but sh' could ruin my life as well as hers an' ah'm not havin' it." Eve and Mary stared at Dru in amazement at what he just said.

"What are ya sayin' Dru?" Mary asked. "Eve's not my favourite, ah've allus loved ya both equal. An' what are ya sayin' about her spoilin' yar life?" Dru appeared very agitated and looked at Eve, then his mother, and then back to Eve. He did not know how to respond to his mother's question and simply picked up his jacket and stormed out of the front door. Eve started to cry again. She was still upset from her traumatic day and now she had to cope with Dru's declaration that she was ruining his life.

Chapter 10

It was a week after Dru's outburst. He and Eve had not had a great deal to say to one another since then. Dru always left the cottage very early in the morning to go to his work and she made herself scarce of an evening, once he returned home. Mary had not discussed the conversations either, so it was a fairly strange atmosphere that pervaded the home like a slightly bad odour. Eve had spoken to Anna about what Dru said that night, and Anna told her not to take it to heart; her brother probably had things on his mind. Eve was to find out soon enough exactly what those 'things' were.

She had gone out late one afternoon, long before Dru came home from his smithy, to deliver some remedies to a farm a couple of miles away and, as she walked there and back, she was gone for some hours. Eve returned home just before supper time. As she entered the cottage, the first thing she saw was a young woman sitting at the table. Eve knew her; she was Alice Mason, a girl from the village. The sight of the woman took her by surprise and for a few moments she was confused. Alice, who was the same age as Eve, had never tried to be friendly towards her in the past, but on this occasion, she smiled pleasantly at Eve as Dru introduced her.

"Alice, ya know mi sister Eve?" he said.

"Aye, ah do," Alice replied sweetly.

"Eve, Alice is my future intended," Dru told her, his face beaming from ear to ear in a silly, boyish grin. Eve was shocked. She had no idea that Dru even knew Alice Mason, let alone that he had been courting her. She smiled a polite smile back and then looked at Dru, who was dressed in his best clothes and was scrupulously clean from top to toe, with well-groomed, combed-down hair. Anna was over the other side of the room, sitting quietly by the range, where Mary was busy cooking a meal. Eve looked around and noticed the cottage was exceptionally tidy with fresh flowers set out in vases on the sills. As she examined Dru sitting next to Alice at their table, Eve felt a mixture of fear, anger, disbelief and betrayal. Her brother had not said anything to her about his intentions towards Alice Mason. How could he not have told her? How could her brother have kept that from her?

"Intended?" Eve finally said.

"Aye, we're to be married," Dru replied. Alice gazed across the table lovingly at him. Eve looked over to her mother and Anna.

"Isn't it wonderful news?" Mary put to Eve.

"Aye," Eve was compelled to reply. "Aye, tis wonderful news," she repeated her mother's words. The entire supper-time was an uncomfortable ordeal for Eve. She found it very difficult to speak to Alice, but tried. Alice had been quite cruel to Eve over the years and every past incident with the girl was brought to mind as she sat looking at Dru's 'intended'. As Eve considered her feelings towards Alice, she deduced that she really did not like her at all. She conceded that she was fairly pleasant to look at, albeit no beauty, but Alice did have a slim body and ample bust. Eve could see why her brother might like the look of her. What she could not understand was why Dru did not realise that Alice Mason, underneath the smiles and sugariness, was actually not a very nice person. It was therefore very hard for her to watch her brother posturing and showing off to the girl. Mary and Anna were also making Alice very welcome and appeared to like her. Everyone in the room suddenly seemed alien to Eve and she felt like a complete stranger in her own home. As soon as she decently could, she left the table and took herself off to her bedroom, only reappearing when Dru had left to escort Alice home.

"That wor rude of ya to go upstairs like that," Mary told her daughter tersely. "Alice wor our company an' our guest. Ya should have stayed an' been polite.

"Ah don't like her," Eve replied plainly. "In fact, ah can't stand her. Sh's not right fer Dru. Ah can't believe he wants to marry her. Alice Mason is a spiteful, cruel and selfish bicce."

"Ya shouldn't be sayin' these things Eve. Sh's Dru's

choice an' he loves her," Mary said. "An' ah want ya to be friendly towards the girl, fer yar brother's sake. Ya'll have to get on wi' her when sh' comes to live wi' us."

"What!" Eve almost screamed. "Sh's nay comin' to live here."

"Of course sh' is," Anna contributed. "Where do ya think sh's goin' ti live when sh' marries yar brother?" Eve was mortified. The thought of having to share her home with Alice Mason made her feel physically ill. How could she ever do that?

"Ah'm not livin' here wi' her," she stated angrily. "If Dru marries Alice Mason an' brings her in to this home, ah'm leavin'."

"Who's leavin'? Dru asked as he came through the front door. Eve looked at the floor and said nothing. "Who's leavin'? Dru asked again insistently.

"Ah will," Eve spoke up. "If that woman comes into this home, then ah'm leavin'."

"Now listen to me, Eve," Dru said angrily. "Alice is to be mi wife an' sh'll be comin' to live wi' me in this home. It belongs to me, an' ah'll decide who lives here an' who don't." Eve stared at her brother. His face and body looked the same, but she no longer recognised him. She took a deep breath, glared at Dru and went upstairs to her bed, without saying another single word.

"Ah'll talk to her," Mary told her son, trying to

rescue the situation. "Sh's a little upset at the moment. Sh'll see things differently tomorrow."

"Sh'd better mam," Dru spat out, "'cause ah'll not have her ruin my relationship wi' Alice."

"Sh'll come round Dru," Anna contributed. "'Tis difficult fer the lass. Alice 'as never been friendly towards Eve, an' now ya're tellin' 'er sh's goin' ti 'ave ti live wi' 'er in 'er own home. Ya must see it from Eve's side," she was appealing to Dru's fair nature. But he was not inclined to be fair to his sister as far as the new love in his life was concerned. His love for Alice Mason had completely consumed him and, after years of work to capture his heart, Alice now truly had total control over it. Eve knew that, and it was why she was expressing such bitterness about their future union. She could also see great unhappiness ahead for her brother.

"Things are goin' to be different around here," Dru told his mother, "an' Eve's just goin' to have to put up wi' it. When Alice is my wife, sh'll be runnin' this home an' Eve'll have to do what sh' tells her to do." Mary decided to say no more about the situation tonight. She would talk to Eve tomorrow, but instinctively, she knew that her family was about to be broken up forever.

Dru's engagement to Alice Mason was announced in church the following Sunday and the banns were to be read for the next three weeks. Dru and Alice planned to get married the month after this, which was November. Dru did not want to leave too great a gap between the banns and marriage, for fear of losing Alice. He was a strong, handsome man and one of property and land, with a good living and excellent future prospects, but he was still descended from the Shetcliffes and was therefore always conscious of being considered as somewhat tainted. Not that Alice Mason cared too much about his lineage. She came from a very large and very poor family, and Dru Jennus was, for her, an excellent catch. She would dismiss all remarks made to her as to his family history; all she wanted, not unnaturally, was some comfort and security in her life, and Dru could amply supply both. The question of whether or not she loved him was not a priority on her list of requirements. She only needed to secure his love for her, and she believed she had done that.

By way of ensuring his constant attachment to her, Alice occasionally played around with Dru's emotions and acted coldly towards him when he wanted his goodnight kiss. She would tell him that she had other admirers in Elmsley, and that she might just decide to take one of them for her husband instead of him. Dru would demand to know who these men were and become upset and agitated. Then Alice would calm him and cajole him by declaring she really only wanted to be his wife and that she was just testing his love for her. Alice Mason had woken up a passionate, jealous and possessive side to Dru's nature that she thought would give her absolute power over him, but the foolish, not-very-bright woman could be playing a very dangerous game.

Mary did speak to her daughter, but Eve made it very clear that she would stand by what she said and leave the home if Dru brought Alice into it. With the wedding planned to now take place within weeks, it seemed like an idle threat. However, Eve was prepared to do anything to carry out her ultimatum.

"Ah'll go into service," she told Mary one evening. "Ah can cook an' look after a house. Ah'm sure ah can get work. There's plenty o' big houses near Ashton."

"Don't be daft," Mary replied. "Nobody would take you on. Ya're forgettin' who ya are, ya silly girl."

"Not everybody knows who ah am," Eve argued.

"An' who's goin' to give ya a reference then?" Mary answered. "Who's goin' to speak fer ya?"

"Ah'll find my own way," Eve insisted. "Whatever happens, ah'll not stay here with that woman. Sh'll be nay good fer Dru an' he'll be unhappy by her. Ah'm tellin' ya mam, ah can see it!"

"Stop it Eve!" Mary told her loudly. "Ya must never tell that to ya brother. 'He'll nay thank ya fer sayin' it. He's getting married to Alice an' that's that. Tis Dru's life an' he has to live it his own way, fer good or otherwise. Do ya understand what ah'm tellin' ya? Ya must never interfere wi' Dru's life, no matter what happens, tis not yar right." Eve was quietened. She heard what her mother had just said. However, tell Dru or not, she was still leaving.

Her whole life seemed to be suddenly changing and not for the best. Eve was rejected by James, who now had another, and her dearest brother was marrying someone she thoroughly disliked. Eve had always hoped that Dru would marry a kindly girl, one that she could call a sister. When they were younger, she and Dru had talked of their futures and how they would all live together in a happy home, looking after each other and caring for Mary in her old age. Now none of that would come true. He was marrying Alice Mason and Eve was leaving the home she was born in.

Faced with her daughter's intentions to leave home, Mary had long talks with Anna about the situation. Mary herself would find it hard to live with Alice, but she knew that Eve could not and most definitely would not, be able to do that. After some discussion, it was decided that Eve should go to live with Anna. The cottage was big enough and it was to be left to Mary on Anna's death, and then to Eve anyway. As Anna was becoming older and could not easily look after the home and the plot of land on which she grew herbs and vegetables, Eve's company and full-time help in the cottage and garden, would be good for her. And so, on the day of Dru's marriage to Alice Mason, Eve moved out of her home and went to live with Anna. She was very upset at leaving her mother however. What would Mary do without her help and caring, Eve questioned herself. Who would look after her? Dru was out all day long at the smithy. Would Alice care for her mother the way that she did? Dru was angry with Eve for leaving the family, but he was also relieved. He wanted to begin his married life in some calm, and with Eve around, given her dislike of his new wife, he knew that would not have happened.

Eve remained upset with her brother for choosing Alice over her, but even she understood that Dru wanted a wife and family, as she might want a husband and children herself one day. And so, Eve settled into Anna's cottage and began to prepare for the winter months ahead, which meant wood-gathering and food-storing and preserving. She usually did this for her mother, as Mary was not quite up to any of these jobs. But this responsibility now belonged to Alice. Eve was therefore very upset, when, on going to see her mother one morning, she found her outside, in the cold, foraging around on the ground.

"Mam?" she called to her. "What are ya doin' out here?"

"We needed some brushwood fer the fires," Mary explained.

"So why are you fetchin' it?" she asked.

"Alice's gone to town," Mary replied, "an' the fires needed to be lit."

"So why didn't sh' light them before sh' left?" Eve asked.

"Ah think sh' wor busy," Mary said. Eve was very unhappy about seeing her mother doing this job outside on such a cold day.

"Go indoors mam," Eve told her. "Ah'll collect the brushwood." Mary went back to the cottage and Eve gathered a large bundle of kindling and took it indoors. Eve had not been to see her mother for three days, as Anna had been unwell and she did not want to leave her for too long. The first thing she noticed when she walked into the cottage was how cold the place was. The second thing was how untidy it was; the table was full of used dishes, the cooking pots were dirty and the floor badly needed sweeping. She said nothing, but stoked up the range and then lit the fire in the other room.

"Ah'll get some wood in fer the burner," Eve said. The wood pile was very low. "Did Alice not fetch in any wood before sh' left fer town?" she asked her mother. Mary mumbled some excuse for Alice not doing it. Eve went outside and carried some wood into the kitchen and set it by the range.

"What's happenin' mam?" she asked Mary. "Why does the place look such a mess?"

"Ah know sweet," her mother said. "Ah try an' keep it tidy, but ah don't feel too well at the moment. Ah'm so tired, ah just seem to want to sit by the burner all day. Ah'm so cold otherwise."

"Tis not you who should be doin' the fires and tidyin' the house mam," Eve replied angrily. "Tis Alice who should be doin' it. Sh' knows ya're not well."

"Ah know," Mary said, "but ah don't want ya to be sayin' anythin' to Dru," she put to Eve. "Ah don't want ya to be interferin' now."

"Who does the cookin'?" Eve asked.

"Ah do...but Alice does some," Mary added quickly. Eve was becoming quite angry by now.

"What does sh' do then, our Alice?" she asked sarcastically.

"Sh' does what sh' can," Mary replied. "Sh's tryin'."

"Tryin'?" Eve snapped.

"Eve," Mary said. "Please don't interfere. Ah know what's goin' through yar mind, but ah don't want ya to make anythin' o' this to Dru."

Eve made no reply but just set to, tidying the place up, cleaning the dishes and pots, and sweeping. She then made a hot meal for her mother. As she was about to leave, Alice walked through the door, dressed up in her Sunday best clothes, and laden down with bags and parcels.

"Oh," she remarked, "tis Eve."

"Aye, tis me," Eve replied crossly.

"What a nice surprise. Ah've just been to town. Ah had to get some provisions," Alice said sweetly.

"Why didn't ya light the fires before ya left?" Eve asked. "An' what do ya mean by lettin' my mam fetch in the brushwood? Ya know sh's not well enough to be out in the cold."

"Ah wor goin' to do it when ah got home," Alice said indignantly.

"An' why is the place so dirty?" Eve continued. "Tis no fit place fer my mam to be. Tis filthy."

"Tis none of your business any more Eve Jennus," Alice rounded on her defensively. "Ah do what ah like in my own home an' it's nowt to do wi' you."

"If my mam lives here then tis my business," Eve replied loudly. "Ya're supposed to be carin' fer my mam, so why aren't ya?" Alice was furious, but knew she was no match for Eve.

"Ah'm goin' to tell Dru about yar busy-body-in'," Alice shouted and rushed out of the door.

"Now see what ya've done?" Mary told Eve. "Now Dru'll be angry wi' me."

"Mam," Eve said. "Ah'm sorry, but ah'm not goin' to see ya do the work in this house whilst that lazy

127

bicce does nothin' but go to town an' shop. Look what sh's come back wi'. Sh' must have bought up half of Ashton." Ten minutes later, Dru came thundering through the door.

"What's all this?" he shouted at Eve. "What have ya been sayin' to Alice?"

"Ah've been sayin' that sh's a lazy bicce," Eve shouted back.

"Ya've nay right to come in here an' speak to her like that!" Dru replied.

"When ah came here this mornin' to see our mam, sh' were out in the field pickin' up brushwood," Eve yelled. "There were no fires lit, the place wor freezin' cold an' filthy. Sh' should be ashamed to leave my mam in the place like it wor, while sh' went out shoppin'."

"Tis none of yar business Eve!" Dru yelled back.

"Sh's supposed to be lookin' after my mam. Ya told me that sh' would take care of our mam," Eve replied, equally loudly. "Ya lied to me Dru. An' it is my business. That's my mam sittin' there an' sh' needs us help. Sh's done enough fer us family. Sh' deserves better." Dru looked around the room.

"This place looks tidy to me," he said.

"Tis tidy 'cause ah just spent my entire mornin' doin it. Ah had to get wood in before ah could even light the fires," Eve argued. "Tell ya lazy wife to do her duty." Alice stood by the door whimpering into her handkerchief.

"Ah'll not put up wi' this Dru Jennus," she complained. "Ah'll not be spoken to like that by her. Ah want to go back to mi mam," she began to sob pathetically. Dru immediately went and comforted her.

"If ya can't be civil to mi wife Eve, then ya're not welcome in mi home," he told Eve. "Ah'll not have ya upsettin' Alice like this again." Eve looked at her brother in disgust and then at his wife.

"Ah'll not be back here again, ya needn't worry," Eve replied. "But my mam's not stayin' here either. Ah'll be back tomorrow to fetch her. Ya can come an' live wi' Anna an' me," she told Mary. "Ah'll bring Joseph to help us wi' yar belongings."

"Ya don't have the right to do that neither," Dru told her. "Mam's livin' here wi' us. Ah'm not makin' her leave."

"Nay, ya're not!" Eve said. "But ah'm takin' her, all the same."

After speaking to Anna and getting her agreement, Eve went back the following day with Joseph and his cart to collect up all of her mother's things. She would need Joseph to help carry a large trunk that held Mary's treasures; those that had been handed down from her mother, Elisa, and all of the Shetcliffe females going back generations.

Dru kept out of the way at his smithy whilst Mary

was being moved from his cottage. He was unhappy that his mother was leaving, but he was also ashamed. Dru knew in his heart that Eve was right, but he did not want to upset his wife. Alice however, stood brazenly in the middle of the room making sure that Eve took nothing from the home that she wanted to keep herself. Eve, on the other hand, made extra sure that all of her mother's possessions went with her.

"Ah want those," Alice said. She was referring to some table cloths that Eve took from the dresser.

"They belong to my mam," Eve said sharply, "an' sh's takin' 'em. Ya can go to town an' buy some more. My brother seems to have plenty o' money fer ya to spend," she told her sarcastically. When all of Mary's things had been loaded on to Joseph's cart, they left.

And so, as Christmas arrived, Anna, Eve, and now Mary, settled down to a quiet day. The cottage was plenty big enough for the three women, and Eve was happy and content to be looking after her beloved mother again, as well as her dearest Granny Anna. Besides it being Christmas day, it was also her nineteenth birthday.

Eve attended church that morning, as she was still obliged to do. Dru made a point of going over to her as she sat down and wished her glad tidings and a happy birthday, which she accepted graciously. Ever since his betrothal and marriage Dru had been attending church himself with Alice, who did not acknowledge Eve in any way. She, in turn, ignored her.

"Ah'd like to come by an' see mam an' Anna tonight," Dru said.

"Ya're welcome to come an' see 'em," Eve told him and they passed a vague smile between them. As Dru moved away from his sister to return to sit with Alice, James Barlow was standing there.

"Happy birthday Eve," he said to her smiling. She was astonished, so much so, she was barely able to thank him for his kindness. He then turned and walked up to the front of the church. Eve watched as he took his seat, not with his mother and siblings, but next to Jayne Addington in the Squire's row. She felt a wave of sickness pass through her stomach. What had begun as a fairly contented birthday was now ruined by the sight of James and Jayne Addington sitting together in public for the first time.

Chapter 11

The winter months passed slowly and with the cold-weather sickness touching many families, Eve was busy making up and giving out her mother's remedies to those who wanted them. It was on one wet and windy Monday morning, when, as she came out of Edna Tasker's home, she finally met Doctor Colin Mason. He was climbing down from his carriage, and he looked directly at Eve. She somehow knew it was the doctor; she recognised him from the description given by her neighbour, Margaret. His hair was as dark as she said it was, and when Eve examined his eyes, they were the darkest brown she had ever seen. Doctor Mason was tall and well built. Not as tall as her brother Dru, or as tall as James, but he was reasonably good looking. He was a little older than she imagined he would be, but pleasant on the eye. The doctor certainly noticed Eve and judging by the way he examined her from head to foot in seconds, he liked what he saw. Eve had her thick winter woollen coat on still, which hid her now shapely body, but her beautiful dark hair was tied up in a roll at the back of her head, as she had taken to doing, and she had not yet put her hat on. Eve's white, porcelain skin was radiant about her cheeks, as she had just left the fireside of Edna Tasker, having sat by it describing the amount of tincture she should give her two children. They had the sniffles and slight temperatures, but were not too unwell besides that.

"So you're Eve Jennus, the medicine lady?" Mason said to her. He saw the puzzlement in her face as to how he knew who she was, and quickly added, "Oh, I saw you go into the house there, and a man walking past told me who you were," he explained lightly. "I'm Doctor Mason madam," he introduced himself, taking off his hat and bowing courteously.

"Pleased to meet you," Eve said in her best voice. She then stood looking at him, not knowing what else to say to the man.

"I've heard all sorts of stories about you," he smiled. Eve liked his smile. "Are any of them true?" he smiled again.

"Ah don't know what ya've heard," Eve replied confidently. She intended to be polite to the doctor, but she was not going to let him see that she was intimidated by him.

"Well, there's the story about you being some sort of witch, who puts curses on people and then damns them to hell," he laughed at this. "Then there's the one about you having a lunatic for a mother, and that is why you are also mad. Then there's the story about you claiming you can cure all sorts of sickness with your mother's home-made, miracle remedies." He stared at her, anticipating an answer. Eve studied the man for some moments, not quite knowing whether he was being friendly or being superior with her. She remained silent whilst thinking of how to respond.

"They is all true," she finally stated boldly. The doctor was taken aback. He had not expected that answer. "Good day to ya Sir," Eve then told him dismissively, as she turned to walk away. She could feel Doctor Mason's eyes staring after her as she did so.

"Er...Miss Jennus," Mason called out and walked sharply to catch up to her. "Miss Jennus," he repeated. Eve stopped and turned directly towards him.

"I am very sorry," Mason stumbled to speak under her stare. "I must have appeared very rude? I hope I did not offend you?"

"Ya were rude Sir, an' ya did offend me," Eve confirmed clearly. She continued to glower at him and he struggled for words.

"I erm...I am humbly sorry Miss Jennus. Please forgive me," he said as if he meant it.

"Ah'll accept yar apology Sir," she told him. "But ah want ya to understand somethin' Doctor Mason," Eve continued. "Ah do help some people in the village when they are sick," Eve was no longer concerned to use her best voice. "Most people livin' here is poor an' can't afford to pay a doctor like you.

Ah don't ask fer money, although sometimes they give me what they can. But ah've never told folks that my mam's remedies are miracle cures, ah just help 'um as best ah can. My mam is not a lunatic, she wor wrongfully put in Paddow House. An' if some people in Elmsley want to think ah'm a witch, then ah don't care. So, if ya'll excuse me Sir, ah have to get home to my mam."

The doctor bowed his head again and politely bid Eve good day. But as she walked away from him, Doctor Mason could not help but gawp after her. He was absolutely bowled over by Eve. As young as he realised she must be, apart from her good looks, she was the most strident female he had ever encountered and she fascinated him. For all of that day and every day over the following weeks, Eve Jennus occupied many vacant moments the doctor had and he wanted to see her again. She was not in his social class of course, but he thought she was intelligent, beautiful and tough, and he found her very attractive. Eve had no intention of telling her mother that she had spoken to Doctor Mason, there was no reason to. Now that she had met the man, Eve had no fear of him either. There had been some earlier anxiety, the experience of Selby still lived with them all, but from her meeting that day, Eve did not think that Doctor Mason would do her any major harm. She thought she had the measure of the man, but knew she still had to remain guarded however.

It was a great surprise to her when, a few Sundays later, Eve saw him at Saint Guthlac Church. The doctor did not sit at the front with the rich and titled, but near to her at the back. Everyone looked curiously at him sitting there, but he simply smiled and greeted them politely. Mason had gone to Elmsley a number of times over the last few weeks and had hoped to bump into Eve on each occasion. However, as that had not happened, the doctor thought he would try the church on Sunday, hoping she would go to the service. He had no idea what he would say to Eve if or when he met her again however, but when he saw her sitting in church, Mason confirmed in his mind that she was as lovely as he thought she was and he had to have her.

Outside the church, after the service, the doctor went over to Eve and tried to engage her in some small talk, enquiring after the well-being of her, and that of her mothers'. Eve's response to him was cool, as she did not understand why he should want to talk to her. As the rest of the congregation filed out of the church, they looked on in amazement at the doctor hovering around Eve. They were shocked that somebody with his social standing should demean himself like that in public by consorting with the likes of her. Mason was planning to ask Eve if he could walk out with her, but he did not get that far.

Dru, aware of the unfriendly attention being paid to Eve from the villagers, made it his business to interrupt the doctor's plans and move Eve away from him. Although still not on the best of terms with her, Dru was, nonetheless, Eve's older brother, and he made it perfectly clear to Mason that he was not happy with his attentions towards her. Mason withdrew quietly and left, telling himself that there would plenty of other days.

It had not just been Dru who registered the doctor's interest in Eve. James Barlow had also noted the man's attentiveness towards her and he did not like it either. For the first time, James looked across at Eve outside the church. She did not look back at him, nor did she let him know that she was aware of his glances, but she was. Eve simply said goodbye to Pastor Bell and left for home. Thinking on the day's events later that night, Eve was not sure if she was pleased at James's reaction to the doctor's friendliness towards her, or if she was not.

A few weeks passed and Mason had not returned to the church, much to Eve's relief. She had found his interest in her embarrassing, especially with much of Elmsley witnessing it. James did not look in her direction again either, and was now sitting next to Jayne Addington every Sunday morning in church. Eve had to resign herself to that spectacle and expected the couple to announce their engagement any day. She dreaded hearing it, but wanted it to be over and done with at the same time. Then it came. At the end of one service, Pastor Bell read the banns for the marriage between James Jonathan Barlow and Jayne Sarah Addington, both of the Parish of Elmsley.

Eve was beside herself with upset when she first heard this news and cried every night for a week. She tried to push James from her mind by busying herself in her work, but every so often, when she least expected it, his face would intrude into her thoughts and she would feel desperate for him again. It was an awful time for her, knowing that week in and week out she would have to see the man she loved in church, sitting next to his wife.

The Barlow marriage was planned for the following April and talk of the engaged couple and the wonderful wedding that they were to have was being spoken about all over the village. Squire Addington was giving the villagers of Elmsley a feast in the school house to celebrate his granddaughter's marriage to James Barlow, now said to be one of the richest wool merchants and woollen cloth manufacturers in North Yorkshire. Eve counted off the days in trepidation as his wedding approached.

It was one afternoon, a week before that occasion, when Ralph Woaton came to ask Eve to help his wife give birth to their tenth child. Woaton owned a farm two miles out of Elmsley. He could have afforded to pay Doctor Mason to attend the birthing, but Emma Woaton only wanted Eve. She herself had been delivered by Elisa, Eve's grandmother, and all of Emma's babies had been brought into the world by Mary, Eve's mother. Eve collected up her bag and went immediately with Ralph to his farm. It was a quick and easy birth and mother and baby were fine. Eve took supper with the Woaton family before making her own way home; she did not want Emma to be left alone by Ralph taking her back in his cart. And, as it was a clement evening, Eve thought the walk back would be pleasant enough, with the smell of early spring coming in across the fields. As she neared the road to Elmsley, she saw James Barlow riding towards her. She panicked for a moment or two and hoped he would just ride past. As he slowed his horse down however, she pulled on all of her confidence to maintain some composure as she watched him dismount.

"Miss Jennus...Eve," he said, stopping and lifting his hat. Her heart was pounding, but her bearing remained calm.

"James," she managed to reply casually.

"How are you?" he asked, slightly breathlessly.

"Ah'm fine," she answered. "How are you?"

"Ah'm well," he said. Eve smiled politely and went to continue on her way. James followed her with his eyes for some moments. "Eve!" he called after her. She turned and looked blankly as him with a hint of annoyance in her gaze.

"Aye, what do ya want?" she said indifferently.

"Can ah talk to you? he asked. "We are old friends."

"Is that what we are?" Eve replied.

"Eve," he said, moving close to her. "Eve...ah'm sorry," James mumbled.

"What fer?" she asked unemotionally.

"Ah'm sorry for us. Ah'm sorry for our friendship. Ah just wanted to tell you that." Eve did not know how to respond to James, so she did not. "Ah just want you to know that ah've always cared for you and ah always will," he continued.

"That's fine," she told him and went to walk off again.

"Eve!" he almost shouted after her. "Ah'm sorry ah'm getting married." Eve stopped and looked back at James.

"Do ya love her...Jayne Addington?" she asked.

"Ah can't answer that," he told her. Eve nodded that she understood. Of course, she should not have asked him such a question, it just came out.

"Tis fine," she said apologetically. James then walked to Eve, put his hands on both of her arms and pulled her towards him. She did not resist. They stood like that for some moments, him wanting desperately to kiss her mouth, and she wanting him to. They were so close they could feel the warmth of each other's breath in the cool evening air.

"Ya have to let go," Eve said quietly to him. "Ya have to let me go." James did. She studied his face. It was a handsome, kind face, she thought, which made it all the worse and her heart ached for him. "Why do ya have to marry her?" she cried. "Why are ya marryin' Jayne Addington?"

"Oh Eve," he sighed, bowing his head. Then he looked at her and took a deep breath. "It is expected of me to marry well. It is not what ah want; not in my heart."

"Well, in yar heart or not, ya're marryin' her," she blurted out. "Now let me go on my way James Barlow, an' get yarself back to yar intended." She turned away and started off for home again. James did not say another word, just stood by his horse and watched Eve until she had disappeared from view. She wept the rest of the way home.

Mary and Anna were sitting by the fire and called to Eve as she entered the front door. They wanted to know all about the birth of the new Woaton baby.

"Sh's well," Eve reported to them, "an' Emma is fine; thankfully it wor an easy birth fer her."

"Eve?" Mary asked. "What's wrong?" She could not help but see that her daughter had been crying. Eve smiled back at her.

141

"There's nowt wrong mam," she replied cheerfully.

"What's wrong?" Mary asked again. Eve sat down.

"Ah saw James Barlow on the way home. We spoke fer a bit, that's all," she said.

"Oh," Mary replied softly, "ya know he's getting' married next week?"

"Aye, of course ah do, how can ah not know. Tis all everyone is talkin' about in the village," Eve said irritably.

"So what did ya talk about?" Mary asked.

"We talked about him gettin' married," Eve told her. "Don't worry mam," she said, anticipating her mother's next question. "Nothin' passed between us."

"Please be careful Eve," Mary warned her. "Don't forget who he's marryin'. They're rich an' powerful."

"Ah'll not forget that," Eve said. She would never forget. How could she? The following week, James Barlow and Jayne Addington were married at Saint Guthlac Church. James was then gone to Eve; he must no longer exist to her as a man. The wedding was followed by a large banquet at Addington House for the Squire's rich and well-placed relatives and friends, and a feast, given in their honour and at his expense, was held in the Elmsley school hall. Every able bodied person in the village attended, young and old, except Eve, Mary and Anna. There was no reason why they should not have gone to the festivities, but neither Mary nor Anna felt up to the task, and Eve had nothing to celebrate. If asked, she said that she had to stay at home and look after her mother.

The next time Eve saw James, was almost two months later at church, after the happy couple returned from their honeymoon trip to Venice. During those weeks, Doctor Mason had been attending the services regularly again and continued in his quest to persuade Eve to walk out with him. Five more times he had asked, and five more times he had been refused.

"Is it true that ya've been talkin' to that Doctor Mason?" Mary asked Eve one evening. "Margaret tells me that he's been attendin' church an' paying' ya some attention afterwards?"

"He has," Eve replied simply, "an' ah've refused his attentions."

"Ya promised me ya wouldn't ever speak to him," Mary said.

"Ah'm not speakin' to the doctor mam, he's speakin' to me. Ah can't help him doin' that can ah?" Eve replied.

"Margaret tells me that he seems to like ya? Ya can't have anythin' to do wi' him Eve," Mary insisted. "Doctors have allus been trouble fer us, an' ah'll wager he'll be nay different."

"Don't worry mam," Eve reassured her. "Ah don't have any intentions o' gettin' friendly wi' Doctor

Mason, whatever he might want or think." She meant that. As far as Eve was concerned, the doctor was only having sport with her. If offered, he would no doubt enjoy the fruits of her body, but there would never be any engagement from him. Eve knew she was well beneath his social standing and that he would never take the likes of her for a wife. But the doctor was not to be easily put off. He continued with his pursuance of her. Many Sundays he attempted to sit near Eve in church and afterwards try to talk to her, but she continued to resist him. Confident that his sister could now manage the man herself, Dru watched the doctor's failed attempts from a distance. By the summer, Mason appeared to have given up on Eve, or at least he was not attending church. James was relieved, but as hard as he tried, he could not help taking sly glances at Eve whenever he had the opportunity. He had even taken to going for regular rides on his horse at different times of the day, in the chance of falling across her. Increasingly, James did not go into his factory either. The truth was he hated being there. He hated the noise, the people, and the grime.

One afternoon, what he was desperately hoping for happened; he met Eve when she was out on one of her errands. He rode up to her then jumped off of his horse.

"Can ah speak with you?" he asked urgently.

144

"What do ya want to speak about?" Eve replied cooly.

"Ah just want to be with you Eve and talk, like we used to do," James told her candidly. Eve's heart sank. She would have done anything to have heard James tell her that once, but not now. He was married and as far as she was concerned, he had turned his back on her.

"There's nowt to say to me," she told him unemotionally.

"Ah love you Eve," he announced shamelessly. "Ah always have and ah know now that ah always will. Ah cannot bear to see any other man even looking at you. Ah cannot bear that doctor talking to you either. Please tell me you will not let him touch you. Ah love you." Eve said nothing. She stared at James, her mind in complete chaos. He moved closer to her. "Ah know you feel the same for me," he said, and before she could react in any way, he put his arms around her, pulled her into his body and kissed her mouth. She melted in his embrace. Eve had never been kissed by a man before and the shock that ran through her body was almost unbearable. She wanted to bathe in the warm, moist pleasure for ever, but then fear tore through her mind as she realised the enormity of what was happening.

"Nay, wi' can't do this," she shouted at James as she pulled away from him. "Tis wrong."

"No, no it isn't wrong," James said and tried to hold her again, but she pushed him away and held him there.

"Ya must leave me alone now James," she told him. "Ya must never try to come across me again like this. An' if ya do, we must be strangers."

"Ah cannot do that," he told her, his eyes showing pain. "Ah should never have married Jayne. Ah cannot love her like ah love you."

"Tis too late James," Eve told him firmly. "Ya did marry her an' ya have to honour that. Ah have to live wi' it, an' so do you." She had already thought through every scenario in her mind. If James had chosen her for his wife, he may have been ruined. Society would have turned their back on him, and his business depended on the social constructs of the class that he belonged to. Whatever she felt for the man, she knew that he could never have taken her in marriage. They could never have been together.

"This must be the last time we speak like this James," Eve said. "Ah've nay intention of walkin' out wi' Doctor Mason, an' he has nay intention of weddin' me. Ah don't care fer him...ah can't. Ah have to tell ya though, one day ah'll meet a good man an' ah'll marry him." James was wretched. He stood in silence as Eve moved back from him then walked away. He wanted to run after her, but he also knew the hopelessness of the situation. He had married Jayne Addington. He allowed his family and hers to persuade him that he loved her and that it was a good match, and now he knew differently. They had nothing in common, and even after so short a time, neither one of them had anything to say to each other. She thought he was common and ill bred, he thought her arrogant, rude, spoilt and selfish. As he got back onto his horse, James could sense the years of unhappy loveless-ness that lay stretched out ahead of him and he was desolate.

Chapter 12

A week passed since Eve had spoken to James and they kissed. She had gone to town with Joseph and returned home to find Dru and Alice in Anna's home. They were standing by the table and Anna and Mary were sitting by the range, and they all watched her as she entered the cottage. Dru and his wife looked grim, Anna and Mary looked concerned.

"So, ya finally done it!" Dru turned around and bellowed at Eve. She had no idea what he was talking about.

"Ah done what?" she asked.

"Ya don't know?" he shouted again. She looked over to her mother.

"What's 'e speakin' about?" she questioned Mary.

"Ah'm speakin' about you, lettin' James Barlow make love to ya," he shouted. Eve was quiet, all kinds of things rushing in and out of her mind. "An' before ya deny it Eve, ya wor seen. Ya wor seen wi' James Barlow. Ah can't believe ya could do that to our family." She remained silent.

"Eve," Mary said. "Tis not true is it?"

"Of course it's true," Dru yelled again. "An' do ya know what they is all sayin' about ya?" he said into Eve's face. "The whole village is sayin' that ya put some kind of spell on him an' bewitched him. None of them is sayin' tis Barlow's fault. They is all sayin' it wor you who seduced him. They is callin' ya a whore."

"We kissed once, that's all," Eve whispered.

"Ah told ya," Alice piped up excitedly. "Ah told ya it wor true. Sh's brought shame on us all."

"What's sh' doin' here anyway," Eve turned on Alice. "Tis nowt to do wi' her."

"Sh's family," Dru said loudly. "Ya've brought shame on us all," he continued at the same volume. "Ah'm goin' to see that Barlow. 'He's not getting' away wi' takin' liberties wi' my family."

"Nay!" Eve shouted back at him. "It wor all my doin'. Ah kissed James. He had nowt to do wi' it. He told me off fer it. Ya can't speak to him. It wor all my doin'."

"Ah told ya sh'd ruin her life didn't ah?" Dru put to his mother. Mary was being comforted by Anna whilst all this fuss was going on.

"This'll all calm down soon enough," Anna said quietly. "It wor a stupid thing ti do Eve, but it worn't so bad. We just 'ave ti stick together as a family until it passes."

"Nay," Dru shouted. "Ah'll not let Eve ruin what ah've been buildin' fer me an' Alice. Sh's wi' child now an' ah can't afford to let Eve bring trouble to our door. Ah'm finished wi' ya Eve. Finished!"

"Dru, ya can't just turn yar back on yar sister," Mary told him. "Ya have a duty to protect her."

"Nay mam," he replied. "My duty's now to mi wife an' unborn bairn." He motioned to Alice to leave and they were quickly gone. Once her brother and his wife had left, Eve sat down and quietly talked to her mother and Anna. She told them exactly what had happened and why she told Dru that it was entirely her fault. She thought that if he spoke to James, James might tell him that he cared for her and that would have been disastrous for him. She accepted that Dru would no longer protect her, but that was going to happen sooner or later anyway, Alice would have made sure of that.

"Ah love him mam," she told Mary, "an' ah don't want any harm to come to him. Ah don't have much standin' in the village anyway, but James does. It doesn't matter what they think of me."

"But they is sayin' ya used some kind o' witchery on 'im and ya tried ti seduce 'im," Anna said, "an' tis not true. Ya have ti defend yarself."

"Nay Anna, ah don't. It doesn't matter what ah say anyhow. Folks round here will believe what they want," Eve replied. She knew exactly what she was doing and what the consequences of that would be and she was prepared to live with them. Mary was upset for her daughter however. She understood what she was doing, but did not agree with it. Within days, the rumours of what had happened between Eve and James Barlow, hugely exaggerated of course, were spreading all over Elmsley. Margaret came to Anna's home one evening and told them in graphic detail what was being said about Eve. Eve's concern was for James however, made more stressful because she did not know what gossip had reached his wife and the Squire, his father-in-law.

In the meantime, James was called to Addington House to answer to the Squire Edmond about the reported liaison with Eve, before the news found its way to his granddaughter. It had been one of his servants who saw the pair together and conveyed the event back to his master. The Squire wanted to question James, and then secure him, to make sure that he said the right things to Jayne regarding the incident. The Squire firstly asked him if it was true that he and the Jennus woman were caressing one another. James sensibly told him it had been merely a friendly kiss; after all they had known one another for many years. He reassured the Squire that he had no feelings for Eve Jennus whatsoever, other than old friendship, and nothing was meant by the kiss. James said that he now realised it was a stupid and thoughtless thing to do. The Squire listened and made up his own mind as to the truth of the matter. After considering what his son-in-law had said, the Squire pointed out a few things to James.

Firstly, he told him of the trouble that Eve had been in when she was younger and how she could have been sent to prison. Then he warned James, emphasising that if he cared for Eve Jennus in any way, then he should stay away and have nothing to do with her ever again. If not, the woman's reputation could be ruined as well as his, and she would also be made more vulnerable, for which he, James, because of his actions, would be responsible. Did he really want that to happen to the Jennus woman? The Squire then ordered him to deny that he had any feelings whatsoever for her to Jayne; she must never know the truth of the affair. He then instructed James to make sure that his granddaughter became with-child as quickly as possible.

James left Addington House emotionally empty. He had denied Eve for the second time and felt ashamed for doing so. Within days he heard the rumours being put around that she had done some witchery by mesmerising him, and he, the innocent party, had been subjected to a sexual attack by her on his person. He was mortified at these reports, but dare not say anything in Eve's defence. When he also heard that she would not deny these accusations against her, James knew that she cared for him more than she cared for herself. He was heartbroken, knowing he could not defend her honour and must never speak with her again or risk both of their ruin.

"Now I know why you would not walk out with me, Eve Jennus," Doctor Mason put to her sarcastically. He happened upon Eve in Ashton, some weeks after the incident had occurred and been duly dissected by the community and the entire blame apportioned to her. "All that time you led me to believe that you were being respectable and high-principled, and what were you doing? You were making love to the Squire's son-in-law. What a fool I have been. You are not a decent woman, you are just a whore."

Eve stared coldly at the man. "Nay, doctor," she replied calmly, "ya're wrong. Ah am a decent woman, but if ah'd have walked out wi' you, then ah would've been a whore." She turned and walked away.

"How dare you speak to me like that," he yelled after her. Eve looked back at the doctor defiantly.

"How should ah speak to you after ya called me a whore?" she shouted back at him. "Ya have nay right to speak to me like that or to call me bad names. Ya're not a gentleman fer sayin' it. Make sure Doctor Mason that ya never speak to me again. Never!" Eve glared at him before storming off.

The doctor was furious with her, but made no other remark. Minutes later, Joseph came by to collect Eve and take her home. She was still shaking from her encounter with Mason and Joseph looked along the High Street for the source of her distress. He noticed the doctor standing some way down the road.

"Is this his doin'?" he asked Eve. "Has he said anythin' to upset ya?"

"He said plenty," Eve told Joseph, "but ah'll forget it soon enough. Please, let's just go home." Joseph drove his cart past the doctor slowly and scowled at him. He decided, having spoken to Dru the day before and heard his intentions to abandon his sister, that he, Joseph, would step in and look out for Eve as best he could in the future, or at least until she found herself a husband to care for her. The likelihood of any Elmsley man taking Eve for his wife was not realistic however. Despite her very good looks, she was far too feisty for most of the eligible males in the village, and then there was her family's history.

With all of the gossip going around about Eve, it was decided that she should stop attending church. Eve would tell Pastor Bell that she was needed at home to look after her mother, which was not so far from the truth, as Mary had been deteriorating health-wise for some months. It was put to the pastor that the Squire might welcome this change himself, in view of the rumours of his son-in-law's adultery, and it would certainly make it easier for his granddaughter not to have to see Eve. And so it was done. Eve was relieved. She hated the weekly scrutinising of her by the villagers of Elmsley, some of whom she knew disliked and disapproved of her. She hated the hypocrisy of it; not having regarded herself as a 'good' Christian, like her fellow worshippers. And with James married, she hated the thought of having to sit anywhere near the man, forever looking at him and his wife.

And so the weeks and months passed. There was growing concern over Mary, as many days she took to her bed and then Eve would have great difficulty getting her to eat very much. Some days she was high spirited and alert, others she was very quiet and sleepy. Anna helped Eve to care for Mary during the day, and Eve did it alone of a night. The old night terrors came back to her mother occasionally and Eve had to sit up with her until they passed. Eve's life became one of caring for Mary and helping Anna. She now did most of the work in the home and on their small piece of land. Joseph was a good and kind friend and helped the women as much as he could. He called every day with fresh bread and cake. Dru visited occasionally to show off his new son Thomas to his mother and Anna. He was a beautiful baby, with a mop of black hair 'just like his fathers', according to Mary. She loved those visits and seemed to come to life when holding her little grandson. Eve and Dru arrived at some kind of a truce. He did not ask her any questions about what she was doing and she did not mention Alice.

Eve occasionally saw Doctor Mason in the village and in Ashton, when she went there with Joseph, but apart from studying her sometimes, he said nothing. With her not going to church, she did not see James Barlow at all. He no longer roamed the lanes and fields looking for her either. Margaret, on one of her visits, reported that the rumours about Eve and him had died down; she had heard nothing on the subject for months. So, although rather dull, Eve's life was reasonably peaceful for some time. Her mother's health went up and down, but they managed well enough. Eve made a small living with the money given to her for the remedies she provided and they survived with the help of Joseph and some meat produce from Dru's smallholding.

It was in her twenty-second year that Eve came across Frederick Addington, the Squire's grandson. She recognised him from the occasional attendance he used to make at church. Eve was waiting outside the sweet shop in Ashton for Joseph to collect her, as Frederick was walking along the High Street. Eve could not help but look at the man. He was dressed immaculately in a dark grey dress coat with grey striped trousers, and a starched, white, high-collar shirt. He walked with a silver-handled walking stick. Frederick was not exactly handsome, but he was striking to look at, with deep red hair and very pale blue eyes. He noticed Eve, a flicker running across his face when he recognised her as being the woman his brother-in-law had once been seen dallying with. Frederick grinned and stopped as if he were going to say something to her. Eve looked straight at him, waiting for his conversation. He did not speak to her however, and, after hovering for some moments, continued on his walk. Eve turned and looked in the opposite direction, in case he looked back.

"That wor the Squire's grandson," Joseph said as Eve climbed onto his cart.

"Aye," she replied.

"Did he speak to ya?" Joseph asked her.

"Nay," Eve answered simply.

"Ya need to be careful of that one," Joseph said. "Ah've heard all sorts of stories about him, an' none of 'em good."

"Aye, but there's plenty of stories out there about me, but they're not right," Eve said.

"That's true. Ah'm just tellin' ya what ah've 'eard," Joseph continued. Eve had been given many bad reports about Frederick herself. Margaret was always coming in with stories of how he had viciously attacked a labourer on the Addington Estate, or swindled a tradesman out of his payment, or damaged a girl's reputation in the village. He was apparently a ladies' man. Rumour had it that at least one young woman had been sent away from Ashton to birth Frederick's bastard child. It was said

157

that old Squire Addington had completely lost control of his grandson, and that Frederick was increasingly becoming a liability to the family. The Squire was also reported as being afraid that when he died, his grandson, the next in line for his title and estate, could not be trusted with his inheritance.

On his return from Ashton that day, Frederick dined with his grandfather, his sister Jayne, and his brother-in-law James at Addington House. James and Jayne had temporarily moved into the big house. Jayne was four months with-child and felt more comfortable staying there, rather than at Stockley House, her husband's smaller estate, where James's mother and some siblings also still resided. After dinner, the Squire retired for the night and Jayne excused herself, leaving the two men to their whiskey and cigars. Frederick, or Freddie, as he is known by family and friends, delighted in telling James that he saw the 'lovely' Eve Jennus in Ashton earlier that day.

"She's certainly a beauty," he said. "No wonder you seduced her; those breasts!"

"Ah did not seduce her," James replied indignantly.

"You do not have to deny it to me brother," Frederick laughed. "I really do not care what you do. If they are ripe, you pick 'em. And she is ripe!" James looked at Frederick in disgust.

"Ah'm telling you Freddie," he argued. "Ah did not touch Eve Jennus. Ah've never touched the woman, ah've too much respect for her."

"Well," Frederick smirked. "If you are not going to pluck that beauty, I think I will." James was sickened.

"If you do anything to harm Eve Jennus, you will have to answer to me," he told Frederick aggressively.

"I see...still sweet on the woman, are we?" he jeered. "Still attracted to the peasant stock? Ah, but then, that is what you came from was it not...brother?" He laughed at James. "It is such a pity that you cannot have her. I can though. I am not married to anyone. Yes, I think the Jennus woman and I will become very good friends."

"Ah mean what ah say, Freddie. You touch Eve and you will pay for it," James said menacingly. Frederick stared at him. He was shocked for a few moments then his swagger returned.

"Are you not forgetting who you are dear brother, and who I am?"

"Ah'm not," James stated bluntly.

"Well then, I suggest you be very careful what you say to me and what you threaten," Frederick retaliated aggressively.

"Ah'm still telling you," James warned him again. "Keep away from Eve Jennus or you will answer to me and ah do not make idle threats." Frederick threw his head back in contempt and walked out of the room, leaving James to finish his whisky alone. James was furious with his brother-in-law and very nervous. He knew Frederick well by now and had been employed by the Squire to get him out of a number of difficult 'situations'. One of these was to arrange the finances for an unfortunate girl in Ashton who had fallen victim to Frederick. She was discreetly sent to complete her confinement many miles away and then have the child adopted before returning to her parent's home. Yes, James knew all about the ways of Frederick. He was therefore naturally concerned for Eve. Whilst he did not think that she would fall for the flattering tongue of his brother-in-law, he had heard Frederick boast often of how had used a 'little bit of force' to 'persuade' the ladies that they really want to succumb to his wishes. 'This method is', according to Frederick, 'always successful for me'. James felt that he should somehow try and warn Eve about Frederick, but could not think how.

Frederick, incensed by the audacity of his brother-in-law's orders to keep away from Eve Jennus, decided to make it his priority to root the girl out. He made it his business to find out where she lived in the village. As the Squire apparent, he was not going to be dictated to by the likes of James as to what he could do and with whom. If he wanted Eve Jennus, he would do all in his power to have her.

Chapter 13

It would not be easy for Frederick to happen upon Eve by chance. She did not leave her home at any regular times, and so he had to find a more devious way of meeting her. Learning that she would visit sick people in the village and local farms with remedies to help them, Frederick induced a farmer, John Plews, to call on Eve and ask her to come to see his sister, saying she had fallen sick. He paid the man handsomely to do this task. Eve obliged Plews and left home that afternoon with her bag to walk the two miles to his farm. She was slightly puzzled, as she had never had any dealings with the Plews family before, but the man was very insistent that she go to his home later that day. Eve was about half way there when Frederick Addington galloped up to her. He smiled and greeted her politely, taking off his hat and bowing his head. Eve did not find their meeting particularly strange in any way, she often saw people out riding or in their carriages when walking the lanes around Elmsley. Frederick stopped and dismounted however, and started to walk towards her, which did make her feel apprehensive. Eve could not think why the man should want to seek out her company or converse with her; he had never done so before.

"Good day Madam," he said jauntily.

"Good day Sir," she replied.

"A fine day to be out," he remarked. "Where are you walking to?"

"Ah'm on an errand to see Mr Plews's sister Sir," she said.

"Perhaps I will walk with you," Frederick told her. "It is rather deserted around these lanes for young ladies such as yourself to walk alone in."

"Thank ya Sir, but ah'm used to these ways. There's no one would hurt me around here," Eve told him.

"No, of course not," Frederick said reassuringly. "I will walk with you all the same." Eve was very uncomfortable at the prospect of the Squire's grandson walking by her side, and for a few moments considered turning back towards Elmsley. However, not wanting to let down Mr Plews and his sick sister, she decided to keep walking towards the farm.

Seven hours later, Eve had not returned home, and Mary and Anna were very concerned. Fortunately, Joseph had been there for some hours, fixing the fencing at the back of the cottage that strong winds had blown down earlier in the week. Eve had already been gone for four hours when he arrived. As the time got later and later, so Mary became increasingly worried for her daughter.

"Tis only two miles to John Plews's place," Mary

said to Anna. "Sh' should've been home hours ago."

"Plews?" Joseph asked. He was sitting at the table eating, having been invited to supper for his kindness in fixing the fence. "John Plews's farm, is that where Eve went?"

"Aye," Anna said. "'E came 'ere this mornin' an' asked Eve ti go an' see 'is sister. Sh's sick, 'e said, an' 'e wanted our Eve to give 'er sommit'."

"John Plews?" Joseph repeated. "His sister? He's only ever had one sister an' sh's been dead fer years."

"Nay," Mary said. "Ah heard 'im myself, tellin' Eve that 'is sister wor sick an' askin' if sh' would go ti see 'er."

"An' what time did sh' leave?" Joseph asked. He was concerned himself now. He knew of John Plews and did not feel easy that Eve went anywhere near his farm. He was a bad lot. His homestead was very run down and his animals were kept in appalling conditions. Many of his neighbours had shunned the man for the way he treated his wife, his children and his livestock.

"Eve went from 'ere at two o'clock," Anna told him. "'Tis nine o'clock now. Sh' should've been back 'ours ago."

"Ah'll go and look fer her," Joseph said, and left quickly. He rode his cart out of the village and westward up the lane leading to a number of farms on the outskirts of the village, John Plews's farm being the nearest. Within fifteen minutes, Joseph had reached it. He saw Plews collecting wood from the front of his cottage and rode through the farm gates and up to him.

"Ah've come to collect Eve Jennus," he shouted to Plews.

"Who?" Plews shouted back.

"Eve Jennus. Sh' came to see yar sister," Joseph told him.

"My sister?" Plews replied. "Sh's been dead fer five years, so why would sh' come ti see mi sister?"

"Ya called on Eve today an' asked her to come here to yar farm. Now where is she?" Joseph demanded, getting more concerned by the second, instinct telling him that something was very wrong. John Plews was playing games with him and he was not going to stand for it. "Where is she Plews?" he shouted angrily. "Ah want to see her now, or I'll be headin' back to the village to bring out the police."

"Ah've not seen Eve Jennus. Sh's not been 'ere!" Plews insisted.

"Ya're lyin' man," Joseph shouted. "Where is she?"

"Ah'm tellin' ya Locke, sh's not been 'ere," Plews yelled back.

"Right," Joseph said. "Ah'm fetchin' the police. We'll see if ya tell them the same story." Joseph started to turn his cart around so as to leave the

165

farm yard. Plews called after him.

"Look, the Jennus woman 'asn't been 'ere, ah'm not lyin'. But ah did go ti 'er 'ouse an' ask 'er ti come an' see mi sister." Joseph stopped his cart.

"So where is she?" he insisted again.

"Sh' wor never supposed ti be 'ere. The Squire's grandson," Plews paused, "Frederick Addington, 'e were meetin' 'er before sh' got 'ere. It wor 'im who wanted mi ti tell 'er ti come ti mi farm. 'E wor meetin' 'er. That's all ah know."

"If anythin' has happened to Miss Eve, ya're in a lot of trouble Plews," Joseph told him and left the farm quickly, riding back along the route to Elmsley. It was now quite dark and he had no idea where to even look. He knew that Eve would not have arranged to meet Frederick Addington, but he also believed that Plews had not seen her. What had transpired, he could not imagine, but his priority now was to find Eve. Every few yards or so Joseph stopped and, scanning the lane and adjoining fields as best he could in the fading light, he called out Eve's name. But there was no answer. The nearer to the village he got, the more Joseph worried. But he decided to go back to Anna's place and see if Eve had returned whilst he was gone looking for her. She had not. Mary was near hysteria by now and almost collapsed with the stress. Anna was holding on to her tightly, having talked Mary out of going to search for Eve herself.

Joseph called on every male he knew in the village who would help him, including Dru and the Police Constable Jowett, and they arranged a search party. Whilst the men combed the fields and lanes from Elmsley to the Plews's farm, Constable Jowett and Joseph paid a visit to Addington House. In the absence of finding Frederick there, the Squire, who had retired for the night, was called upon to speak with the constable. James accompanied the Squire to the Great Hall, where Constable Jowett and Joseph were waiting. The story was told, but neither the Squire nor James had seen Frederick all of that day and they did not know where he might be found either. James looked into the eyes of Joseph and a knowing passed between them.

"Ah'll see Constable Jowett and Mr Locke out," he told the Squire. As Joseph was leaving, James put his hand on his arm. "Ah'll find Frederick," he said. "If he has had anything to do with this, he will be called to account for it, ah can assure you."

"Ah'm not interested in Frederick," Joseph replied. "Ah just want to find Eve. Her mother's in a dreadful state an' ah promised ah'd find her." James nodded that he understood. When Joseph and Jowett had left, he returned to the Squire, who was standing looking out of one of the hall's large windows into the night.

"I want you to take Hardaker and Crabbe and go and find my grandson," the Squire told James sternly. "Hardaker might know where he is, he has found him before. Bring Freddie back here. If he will not return willingly, you have my orders to use force. But bring him directly to me. I will wait here for you." The Squire returned to his seat and sat staring straight ahead. He had warned his grandson time and time again about interfering with the girls from the village and local town, and was deeply shocked to hear that Freddie might have something to do with the disappearance of Eve Jennus. James called upon Hardaker and Crabbe, both burly labourers on the estate. Upon questioning, Will Hardaker revealed that he had often collected the Squire's grandson, drunk, from a brothel in Farnleydale, a town some five miles north of Ashton. This seemed like a possible place for Frederick to be, so the three men rode there at some haste. When they reached Farnleydale, Hardaker led them to the brothel and Frederick was found, face down in a drunken stupor in one of the 'better' rooms upstairs in the establishment. The Madam there refused to let her client go without payment being made, so James settled Frederick's debt, whilst Hardaker and Crabbe carried him downstairs and threw him over his horse, securing him against falling off on the journey back to Addington House.

On arrival, Frederick was carted, feet dragging along the floor, in front of the Squire. He had begun to regain some of his senses by now, having vomited up much of the ale he had drunk earlier, on his rough ride back. The Squire looked at his grandson in disgust as he was manhandled into the Great Hall.

"Did you interfere with Eve Jennus today?" the Squire asked Frederick.

"Err, what?" Frederick mumbled, trying to keep his head erect. The Squire rose from his seat, walked over to his grandson and threw a large glass of water into his face.

"Did you have anything to do with the disappearance of Eve Jennus?" he repeated loudly. "Do you know where she is, boy?"

"No," Frederick replied cockily. He had quickly pulled himself together and struggled out of the clenches of Hardaker and Crabbe to try and stand on his own two feet. "I'll deal with you both later," he threatened the men as he straightened up his clothing.

"You will do no such thing!" the Squire shouted at him. "I will ask you again. Do you know where Eve Jennus is?"

"What do you care?" he directed at his grandfather. "She's just a whore. She offered herself to me for money," he bragged.

"You are a liar," James screamed at Frederick and grabbed him around the throat. "What have you done with her?" he yelled, throttling him.

"That is enough!" the Squire shouted and motioned to his workers to make James unhand his grandson. They pulled him off.

"This is wasting time," James shouted in distress. "He knows where she is. She could be dying out there somewhere," and he lunged at Frederick again.

"The last I saw her...when I left her, she was by the lane leading off to Fellows Farm," he shouted back to James, diving behind Hardaker for protection. James turned and ran from the hall, down the stairway and out of the main door to where his horse was waiting. He mounted it and raced out of the estate and onto the road back to Elmsley. Fellows Farm lay east of that road and that is where, if he was to be believed, Frederick said he had left Eve. As James frantically rode, he prayed for her safety. He turned at the crossroads and galloped towards the lane leading to Fellows Farm. Ahead, he could see lanterns alight, and as he drew closer, James saw Joseph Locke and two other men carrying Eve. He jumped from his horse and ran over to the party, shouting her name. Constable Jowett stopped him, standing between him and Eve.

"Is she all right?" James cried, trying to look past Jowett. "Can ah see her?"

"Now then Mr Barlow," Jowett said. "Miss Eve is in a bad way. We have to get her home as quickly as possible. There's nay time fer ya to be seein' her. Not now." Jowett turned back to Joseph and watched as he and the men carefully carried Eve onto his cart and laid her gently on the blankets that Joseph had brought with him. When she was settled, he covered her. One of the men climbed up to look after Eve on the journey home, cushioning her head, and the third man and Joseph climbed onto the front of the cart and they rode off. James stood looking on in anguish.

"Ah just wanted to make sure she was unhurt," he told Jowett.

"Well, we don't know what her injuries are till we get her home," Jowett said. "Ah have to ask ya Mr Barlow, how come ya knew Eve wor here?"

"We found Frederick and he told us that this was where he met Eve today," James stated. "Ah just rode here by chance. Thank God she has been found."

"Aye, an' none too soon either," Jowett said. "Ah'll be up at Addington House in the mornin' to speak to Mr Frederick. Ah'd be obliged if he's there when ah come. Ah don't want to have to go search fer him."

"He will be there," James reassured him. "Ah'll make sure of that. But ah want to go to Eve's home now to see if she needs anything. Ah've got to find out how she is."

"Ah don't think that's a good idea Mr Barlow," Jowett told him. "Dru Jennus will no doubt be there wi' his sister an' ya'll not be welcome. Ya know how he feels about yar family."

"Then ah'll ride back to Farnleydale and speak to our doctor," James said. "Tell Eve's mother that the Squire's doctor, Doctor Botheroyd, will be calling on them first thing in the morning to see Eve."

"Ah'll tell them," Jowett replied. Joseph arrived back at Anna's cottage, and Dru, having been given the news of Eve's finding and returned there to meet them, came out immediately and lifted his sister from the cart. He carefully carried Eve indoors and Mary gasped in horror at the sight of her daughter.

"Oh God," she yelled. "Eve!" Mary touched her face. "Take her upstairs," she ordered her son. Dru took Eve up and laid her gently on her bed. Joseph stayed waiting anxiously downstairs. Mary went to her daughter's side.

"Anna, get a bowl o' hot water an' some cloths," she told her. Between them, Anna and Mary undressed Eve and cleaned the dirt and blood from her face and hands. Mary then checked her daughter's body for trauma and for any signs of rape. She had not been sexually violated, but had a wound on the back of her head. Once her face and neck had been carefully washed, new bruising could be seen about her cheeks and mouth. She had clearly been struck. Eve was unconscious, but breathing steadily. Mary checked her eyes, which showed that she was not deeply unconscious, so she was hopeful that her daughter would not die.

"How is sh'?" Joseph asked Anna. He had been waiting downstairs with Dru for the last hour.

"Sh's comfortable," Anna told him. She had come down to fetch more hot water. "Mary's given 'er some remedy an' dressed 'er wounds an' now sh' seems peaceful."

"Do ya think sh's goin' to be all right?" Dru asked Anna. He was deeply shocked and clearly upset. Joseph put his hand on Dru's shoulder to comfort him.

"Ah think so. It all depends on how long sh' stays unconscious fer," Anna replied optimistically, trying to hide her fear and concern. "Mary seems ti think that sh'll be out o' it soon an' sh's probably right. Sh' usually is wi' this sort o' thing." There was a knock at the door and Joseph answered it. Constable Jowett was enquiring as to how Eve was and Dru told him her condition, as far as his mother and Anna could comprehend it. Until Eve could say what had actually happened to her, the constable told them, he could take the matter no further. While he was there, Jowett passed on the message from James Barlow regarding his sending the Squire's doctor to examine Eve in the morning.

"Ah'm not sure how Mary would find that," Anna told him.

"Surely it can't hurt to have the doctor just look at Eve?" Jowett commented.

"Ya don't know Mary," Anna replied. "Sh' 'ates doctors...all o' them."

"Well, ah'm just passin' on the message as it wor given to me by Mr Barlow," Jowett said, "Personally, ah think it's a very generous offer from the man. Tis not everyone gets to be seen by the Squire's personal physician."

"Considerin' tis the Squire's grandson who might 'ave done Eve's injuries, it don't seem so generous does it? Frederick is Barlow's brother-in-law." Dru spoke up angrily.

"Now then Dru, we don't know anythin' fer sure yet, do we?" Jowett said. "It might be best to reserve our judgement till ya sister tells us what happened."

"Well, ah'll say to ya now," Dru told Jowett. "If Frederick Addington touched my sister ah'll make him suffer fer it."

"That's no way to be talkin' Dru," Jowett warned him. "Ah can understand ya anger, but if Mr Frederick did this to Eve, Squire's grandson or not, he'll face the law, ah can promise ya that. But tis not fer you to be takin' the law into yar own hands. Anyway, ah'll bid ya good night. Ah'll call in the mornin' to see how Eve is."

"Aye, an' thank ya Samuel fer yar help. Bless ya fer comin' out so quick an' 'elpin' us find Eve," Anna said. Joseph nodded in acknowledgement.

"Ya're more than welcome," he replied. "Ah'm just sorry fer yar family. Tis a terrible thing that's happened to Miss Eve." After Jowett had gone, Anna told Dru and Joseph to leave as well. There was nothing else to be done for Eve this night, other than what Mary and she were doing. Dru had a wife and young baby to see to and needed to go home, but Joseph asked if he could stay, 'just in case', he said. If anything happened, he could quickly get Dru, and besides, he would not be able to sleep for worrying. And, as he was there, might he not help with boiling water up and making drinks for those nursing Eve? Anna agreed and was glad of Joseph's offer.

It was a long and stressful night. Mary and Anna took it in turns to watch over Eve. She did not move or make a single sound, until daybreak. Mary was dozing in a chair by the side of her bed when Eve's head moved very slightly and she made a faint murmur. Mary sat up sharply.

"Eve," she said quietly. Mary stroked her daughter's hair to encourage her to wake up. Eve responded to her mother's voice and touch, and moved some more. "Eve, my sweet child. Eve," Mary said softly. Eve slowly and hesitantly opened her eyes. Once she could focus, she looked at her mother. Mary was crying and continued to gently stroke her daughter's hair. "Eve," she said again, and kissed her face.

"Mam," Eve mumbled and tried to smile. Anna must have been sleeping lightly, because she came directly into the room and over to Eve. She did not say anything to her, just touched her forehead gently, brushing away some strands of hair, and smiled a very relieved smile.

"Ah'll fetch some fresh water ti drink," she told Mary. Mary nodded. Anna woke Joseph, who was sleeping upright in a chair by the range. She told him that Eve was conscious and he and Anna cried into each other's arms in sheer joy. Joseph had to go to his bakery, but told Anna he would come by later to see how Eve was recovering.

Chapter 14

Doctor Botheroyd, as directed by James Barlow, called at seven o'clock at Anna's cottage the following morning. Mary had been told during the night that the Squire's physician had been instructed to see Eve. Anna very carefully slipped the news in during a conversation. Mary was silent on the telling, so Anna had no idea how she would be when the doctor called.

"Good morning," Botheroyd said chirpily as Anna opened the door to him. "I'm Doctor Botheroyd, and I've come to see the patient, Eve Jennus." Botheroyd took off his hat. He was a small, wiry man with a very large nose, over which sat a pair of spectacles. Anna looked behind her, where Mary was sitting warming her hands by the range; she was feeling cold from her sleepless, night time vigil. Mary motioned for her to let the doctor come in. Surprised, but relieved at Mary's gesture, Anna invited him into her home.

"Ah'm Eve's mother," Mary said, rising to her feet. "Ah wor told that Mr Barlow instructed ya to see my daughter. Before ah let ya see Eve, ah want to know what ya think ya will be doin' fer her." Anna noted that Mary's tone of voice was stern, but not too unfriendly.

"Well," Doctor Botheroyd began. He had been given

very strict orders to be respectful and non-confrontational to Mary Jennus. The doctor was clearly adhering to those orders. "Mrs Jennus. I would like to examine your daughter to firstly ascertain any injuries. Then, I will talk to you about possible treatment. I was told that Miss Jennus was unconscious when she was found last night. Is that correct?"

"Aye," Mary replied. "Sh' was, but she opened her eyes this mornin', so sh's out of immediate danger." Doctor Botheroyd wanted to disagree and quote all kinds of medical facts to Mary, but he kept his own counsel. Sensing the doctor's refrainment, and respecting his humility, Mary agreed to let him examine her daughter. Eve was surprised to see a strange man enter her bedroom and more surprised to find out that the man was a medical doctor. He explained however, very kindly and very courteously, how he had been engaged by James Barlow to come and see her and, if required, treat her for any injuries or trauma she had suffered. This was an entirely new experience for Eve, being seen and handled by a doctor, but she agreed and spoke candidly about what pained her and how she felt. Mary remained in the room, guarding her daughter. The doctor examined the back of Eve's head and, although the gash on it was obviously the cause of her being unconscious, agreed with Mary, that it did not appear to be life-threatening. The injury, he said, caused a concussion, which she was slowly recovering from now. Botheroyd was satisfied that the wound had been dressed very well by Mary, and said so. Eve's speech, sight, hearing and limb movements were then tested and found to be normal. The injuries to her face were superficial, he told her, even though painful, and would heal fairly quickly. Doctor Botheroyd then gently broached the subject of rape, and Eve told him confidently that she had not been sexually assaulted or violated. Did she fully understand what 'rape' was, the doctor asked her, accepting that Eve was still a virgin? She assured him that she did. He then felt her pulse and listened to her heart, reporting to Mary that her daughter was a healthy and strong young lady, and that he thought she would recover fully from her ordeal. Botheroyd said however, that she should have complete rest for a few days and then slowly take herself into her normal life's duties. Doctor Botheroyd concluded his examination, smiling and graciously. Mary and Anna thanked him and the doctor left, telling the ladies that should Eve still feel unwell in a few days, then he would, of course, call again to see her.

Once Botheroyd had gone, the women talked about his visit. Mary knew that he had no doubt been told how to behave with them, but admitted that it helped her to have his opinion on her daughter's condition. Anna remained astounded that Mary even let the man into the home, and Eve felt comforted that James cared about her and was responsible for the visit from him. Doctor Botheroyd had to report back to the Squire and James Barlow on Eve's condition, and arrived at Addington House at the same time as Constable Jowett, who was there to interview Frederick. The doctor and constable were shown into the Great Hall, where the Squire, his grandson Frederick, and James were sitting waiting. After the usual greetings were exchanged between them, Doctor Botheroyd was called upon to give his account of Eve Jennus's condition. James had slept little that night and was very apprehensive waiting for this news. He had to appear calm however.

"The Jennus woman has regained consciousness," the doctor reported. "In my opinion, she will make a full recovery."

"Thank God!" James said, expressing his relief and looking very happy to hear this news. Jowett smiled as well. The Squire made no comment and Frederick looked totally uninterested.

"Ah would like a full statement from you doctor regardin' Eve's injuries," Jowett told him. "Did sh' tell ya how sh 'got them?"

"No constable, she did not tell me, and I did not ask her," the doctor testified. "I rather felt that was your job Sir. What I can say is that the wound to her head could have been made by any number of things, and by a number of ways. It could have been made from a blow by something blunt or a fall onto something blunt. Miss Jennus also had some injuries to her right cheek and around her right eye, which are consistent to a blow about the face, but again, could have occurred during a fall. There were various other bruises and cuts on her body, arms and legs, but these were all superficial and not life-threatening."

James stared across at Frederick hatefully, knowing he had done this damage to Eve. Frederick sat examining his finger nails the whole time, seemingly uninterested and unconcerned about the account just given by Doctor Botheroyd of Eve's condition. He did not look up once from his preening.

"Was the woman violated?" the Squire asked the doctor pointedly.

"No Sir," he replied, "although I did not examine the patient. I doubt if her mother would have allowed me to. But Eve Jennus, when questioned, told me that she had not been assaulted sexually in any way, and seemed to fully understand the meaning of that act." The Squire, as well as James, appeared relieved at this report and James murmured something under his breath. Jowett had been taking notes of this conversation and turned to Frederick.

"Ah have to ask ya Mr Frederick," he began, "what happened when ya met Eve Jennus yesterday. Ah would like ya to tell me what ya did."

"I did not do anything," he replied arrogantly. "I went out riding in the afternoon and happened upon the woman walking along the lane just outside Fellows Farm. I merely said 'good morning' to her. I made no other conversation and went on my way."

"Ya did not say anythin' else to Miss Jennus or touch her in any way?" Jowett asked him sternly.

"Why would I want to speak to that woman...or touch her?" Frederick sneered. "She is a peasant for God's sake!" he added indignantly.

"Last night you told us that she offered herself to you for money," James spoke up angrily.

"Last night I was drunk," Frederick answered bluntly. "I cannot remember anything I said."

"John Plews told me that ya paid him to get Eve Jennus to go an' see his sister, so that you could meet her on the way. What do ya say to that Sir?" Jowett asked.

"I did give Plews some money to get Eve Jennus away from her home. I had some notion of meeting the woman," Frederick admitted casually. "My dear brother–in-law over there seemed to find her attractive, and I was merely interested to find out why. Let's be honest gentlemen, one cannot pass up a chance of enjoying a pretty lady, now can one?" he laughed, as his grandfather and James looked over at him in disgust. "But when I saw her, I was fairly disappointed. She is very plain, very plain indeed. So what did the Jennus woman tell you constable...lies no doubt?"

"Ah haven't spoken to Miss Eve yet. But ah shall do, an' then ah might be back to speak to you again Mr Frederick," Jowett told him.

The doctor and the constable were thanked and shown out of Addington House by James. Doctor Botheroyd returned to his surgery and Constable Jowett made his way to Anna's cottage. Upon his arrival, he informed Mary and Anna that he had spoken to Doctor Botheroyd, who had told him of Eve regaining consciousness. Jowett added that he was very pleased to hear the good news. Mary felt it was too soon for Eve to speak with him however, so he went on his way and arranged to go back the following day to interview her.

After the doctor and Constable Jowett had left, the atmosphere in Addington House was unpleasant. The Squire was angry and disturbed, but he was also tired. He had spent a lot of money and much of his goodwill trying to keep his grandson out of the hands of the law. He was sickened with the behaviour of Frederick and was in no doubt that it was he who had injured Eve Jennus. Before his grandson could leave the hall and disappear for the day, the Squire demanded he speak with him.

"I now want you to tell me the absolute truth about what happened yesterday," he ordered Frederick.

"I have told you Sir," Frederick replied indifferently. "I did see Jennus, but I did not touch her."

"I do not believe you Freddie," the Squire told him. "But I want you to hear me and hear me well. Eve Jennus's great grandfather, Jabez Bowlin, did a service to the Addington family many years ago. We therefore owe his family a debt. If you ever go near Eve Jennus again, I will tell Constable Jowett about the scratches you have on your chest and neck, the scratches you have hidden underneath your cravat." Frederick stared at his grandfather. He wanted to ask him how he knew, but resisted the temptation. He then thought that he would say he got them at the brothel where he went to last evening. Instead, he said nothing, just turned and began to leave. "I mean what I say Freddie," the Squire called out to him. "I also intend to make sure that other people know this information as well, so that when I die, Eve Jennus and her family will remain safe from you. Do not ever forget this conversation."

The following afternoon, Constable Jowett returned to speak to Eve. She was sitting up in bed now and beginning to feel quite her old self. She had taken some soup and a slice of the bread from the loaf that

Joseph had brought around early that morning, straight after baking. Eve had already seen a number of visitors to her sickbed that day. Margaret had called with some flowers from her garden and the latest gossip. That cheered Eve up. Joseph had seen her briefly and Dru called on his way to his smithy. For the first time in months, Dru and his sister held one another and promised never to argue and become estranged again. He thought he was going to lose Eve, and it shook him. She felt vulnerable and weak and it was assuring to know that her big brother was back in her life. Mary was exhausted by the whole affair and Anna was concerned that she should rest more. But Mary told her that she would rest when Eve was fully recovered. The constable was invited in and taken up to Eve's bedroom.

"Now then lass," Jowett smiled at her. He was genuinely pleased to see Eve looking so much better than when they found her, lying behind the stone wall, just along the lane from Fellows Farm. Jowett had already spoken to the Bateson family who lived there, but they did not see or hear anything unusual the evening Eve was injured.

"So Miss Eve, can ya tell me what happened to ya?" Jowett asked her.

"Aye," Eve began, taking a breath. "Ah was walkin' along an' ah fell. The next thing ah knew, ah was in bed at home." Jowett was very surprised and looked across to Mary, who said nothing and gave no reaction.

"Ya fell?" he asked Eve. "Did ya meet Frederick Addington on the way to the Plews's farm?"

"Ah don't remember," she replied.

"Ya don't remember seein' anyone?" Jowett continued.

"Nay," Eve answered simply. "Ah can't remember much of the whole day." Jowett sat there, waiting for and actually wanting something more. He had been convinced that Frederick was lying when he said he had not interfered with her. But he looked into Eve's face and she showed no signs of dishonesty herself. He was unconvinced by her account however, and did not want to let the interview go there.

"Fine," Jowett said cautiously. "If ya say ya fell then ah have to take that as bein' the facts." He studied Eve for some moments. "Is there any reason why ya would be tellin' me a lie Miss Eve?" he asked her. "Ah can't help ya if ya don't tell me what really happened."

"Thank you Constable Jowett," Eve smiled at him." Ah know ya're concerned fer me, but that's what happened." Jowett had done all he could. He had to accept what Eve was telling him, even though he completely doubted her story. He thanked Mary, wished Eve a speedy recovery and left.

"Ya did the right thing," Mary told Eve. "Ya'll nay get justice anyway, an' all ya would've done is upset Mr Frederick. When the old Squire's gone, Frederick will be the new Squire an' we'll all have to live under his rule. Tis better that he knows that ya didn't tell on him." Eve carefully laid her head back into her pillow. She knew her mother was right, but she was still very upset and angry with Frederick Addington. She thought back on the events of the previous evening.

After he had dismounted, Frederick walked with Eve as far as the top of the lane heading down towards Fellows Farm, questioning and becoming increasingly familiar with her. She felt embarrassed by some of his curiosity and refused to answer him. He pressed her about James and what she had done with him, insinuating that they had been lovers and he made explicit sexual remarks to her. Eve refused to respond to his increasingly vulgar prying and told him that she did not want his company and asked him to leave her. Frederick became agitated and then furious with Eve for having such audacity. She was being disrespectful, he told her, and how dare she speak to him in such a way, a man of his birth and station. When he took hold of her arm, she struggled to free herself, and when he attempted to kiss her, Eve screamed and fought with him. Frederick slapped her face hard and she fell to the ground. He tied his horse to a gate and stood over her as she lay in the dirt.

"I am going to show you what a real man is," he told her. "Not like that weakling James. Now lift your skirt woman." Eve told herself to stay calm, and then, with a quick move, managed to pick herself up from the ground. She attempted to run from Frederick, but her grabbed hold of her hair and pulled her back. She struggled again, but as he turned her around towards him, she lashed out with her fingernails, clawing his neck and ripping through his shirt to his chest. He yelled out in pain and slapped her so hard she spun around and fell backwards, her head hitting the stone wall that bordered the lane. Eve crumpled in a heap at the bottom of the wall, a large gash opening up in the back of her head that immediately bled profusely. Thinking he had killed her, Frederick picked Eve up and threw her over the other side of the wall and left as quickly as he could, riding hard to Farnleydale.

"What if he attacks me again?" Eve asked her mother.

"Ah doubt if he'll ever have the nerve," Mary told her. "In any case, it won't be forgotten, what he did. Frederick Addington will regret the day he did that to you. He'll get what he's due in time." Then she asked Eve if she felt well enough to talk to her about the future. Eve said she was.

"Is there nay man, apart from James Barlow," Mary asked, "that ya could love?" Eve was surprised at the question but answered honestly.

"Nay, there's nobody ah would ever want. Ah told ya mam. Ah love James an' that's it," she said.

"But he's married Eve, an' now his wife's carryin' his child," Mary replied. "He'll never be yours my sweet, ya know that don't ya?" Eve nodded. She knew that she would never be with James.

"Ya can't just sit yar life out. Ya have to find someone else," Mary told her.

"Why do ah?" Eve asked.

"'Cause, when Anna an' me is gone, ya'll need someone to look out fer ya. Dru's got his own family now an' his duty is to his wife an' bairns, not to you, or even me. An' what about children of yar own?"

"Ah know mam," Eve said. "Ah know what ya're sayin', but ah can't think on another man while ah love James. An' who would take me fer 'is wife anyway?"

"Ah know someone who would," Mary told her boldly. Eve looked at her mother in total astonishment and laughed self-consciously. Mary had never spoken to her about husbands before and she felt a little shy about the whole conversation.

"Go on then," Eve said mockingly. "Tell me who ya think would take me fer his wife."

"Joseph," Mary said.

"Joseph?" Eve almost shouted.

"Aye, Joseph," Mary repeated. "Joseph's loved ya fer years."

"Nay, he doesn't love me," Eve laughed, "an' Joseph wor my father's friend mam. He's not a young man. He's years older than me," she argued.

"He's older than you, tis true, but there's nay better man neither in this village nor beyond it," Mary told her daughter. "Joseph Locke would lay down his life fer you. Ah know he would." Eve had never thought of Joseph as a man or a suitor. He was always her father's friend, her mother's friend, her and Dru's friend.

"Ah can't believe ya're serious mam," she told her. "Ah can't believe ya think that Joseph loves me and that ah could love Joseph."

"Ah know he loves ya. As fer you lovin' him, well, maybe ya can't, but that doesn't mean ya shouldn't marry him," Mary told her. Eve was astounded by the whole discussion she was having with her mother and wanted to end it. She loved James and was prepared to live alone for the rest of her life, as long as she believed he loved her. She had accepted that he was married to Jayne Addington, but was content to know that he did not love her. They were expecting their first child, but Eve understood that James would have to perform his husbandly duties. That did not mean he loved his wife. The more she told herself these things, the more she believed them. Mary and Anna decided that they would try and convince her differently at every opportunity they had however.

By the following week, Eve was feeling much improved and had taken the odd stroll around the village. Surprisingly to her, a number of people she met whilst she was out, expressed their sorrow at the accident and wished her a full recovery. Joseph called as he usually did every morning, with bread and cakes, but Eve found herself being slightly cool with him. And now it had been suggested by her mother that Joseph loved her, Eve found it difficult to be in his company alone. She only went to Ashton once a week with him and spoke very little on the journey there and back. Poor Joseph did not understand what he had done to offend Eve and was visibly upset by her stand-offish-ness. One morning, when Eve had gone out to deliver a remedy in the village, he casually mentioned her behaviour towards him to Mary, trying to see if she knew why.

"Tis because ah suggested that sh' get married to you," Mary said plainly.

"What?" Joseph asked. He was taken a-back. "Ya said that to Eve?"

"Aye, an' don't go pretendin' that ya've never thought of it yarself," Mary replied bluntly. "Ah know ya love her. Ya've allus had a soft spot fer our Eve."

"Aye, tis true ah do care about her, but ah never thought of Eve as my wife. Ah'm far too old fer her. Nay wonder sh's been upset. Ya've put me in a difficult place Mary. What can ah say to her?"

"Just ask her to marry ya," Mary told him. Joseph laughed nervously. He was embarrassed, stunned and flabbergasted. There was absolutely no possibility that he was going to ask Eve to marry him, and it was the furthest thing he would ever believe could happen. Eve came through the door at this moment and knew she had interrupted a conversation about her. Joseph could not look her in the eye and quickly excused himself.

"What have ya been sayin' to Joseph mam?" Eve asked her mother.

"Ah told him to ask ya to marry him," she replied.

"Mam!" Eve said loudly. "Ah'm not goin' to marry Joseph Locke. Please stop embarrassin' me an' embarrassin' him."

Chapter 15

Over the following weeks, Eve returned to good health and resumed her normal life of helping mothers with their birthing, making remedies and curing pastes with Mary, and administering them to her neighbours, as well as doing the household chores and looking after the garden. Once Eve had fully recovered however, Mary seemed to weaken and Eve was spending more of her time now caring for her. Mary then had a particularly bad bout of illness, which did not respond to any of Eve's tinctures and she even contemplated calling in a doctor for her, perhaps Doctor Botheroyd, she suggested to Mary, but she would have none of it. Eve's concern was that her mother's resistance was now very low and the slightest exertion was making her breathless, which would be made worse by the approaching cold weather as the winter months began to take hold.

Eve took the opportunity of going into Ashton one afternoon with Joseph to buy some provisions, leaving Anna to watch over her mother for an hour or so. With her daughter's twenty-third birthday coming up soon, Mary suddenly wanted to bake a special cake for the occasion. Anna ran around the village borrowing ingredients from different neighbours and Mary stood enthusiastically making up the mixture. The cake was to be a surprise for

Eve and they would eat it Christmas evening. Until then it would be hidden away. Mary finished baking and lovingly wrapped the cake up and set it in a large tin, which she pushed to the back of the larder's highest shelf, hopefully out of sight from Eve. As Mary stepped back down from the stool, she collapsed and fell, taking some storage jars from the lower shelf with her to the ground. Anna heard a crash and ran to see what had happened.

She found Mary on the floor of the pantry, seemingly unconscious. Anna felt for a pulse and then checked her breathing, but she had neither. Mary was dead. Anna screamed. Not knowing what to do, she sat and held Mary tightly in her arms on the cold, stone floor of the pantry until Eve returned home a short time later. When Eve came in and found her mother being supported in Anna's arms, she was at first confused and unsure of what was happening. But as she began to comprehend the situation, and realised that her mother had died, Eve's legs gave way in the shock, and she fell, hysterically crying and shouting out for her. Anna opened her arms to Eve, and they both cradled Mary between them.

"What happened to me mam?" Eve cried.

"Ya mam's 'eart, it must 'ave finally given up," Anna told her in between tears. "Sh' just went. It wor obviously 'er time Eve. We 'ave ti let ya mammy go mi sweet." They both sat holding Mary for the next hour, talking to her, kissing her and crying.

"Go an' fetch Dru," Anna eventually told Eve. "Ah'll stay 'ere an' look after ya mam while ya go an' get yar brother." Eve went to Dru's home and brought him back. He was beside himself with grief when he saw his mother, and sobbed loudly as he picked her up from the floor, out of Anna's arms, and carried her body to her bed, gently laying Mary out on it. Eve and Anna then left him to be alone with her.

"Ya 'ave ti be brave now Eve," Anna told her. "Ya 'ave ti be brave an' strong." But Eve felt neither. She felt afraid, sick to her stomach and lifeless. Her whole being was empty. That night saw a series of visitors to Anna's cottage. Dru's wife, Alice, had told Joseph, and he was the first to come. Joseph was dreadfully upset and asked if he could see Mary. He went to her side and sat talking to her for some time, holding Mary's hand and kissing it. Eve entered her mother's room to tell Joseph that Dru wanted to speak with him and was moved to find him kneeling beside her, crying.

"Ah'm so sorry Eve," he told her. "Ah cared very deeply fer yar mam. Sh' wor allus so kind to me. Sh' wor a special woman. A very special woman." Eve did not reply but nodded an acknowledgement at what Joseph had said. "Yar mam's wi' yar father now an' yar Nanna. No one can ever hurt her again," he told her. Eve could not say anything, she just began to sob and Joseph held her. "Come on lass," he said after some time. "Let's go an' see what yar brother wants."

Dru was sitting with Anna. He looked shocked and exhausted. Anna had told him what had happened with his mother, and how she had just simply gone, but he still seemed confused. Dru turned to Joseph as he came down the stairs.

"Ah need ya to help me Joseph. Ah don't know what to do now," he told him.

"Well, the first thing is, ya go an' tell Samuel Jowett," Joseph said calmly. "He'll probably call on a doctor to come an' look at yar mam."

"What fer, why would we need a doctor?" Dru asked.

"Just so he can say that yar mam died a natural death," Joseph replied. "Look, ah'll go an' fetch Jowett." Joseph went to the police house and returned with the constable very soon after. Jowett looked shaken at hearing of Mary's sudden passing and respectfully took his hat off as he entered the cottage. As indicated by Joseph, Jowett told them that he would be calling upon a doctor to examine Mary. It was nothing to worry about, he assured them, just procedure. Their mother was not very old and therefore a doctor's examination was required by law.

Three hours later, it was Doctor Mason who called at the cottage. Eve withdrew to her bedroom whilst the man was there, and Dru and Joseph dealt with him. Thankfully, he was satisfied that Mary had died from heart failure and her body was therefore allowed to stay with her family. Mason inquired after Eve's whereabouts and health as he was leaving, which was met with a curt response from Dru. The doctor seemed to find that amusing and he grinned superciliously, which led to an abrupt reprimand from Joseph. He told Mason to remember why he had been called out and to show some respect for the grieving family. The doctor turned to leave enraged at his telling off, and sharply informed Dru that he would be sending his bill to him within the next two days. When Mason had gone, Jowett apologised for the man's behaviour. He had been dismayed by it and assured Dru that he would not be calling on Doctor Mason to come to their home again.

Mary was laid to rest next to her husband Thomas in St Guthlac's churchyard four days later. It was a simple and quiet affair. Dru was very upset but Eve was inconsolable; she was finding it hard to accept her mother's death. Anna had been trying to alleviate Eve's grief by spending the last few days telling her of the miracle that Mary lived as long as she had done. She told Eve how three times, as a very small child, Elisa had nearly lost her, but Mary fought for her life each time and won. It all took a toll on her heart however. She was left a frail child, susceptible to illness and had it not been for the great care of Elisa, Mary might have been taken long before she became a woman. Anna also told Eve that it was a wonder that she birthed two babies with such a weak heart and that Eve should therefore give thanks that she had her mother for as long as she did. Anna also reminded her how Mary had survived being sent to Paddow House and how easily she could have died in there. 'The angels must have been looking after 'er', Anna said. Eve had not really known much about her mother's weak heart before. Mary had certainly never made much of it to her and hearing about this from Anna helped Eve to cope with her loss. But how was she to carry on? How was she to live without her dearest mam?

"We all 'ave ti live wi' loss Eve," Anna told her. "At least ya've got memories ti keep. Ah can barely remember mi mam or father, or mi two older sisters. Ah lost 'em all, an' that wor that." Eve had forgotten that Anna's whole family had died when she was a very young child. "Ah still miss 'em though," Anna said. "Even though ah can't remember 'em, ah've missed 'em all o' mi life. Ya've got ti get on wi' yar own life now Eve an' take on yar destiny. Tis now yar time an' Mary gave mi instructions to speak plainly ti ya if sh' wor ti die. Ah think sh' knew 'er time wor coming."

Over the weeks after her mother's passing, Eve received a number of letters. One was from James Barlow, expressing his sorrow for her loss. She was glad that he troubled to do that and put the letter away in a safe place for keeping. As best as she could, Eve carried on as normal. The awkwardness between her and Joseph seemed to have dispelled, and she no longer felt uncomfortable in his company. It was as if some kind of unspoken understanding had passed between them, and their friendship became as it used to be. Joseph was a great comfort to Eve and Anna after Mary's death, and Eve knew that he supported Dru emotionally as well; Joseph had become a second father to him over the years.

Eve now took possession of the books belonging to her mother. On the last page that Mary wrote in one of the books, she referred to two letters, folded behind that page; one was to Eve and the other to Dru. Eve opened and read her letter.

To my dearest, sweetest Eve,
When you read this letter I will have passed. I know that you will be fine without me, daughter. You are a strong and clever lass and I trust Joseph to protect you now. Although you may miss me, I want you to

know that I will always be with you in everything you do, and everywhere you go.

As well as a little money I have saved to give you and Dru, I leave you three books. They are all treasures beyond price that have been handed down through the females in our family for many generations. One of the books you already have, and it holds everything you need for making the remedies and cures.

The second book tells you other things that you must learn about as well, so that you can protect yourself and help others. These are things you have not needed to know about until now. Use this knowledge carefully.

The third book is the history of our family. You are now the guardian of it. In time, you must record your own life in its pages. What was written in this book by your ancestors bears witness to their lives and is a testimony of the truth. Their history is for your eyes only. As you read through your grandmothers' stories you will understand why our family has always been feared, loved, misunderstood and misjudged at times. Your ancestors, including me, have done many things in their lives that you might not understand, but you must never sit in judgement over any of us.

I know you will look after Anna and care for Dru as much as you can. I fear for your brother, but he has to walk his own path. I know you will do your best for him and little Thomas. Above all else, please take great care of yourself. You are our future.

I have been very fortunate in my life. I have known a wonderful grandmother, a beautiful mother, a good, true husband, two perfect, loving children, and of course, our special Anna. I have received kindness from some dear friends, especially Joseph, as well as pain in my life, and I am content to leave the world and join my precious husband, Thomas, and my own precious mam. I have arranged where I want to be laid to rest; Pastor Bell has my instructions.

Always remember that I love you.

Your mother, Mary Elizabeth Jennus, proud daughter of Elisa Maria Shetcliffe, granddaughter of Maria Eve Shetcliffe, great-granddaughter of Elyse Mary Shetcliffe and descendent of Esobel Eve Shetcliffe.

Eve read the letter from her mother many times over the weeks following her passing. She set about the hard work of becoming an expert in her trade and reading the family history. There was much to learn, and a great deal to find out about her ancestry. Grandmothers, going back through generation after generation, who were known to Eve by name only, suddenly came alive to her through their life stories, which they had written themselves. Their words, their thoughts and their actions throughout their lives were all recorded in great detail. Eve found herself submerged in her family's incredible history as she read through the pages of the book. She was astounded, surprised, and excited to read some of the revelations of her grandmothers, but above all else, she was proud to be her family's future and to have the privilege of setting down her own life accounts after theirs.

Of the many things that fascinated Eve from each of her grandmothers' 'stories', were the lists of peoples' names. Next to the rolls of names were dates of their deaths and what they apparently died of. Eve wondered why such inventories were in the book. She found a similar list in her mother's story, which had three names set down in it, all known to her.

The first was that of Jonathan Barlow, with the year of his death and how he died, which was not as instantaneous as was rumoured at the time, according to Mary's record. She wrote that he laid for a number of hours with a broken neck before he died, unable to move. Barlow's entry was followed by the name of Doctor George Selby, with the year of his death and how he died, which Mary stated as being 'rather' unpleasant. She wrote that Selby contracted an internal infection that he suffered painfully and violently on his body, until death followed slowly, some days later. The last name on the list was Frederick Addington. Mary recorded the year and cause of his death as well. But Eve was confused, because Frederick was still alive. Mary's notes said he 'died' of syphilis, the date of death being twenty years from then. During this time he apparently suffered with dreadful recurring bouts of illness from the disease as it slowly ate away at his body. Eve asked herself what these registers could possibly mean, and then a slightly uncomfortable thought crept into her mind.

"He'll get what he's due in time," Eve whispered. She remembered her mother's exact words, and then she understood.

During the weeks after Mary's death, Eve began delivering remedies herself again. Joseph had been doing this whilst she was recovering from her injuries and then whilst she grieved for her mother. He wanted to carry on doing it as he hated the idea of Eve walking alone outside of the village, but she insisted on not changing her ways. Joseph had always believed that she lied about Frederick Addington, and was concerned he might attack her again. But Eve being Eve, would have none of it. She felt perfectly safe walking the lanes alone and was no longer concerned about Frederick Addington. He would not touch her again.

Eve's life soon became very busy. She took on all of the household and garden chores and looked after Anna. Margaret called regularly with the latest news in the community and Joseph visited daily. She studied her book of remedies well and went about her business quietly, becoming the unofficial, but trusted midwife in Elmsley. Through her work, Eve's life took on a meaningful existence.

The following years passed by with few major events, except two. The old Squire, Edmond Addington died, and his grandson, the arrogant and callous Frederick, took his title and place in the community as Justice of the Peace, much to the disquiet of Eve and many other folk in Elmsley. The second event was the birth of another child to James and Jayne Barlow. Eve rarely saw James now, except on the odd occasion in Ashton or Farnleydale. Even then, it was always at a distance and he never acknowledged her being there. She still found her heart beating that bit faster for days after she had seen him though; she still loved him. Eve seldom happened upon Doctor Mason, fortunately, but when she did, the man was polite enough and even took his hat off to her in greeting, much to Eve's surprise. They never spoke however.

Little Thomas was growing up fast and Eve did manage to see the boy when Dru brought him to Anna's cottage, unbeknownst to Alice of course. The child always seemed to have the sniffles and an unhealthy pallour, and Eve would sneak some tincture to him when Dru was not looking, following it up with a sweetie from her 'special' jar. It was a secret that Thomas and she shared, and as young as the lad was, Thomas did not tell on his aunt.

Chapter 16

It was the late summer of 1892, Eve's twenty-eighth year. Dru had recently taken to calling at Anna's cottage more frequently of an evening and staying longer and longer, sometimes even eating there. He was welcome of course, but Eve knew there must be reasons why he was not spending that time at home. Eventually, she managed to bring the subject up with her brother. After some initial denial, he opened his heart and spoke of his total frustration, disillusionment, and anger with his wife. He told Anna and Eve that Alice did little cleaning and cooking around the home, nor did she look after his son properly. Their own relationship had little love in it either, he confided in them. Dru complained bitterly that Alice was also spending his income almost as quickly as he was earning it. Eve told Dru to put his foot down and control his wife, but he said he had tried and they just ended up having terrible rows. He was at his wits end and very unhappy. Eve made no comment, but she did not need to.

"Ya were right Eve," Dru told her. "Ya tried to warn me, but ah was so in love wi' her. Ah still am, but ah can't live like this. Some days, ah get home from mi work an' have to feed the little'un myself, 'cause Alice 'as been out all day an' says sh's too tired to

206

cook fer us. Most of the time, she leaves little Thomas wi' mi next-door neighbour. Tis like sh' don't want to be a mammy to him, or a wife to me." Eve felt no glory in being proved correct and was upset for her brother. "If sh' doesn't change ah'll throw her out," Dru said angrily.

"Ya can't do that," Eve told him." Ya just have to keep tryin' to make it work."

"Aye," Anna joined in, "ya 'ave ti keep yar family together for Thomas's sake." But Dru was stubborn and bloody minded. Eve knew that her brother was miserable and not coping very well, but she could do little to help him, other than be there and let him talk whenever he needed to.

Dru had not been to Anna's cottage for a couple of weeks, but he arrived late one evening looking tired and strained. The first thing he grumbled about was that people seemed to be taking their business into the smithy and forge near Farnleydale instead of coming to him.

"They are just not givin' me their work," he blurted out. "As if ah don't have enough problems, now ah'm losin' mi livin' as well."

"Dru, what are ya sayin'?" Anna asked him.

"Mi business is nay doin' well Anna," he told her. "An' Alice is on me back the whole time fer money an' ah don't have any to give her."

"Ah'm sorry to hear this Dru," Eve told him. "Just

give it a bit of time. They'll come back to ya."

"Ah can't wait," he said. "Ah don't have anythin' to give mi wife."

"What about the money mam left ya?" Eve asked him. "Didn't ya put it away fer such times as when it wor needed?"

"We've already spent that," Dru told her.

"Ah'll give ya the money mam left fer me," Eve said and went to her room to fetch it.

"Dru Jennus," Anna said. She was more than annoyed with him. "Did ya not save any money? Ya've been doin' so well over these past few years. Ah don't understand why ya 'ave ti take t' only money Eve 'as in t' world."

"Alice is nay good wi' our finances!" Dru replied tensely. "Ah told ya that! Sh's spent everthin' we've had. Ah can't seem to stop her from spendin' my money. Ah don't even know what sh' spends it on. There's nowt food in the house an' Thomas is allus in need o' clothes. Ah just don't know what else to do wi' her."

"Oh Dru," Anna sighed. "Well, when yar work picks up again, make sure ya give Eve back 'er money cause that's all sh's got."

"Ah will," Dru told Anna. Eve came downstairs and gave Dru the small amount of money that Mary had left to her. That and her mother's wedding ring and a few other pieces of jewellery left to her from her grandmothers, were all she had of any note.

"Thank ya Eve," Dru said gratefully. "Ah'll get it back to ya as soon as ah can." He left and Eve drew the curtains and lit the lanterns for the night. Not an hour later however, Dru returned with his son, Thomas, sound asleep in his arms.

"Alice left 'im wi' Sally next-door, an' told her sh' wor goin' into Ashton wi' her sisters," Dru said angrily. "But that wor hours ago an' sh's still not returned. Sally has to see to her own family an' asked me to take little'un." Eve held out her arms and took the sleeping child from her brother.

"Ah'll put Thomas in my bed," she told him and took the boy upstairs.

"Ah'm goin' into town to find Alice," Dru told Anna. "Look after Thomas till ah get back." Dru had gone by the time Eve settled the child in her bed and returned downstairs.

"Where's Dru?" she asked.

"'E's gone ti Ashton ti find Alice," Anna replied. Eve was concerned to hear that.

"He would've been better off waitin' at home fer his wife," she said. "What's he thinkin' of, goin' in to town after her. Ah don't understand what's happenin' wi' them two. What does Alice do in town anyway? An' who takes her there?"

"Ah've 'eard sh' goes in wi' friends of 'ers who've got a carriage," Anna told her.

"Well ah blame Dru. He should have stopped her before it got to this. He's been too soft on Alice," Eve said.

Dru took his cart to Ashton and rode it slowly along the main road running through the town, searching for Alice. After an hour of looking, he saw her come out from one of the local inns. She was not alone, but in the company of a number of other people. He recognised some of the women, but not all of the men. The one man's face he did know well however, belonged to Frederick Addington, now the Squire Addington. The group were all laughing and generally being jovial, until Dru pulled up alongside them. He was seething with temper and shouted to Alice to get up onto his cart. She looked completely shocked to see her husband and stood speechless and mortified.

"Get yarself up here Alice," Dru shouted again, louder this time.

"Who is this man?" one of the men in the company asked, stepping forward.

"Ah'm her husband," Dru told the man aggressively. "Who are you?" The man looked sheepish and withdrew.

"Did ya not hear what ah said?" Dru ordered Alice again. "Ya can get home to yar son. Now move!" Alice had gotten over her shock and was now furious with Dru for showing her up in front of her friends.

"There really is no need for you to be talking to Miss Alice like that," Frederick Addington piped up.

"Sh's nay 'Miss Alice'," Dru bellowed at him, "Sh's Mrs Jennus, my wife, an' ah'll ask ya to be mindin' yar own trouble."

"Do you know who you are addressing Sir?" Frederick asked haughtily.

"Aye, ah know who ya are, an' it doesn't bother me," Dru told him. "Ah'm talkin' to my wife. Ah'm not addressin' you, Sir." Alice moved towards Dru as if she were going with him, then Frederick took hold of her arm, preventing her from climbing up onto the cart. Dru was incensed at the sight of Frederick touching his wife, and leaped from his seat. He grabbed Frederick by his shoulder and violently pulled him away from Alice. She screamed and shouted at Dru to stop. Frederick made some sort of feeble attempt to remove Dru's hand, but he had a vice grip on him and Frederick was unable to free himself. Alice screamed at Dru again to let go of him.

"Get on the cart," he shouted back to her and she did as she was told this time. Dru then threw Frederick onto the ground, yelling, as he stood over him, that he should consider himself to be lucky this day. Dru said he already owed him a beating for harming his sister and warned him that if he even spoke to his wife again, he would kill him. With Alice on board, Dru whipped his horse and drove the cart like a madman out of Ashton. Alice clung on to the side of it for dear life, screaming at her husband to slow down. But Dru was crazed, and kept on whipping the horse to go even faster. Of all the men she could have been seen with that late evening, the new Squire, Frederick Addington, must have been the worst one for Dru. His mind exploded and his rage took over his entire being.

The cart was veering manically from side to side and the wooden wheels shuddered under the strain of the speed at which they were being driven on. Dru took the cart around the bends of the winding lane at a frightening pace, made more dangerous in the failing light. Something then happened; a wheel hit a stone, or a ditch, or nothing, then the whole cart exploded into the air, sending parts of it in all directions. Dru was thrown yards ahead along the lane and Alice was hurled into a bordering tree.

It was getting very late and with no return of Dru, Eve knew something awful must have happened. She settled little Thomas for the night and made sure that Anna had all she needed to look after him for a few hours. Eve secured the cottage then made her way to Joseph's bakery, at the back of which she found him setting out the trays for the next morning's baking. She explained what happened earlier and where Dru had gone. He harnessed his horse and cart and they set off towards Ashton. They first found Dru's horse, which stood eerily by the side of the lane, part of the wooden cart still attached to its shafts and traces. Eve looked feverishly around. It was very dark, but Joseph had brought a torch with him, which he lit for the search. They walked the rest of the area, calling out Dru's name. Joseph then saw him lying face down some yards away and ran to him. He gently turned Dru over. Although bloodied, he was just conscious. Joseph called to Eve for some blankets from the cart and he covered Dru with one and put another underneath his head.

"Ah'll not be able to lift him on my own," he told Eve. "Ah'll have to go an' fetch some help."

"Ah'll stay wi' Dru while ya go," she said. Joseph then left to bring other men to help him get Dru into his cart. Eve sat stroking her brother's head. "What foolish thing have ya done now Dru?" she whispered. "Ya shouldn't have come into town tonight." A short time later, Joseph returned with three helpers, one with his own cart, who brought Constable Jowett with him.

"Was Dru on his own?" Jowett asked Joseph.

"Ah don't know Samuel. He went into Ashton to find Alice, but we don't know if he did," he replied.

"Well, we ought to look around here, just in case," Jowett said. While the other two men were helping Joseph get Dru up into his cart, Eve and the constable searched around the area. After a short while, Jowett found Alice further back along the side of lane, at the bottom of a large tree, half hidden in some dense bushes. He carefully removed the undergrowth around her, holding his lighted torch to see more. One look at Alice's face and Jowett knew she was dead. Eve approached and was told to keep away and go back with Joseph and her brother. She knew from this command that Alice must be badly hurt. Jowett then came over to Joseph and Eve and informed them that he and another man would be staying to see to Alice, who he then confirmed to them, was deceased. Eve was shocked and horrified by the whole episode and was silent on the journey back with Dru to Anna's cottage. By the time they reached there, Dru had come fully to. He was able, with support, to walk indoors and go upstairs, where Joseph helped settle him on the bed. He was clearly very confused and the decision was made to avoid telling him about Alice just yet. Joseph began to clean his wounds; he was badly cut around his face and chest.

Jowett called at Anna's cottage on his return to the village, and told Eve that he would speak with Dru in the morning, but he gave instructions that he was not to leave the cottage. Eve asked him where Alice had been taken and Jowett told her that she was laid out in a room at the back of the police house.

The doctor was going to examine her body in the morning. When the constable had gone, Eve went to help Joseph see to her brother.

"Where's Alice?" Dru asked Eve as she entered the room. Joseph was sitting next to him by the bed. "Sh' wor wi' me. Is sh' all right?" Eve and Joseph looked at each other, not really knowing what to do. "Joseph," Dru turned to him. "Where's Alice?" he asked again.

"Sh's been hurt," Joseph told him.

"If sh's been hurt, then who's lookin' after her?" Dru asked, gazing at Eve this time. "Why aren't ya lookin' after her?"

"Dru," Eve said, taking a deep breath. "Alice is dead." She had studied her brother and knew that he would not be easy until she told him the truth. Dru stared at her for some moments.

"What? Nay, sh' can't be dead," he said. "Where is sh'?"

"Sh's at the police house," Eve told him. "A doctor will be seein' her in the mornin', Jowett said." Dru laid in silence for some time looking vacantly at the ceiling, then let out an awful yell. Eve tried to quiet him, telling her brother that his son was asleep in the next room and that he would wake him up. But Dru was not hearing anything. He flayed around on the bed for a moment or two in anguish, and then forced himself to sit up. Joseph tried to calm him, but Dru pushed him away and he fell to the floor. Eve told her brother to calm down. She had some idea of what was going through his mind. Dru stood up and tried to steady himself on his feet. Even though he was still clearly concussed, Eve knew exactly where he was planning to go.

"Jowett said ya have to stay here Dru," she told him.

"Nay, ah have to see Alice," he shouted back. Joseph had got up from the floor by now and was begging Dru to remain still, telling him that he had been hurt and should not move around. "Ah have to see Alice," he repeated and pushed both Eve and Joseph aside and went from the bedroom. There was no way that they could stop him. Dru was a big, strong man and out of his mind with shock at the moment. Eve motioned to Joseph not to get in his way, as, even though he loved him, Dru was not responsible for his actions right now. Eve saw a terror in her brother's eyes that she had never seen before and she was frightened for him. Dru stumbled down the stairs and headed for the front door.

"Dru," Anna called to him. "Where is ya goin' lad?" but he did not reply to her. She moved towards him to block his path, but Eve intervened and moved Anna aside, telling her with her eyes not to stand in his way. Joseph and Eve then followed Dru out of the cottage and up the lane to the police house. They had no idea what Constable Jowett would do, seeing Dru at his door, but Eve had to hope that he would judge the condition of her brother and act accordingly. Once he reached the police house, Dru thumped on the door. Jowett answered it, putting on his police jacket. He did not seem surprised to see Dru, but still looked slightly apprehensive. Jowett was a large man himself and no more than ten years Dru's senior, but he was still no match for him physically.

"What are ya doin' here Dru?" he asked calmly.

"Ah want to see mi wife," Dru cried. "Please Samuel ah've got to see Alice." He seemed quite lucid and Eve was encouraged that he sounded more together mentally. Jowett looked behind Dru and noted Eve and Joseph were with him.

"Alright Dru, ah'll let ya see Alice," Jowett told him gently. He then took Dru through the police house, past the cell and on to a locked room at the back of the building. It was dark in there, so he lit a lantern and set it on a small table at the side, by the wall. There was nothing else in the room accept a long bench in the middle, upon which Alice was laid out, covered completely in a pure white cloth. The room was windowless and cold, with a bare stone floor. Dru stood in the doorway, his eyes fixed on the shrouded form in front of him. He froze and then began to weep uncontrollably.

"Oh God, ah've killed her," he cried. "Ah killed my Alice." Jowett put his hand on Dru's shoulder and guided him into the room and over to the bench. Dru allowed himself to be led like a small boy and stood with his head bowed in front of it.

"Do ya still want to see Alice?" Jowett asked him kindly. Dru did not answer, but nodded. Jowett pulled back the cloth from Alice's face and Dru slowly looked up and at her. She looked peaceful, as if asleep, and there were no injuries to be seen. Dru stared at his wife for some time, his body rocking slightly from side to side. He had stopped crying and stood motionless and silent by the bench. After some time he put his hand to Alice's face and held her cheek, very gently, so as if not to move her.

"Ah'm sorry Dru," Jowett told him. "Ah'm right sorry fer yar loss."

"Ah killed her," Dru said again, only more calmly.

"Nay lad, it wor an accident," Jowett replied. "Yar wheel must have hit sommit an' the cart threw ya both off. One of yar wheels wor smashed up right badly. We brought back yar horse. Ralph Pullen put him away in yar stable. He took off his harness an' settled him in fer the night." Jowett then left Dru alone with Alice for over an hour, returning later to see him out of the police house and back to Eve and Joseph, who were waiting outside. They supported Dru as he joined them and slowly walked him back to Anna's cottage. He was just managing to hold himself together, but when they got back, he wanted to see Thomas. As he stood watching his sleeping child, Dru broke down again and sobbed bitterly for hours.

As the day began to break, Eve finally managed to persuade him to take one of her tinctures and he lay down and went to sleep. She realised that this new day was going to be a difficult one for her brother and he would need all the sleep he could get.

Chapter 17

Constable Jowett was called to Addington House very early the next day to speak with Squire Frederick Addington. He was summoned there to inform him of the circumstances surrounding the death of Alice Jennus. News had reached Frederick that she was dead. After Jowett gave the Squire the details of how and where she was found, and reported on the condition of Dru's cart, Frederick ordered him to arrest Dru Jennus on a charge of murder. Jowett was stunned by this command and described the broken wheel on the cart again in greater detail, telling him that in his opinion, this was a tragic accident. The Squire would have none of it and told Jowett that he himself was with Alice Jennus not long before her death. He had heard Dru Jennus telling his wife that he was going to kill her. Frederick told Jowett that there were other witnesses who heard him say this also. The Squire said that when Jennus drove his cart up to his wife, he had murder in his heart.

Jowett respectfully disagreed with Frederick and told him that Dru Jennus was no murderer and would never have killed his wife. But the Squire was adamant, and told the constable that as the local Justice of the Peace, his orders were to be carried out. Dru Jennus must be arrested and charged this day with the murder of Alice Jennus. Frederick then dismissed the constable and told him to get to it. Jowett was shocked and bewildered. He had not expected the Squire to issue those orders and he left Addington House in a state of complete dismay and upset. How can he arrest Dru? He had known him since he was born, and liked him. He knew that Dru was no killer. How can he go to Anna's home and perform this terrible task?

"Mornin' Samuel," Anna said as she opened her door to Constable Jowett. "Ya're early ti be 'ere."

"Mornin' Anna," he replied. "Aye, ah'm early. Ah'm sorry fer that. Is Dru awake yet?"

"Nay, 'e didn't put 'is 'ead down till it wor getting' light this mornin'" Anna told him. "Eve gave 'im one of 'er drafts ti make 'im sleep a while. 'E wor in such a state, sh' thought it better 'e slept some. Would ya like a cup o' tea while ya're waitin' ti talk ti Dru?" Anna had just made herself and Thomas a drink. They were sitting eating their porridge at the table.

"Er...nay, ah don't think so," Jowett replied, looking at little Thomas with concern. Eve came downstairs and saw that the constable had arrived.

"Ya're early Samuel," she remarked, surprised to see him calling at such an hour. "Dru's still asleep. Ah gave him sommit to make him take some rest."

"Ah told Samuel ya did," Anna said.

"Ah've just come from speakin' wi' the Squire,"

Samuel told Eve with some difficulty in his voice. She immediately picked up on that.

"There's nowt wrong is there?" she looked directly at Samuel, who averted his eyes. She now knew there was. "What's wrong Samuel?" she asked him pointedly. Her heart sank into a deep pit, because she knew exactly what the constable was going to say next. "Anna, can ya take Thomas into the garden please?" she asked her calmly. "Go wi' Anna, Thomas, an' see if ya can find some nice flowers to pick fer me," she said, and gave him a sweet from her jar to take with him. Anna looked baffled by the conversation, but took Thomas's hand and led him outside, chatting happily to him.

"Ah...ah don't know how to tell ya this," Samuel looked uncomfortably at Eve, who was bracing herself to hear bad news. "Ah'm afraid ah have to arrest Dru and take him into custody," he said very softly.

"Ah see," Eve replied. She felt sick to her stomach. "What's he bein' charged wi'?"

"He's to be charged wi' murder," Samuel barely managed to say. "Ah'm right sorry Miss Eve. Ah don't know what to say to ya. Ah just don't have any choice. Tis not my doin', but ah have to carry out my orders." Eve could not think of what to say, she was shocked to her core. "Ah have to take Dru now Eve," Samuel told her. "Can ya please wake him up?"

"He's in no fit state to go anywhere yet Samuel, ya know that," Eve pleaded.

"Ah know what yar sayin, but he has to come wi' me now. Ah'm right sorry," Samuel apologised again.

"Aye, ah'll go an' do it," Eve replied steadily. She went to Dru and roused him from his deep sleep. It took him some time to come around and Eve was concerned that he was still suffering from his head injuries, but she could only give him another one of her tinctures later in the day. When he was fully awake, Eve did not skirt around the issue. She told her brother straight that Samuel Jowett was downstairs and that he was here to arrest him. She thought it better coming from her, rather than him. Dru sat in silence for some moments considering what his sister had just told him. He did not protest or seem afraid. Eve must have looked terrified however, because Dru's first reaction was to assure her that he was fine and that he was resigned to his fate, and she must not worry for him. She started to cry and held onto Dru tightly, telling him that she loved him and would stand beside him all the way ahead. Dru told Eve to wait downstairs whilst he dressed; he would be down shortly. As she left the room, she turned back to Dru and a gentle smile of love and kinship passed between them. They both knew that this could be the beginning of a very dark time for Dru.

"He'll be down soon," Eve told Samuel. He nodded. A few minutes later, Dru came down the stairs. He looked exhausted and ill, but not angry or desperate. Samuel greeted him as a friend.

"Dru," he said. "Ah'm right sorry about this. Tis none o' my doin', but ah have to take ya to the police house and charge ya. Ya understand what ah'm sayin', don't ya?"

"Aye," Dru replied simply. "Can ah just have a minute to speak to Thomas," he asked.

"Of course ya can," Samuel told him.

"Thomas is in the garden," Eve told her brother, and he went to see his son.

"Ah'll testify fer Dru," Samuel told Eve. "Ah'll do all ah can fer him, ya know that don't ya?" Eve faintly smiled at him; he was a good, kind and fair man.

"Thank ya Samuel," she replied. "Please take care of Dru fer us." He nodded. Dru returned from speaking to Thomas and told Samuel he was ready to go with him. He would leave his son in the capable hands of Eve and Anna.

"Ah'll bring some clothes and food down to ya later," she told her brother as he left with Samuel. Constable Jowett did not feel the need to put handcuffs on Dru, and the two men walked calmly out of Anna's cottage and through the village to the end of the high street, where the police house stood. It was hard for Dru to return there and be put in the cell so near to where his wife lay, silent and alone.

Later that morning, Joseph called at Anna's cottage. He was horrified to hear the news about Dru, and told Eve that he would go and find out all he could from Samuel. Upon his arrival at the police house, Joseph first spoke to Dru in his cell and he told him the whole story. Joseph tried to reassure his friend that everything that could possibly be done for him would be. But Dru knew where the order for his arrest came from and warned Joseph not to be very hopeful of a positive outcome from this. After speaking with Dru, Joseph talked to Jowett, who told him that Squire Addington and his friends would most likely testify against Dru, saying that he heard him threaten to kill Alice. Joseph argued that the Squire had lied, and was obviously enlisting his friends to do the same. But Jowett warned Joseph that if a jury heard these testimonies, true or not, then Dru would be hanged for certain. Joseph dreaded taking this information back to Eve and Anna.

"Ah'll go an' see the Squire an' ask fer his mercy," Joseph told the women.

"Nay," Eve said. "That won't make any difference to the man. We need to talk to James Barlow."

"Barlow?" Joseph asked. "Why Barlow?"

"Ah just know we have to talk to him," Eve replied. "He's the closest to Frederick. James will speak to him fer us, ah know he will." Joseph did not agree with Eve's idea, but he had said he would do whatever he could to help, so he did. That evening, he drove to Stockwell House and left a message there for James Barlow, as he was not home at the time. Joseph asked him to come to his bakery in Elmsley, to speak on a matter of great urgency. That night, a messenger was sent by Barlow back to Joseph, to say that he would be at his bakery at 7 o'clock the following morning. James had heard the news of Alice's death himself by now and guessed Joseph's call concerned this. Upon receiving Barlow's note, Joseph relayed the message to Eve. She did not know whether to be present at this meeting herself; she had not spoken to James for some years and suddenly felt sick at the thought of it. But Eve decided that her brother's life was more important than her apprehension and embarrassment. She got to Joseph's bakery very early and waited for James. As he walked through the door and saw Eve standing there, he looked startled. He had clearly not expected to see her.

"Eve!" he said. "How are you?"

"Ah'm troubled," she replied. "We need yar help James." He nodded.

"Is this trouble concerning your brother's wife's accident?" he asked. "Ah'm very sorry for him. Please convey my sympathies to Dru. But, how can ah help?"

"We need ya to talk to Frederick," Eve replied. "He's lyin' an' we need ya to talk to him." James looked puzzled.

"Ya do know that Dru's been arrested fer murder, don't you?" Joseph spoke up. James looked stunned. He clearly did not know.

"No," he replied. "Ah don't understand. Why would he be arrested for murder? My footman told me that Alice Jennus died in an accident."

"Dru's been arrested fer murder because the Squire lied an' told Constable Jowett that he heard my brother tellin Alice that he wor goin' to kill her," Eve explained. Joseph then told James the whole story, as Dru had communicated it to him, and he also gave James the account of the meeting that Samuel Jowett had with Frederick.

"Tis Frederick that ordered Jowett to arrest Dru fer murderin' Alice," Joseph told him.

"Ya're the only one who can help us," Eve told James. "Ah'm not askin' ya to do anythin' fer me. Ah'm askin' ya to see that Dru is treated fairly. He did not murder his wife. He's a fool, but he's nay killer." James stood assimilating the information he had just been given.

"Ah'll see what ah can do," he told Eve cautiously. "Ah'll certainly talk to Frederick, but ah cannot promise that he will change what he said."

"He's lyin'," Eve said loudly. "An' he wants to see my brother on the gallows. Ya have to talk to him. Ya have to help us James." She began to cry. James looked at Eve sympathetically and with love. He wanted to hold her, to console her, but he could not. Joseph was there, and James was trying hard not to let down his guard, one that he has fought hard to maintain for many years.

"Ah'll do my best," James said gently, trying to comfort Eve. "Ah promise ah'll do what ah can to help Dru." Eve seemed heartened by this promise and controlled her crying. She wiped her eyes and looked at James to assure herself that he meant it. He was studying her face, her eyes, her hair and her mouth. Eve suddenly felt embarrassed by his attention, especially with having red eyes from crying.

"Thank you," she said matter-of-factly, in an attempt to break his gaze. James continued to stare at her however and Eve seemed to be in jeopardy of losing her confident deportment. Joseph also suddenly felt awkward. He was filled with the overwhelming sense that the two people in the room with him cared deeply for one another. He knew that James Barlow had at one time been sweet on Eve, but now he realised that those feelings went far deeper than that. He had also not fully grasped the fact that Eve loved James either, and now he

228

recognised that, his heart sank. Mary had been right when she said that he loved Eve. He did. Not that he ever thought that she loved him. But as the years passed and Eve had not found a husband, and she had come to rely on him more and more, Joseph did harbour a faint hope that she might come to care enough for him to consent to be his wife. That hope faded very quickly, as he stood watching James and Eve in the presence of one another. It was obvious that the pair of them shared a deep, passionate love, and Joseph found that difficult to witness. He just wanted to leave the room.

"Ah'll be outside if ya need me," Joseph told Eve, and before she could protest and make him stay, he left. Now they were alone, James awkwardly fumbled around for some words.

"It is good to see you Eve," he finally told her, smiling softly. "You have not changed. You are still the most beautiful woman ah've ever seen. Ah still love you." James could not help himself.

"Why are ya talkin' like that?" she asked him. "Ah don't appreciate ya sayin' that ya love me."

"Ah know," he replied, "but ah wanted to tell you that ah still do." Eve stared at James. She still loved him, but she was not going to tell him that. And he was still the most handsome man she had ever seen. His hair, a little darker now, still curled boyishly around his neck. His smile was still captivating and his eyes still lovely. How could she stop loving him?

"Please help my Dru," she asked him calmly.

"Ah will," he replied.

"Ya have to go now," Eve told James. He nodded and reached out, slightly touching her hand before moving towards the bakery door. He turned back as he passed through it and smiled at Eve.

"Ah'll speak to Frederick and then ah'll come and tell you what he says," he told her, and before she could answer him, James had gone. Joseph came back into the bakery and they talked about the meeting and what they believed might be the outcome of James's talk with Frederick. Joseph was unconvinced about any help Barlow might be able to give Dru but Eve was hopeful that James could influence the Squire. What Joseph was unaware of, was that Eve had not 'seen' her brother being hanged, although she did believe he would have to answer for Alice's death in some way. She told Joseph that if anyone could help Dru now, it was James Barlow.

James rode to Addington House directly from Joseph's bakery. Frederick was at home and James asked to speak with him. The two men sat down to breakfast together.

"Ah heard about your order to have Dru Jennus arrested for murdering his wife, Freddie," James said.

"Yes?" Frederick asked. "But why should you bring this up at my breakfast table brother?"

"Because it is not true, and you know it," James replied bluntly.

"It is true. We all heard Dru Jennus threaten his wife," Frederick said irritably. "The man threatened to kill her and then he did, and he will hang for it!"

"No Freddie, he will not," James told him.

"How say you?" Frederick asked. James calmly finished drinking his tea.

"Because you are going to say that you made a mistake and then your friends will agree and say the same, and Dru Jennus will be let out of prison and the charge of murder will be dropped," James demanded. "Jennus did not murder his wife and you know it. You lied to Constable Jowett, because you did not hear the man threaten his wife. Dru Jennus threatened you."

"How dare you call me a liar?" Frederick shouted and stood up angrily from the table. "How dare you question my word?" James remained seated and calm.

"My dear Freddie," James said. "Ah call you a liar because you are a liar. You will rescind your statement to Constable Jowett immediately."

"I will do no such thing," Frederick protested loudly.

"Ah'll repeat what ah just said," James told him.

"You will withdraw what you told Jowett. Your father left me with some information about you and the unsavoury things that you have done that you would not want to be spread around the county...Squire Addington. Some of it concerns Eve Jennus. If you do not change your statement ah will make sure that this information is heard by everyone."

"That Sir is blackmail," Frederick said angrily.

"Yes Sir, it is," James replied and left the table and then left Addington House.

Chapter 18

As Dru was settling himself to spend another night in his cell, Samuel Jowett unlocked the door and told him to step out. Dru did as he was asked and as Samuel walked back into the front of the police house, he followed. Dru was then told to put his signature in a book that lay open on the desk. Samuel handed him a pen and inkpot.

"What's this fer?" Dru asked.

"Tis fer yar release," Jowett told him. "Ya're free to go." Samuel smiled at Dru.

"How's that?" he asked Samuel, looking completely confused.

"Let's just say that Squire Frederick Addington realised that he had misheard what ya said about killin' yar wife," Jowett told him. "He called me to Addington House this afternoon an' told me he wor mistaken. Ya won't be charged fer murder, Dru, but there will still be an inquest. Ya know that don't ya? The doctor came here yesterday an' examined Alice. He said it wor a terrible blow to the back of yar wife's head from the fall that caused her death. He found wood splinters from a tree embedded deep into her scalp, so ah believe that the inquest will find a verdict of accidental death, but ya can never be sure."

Dru was completely shocked. He was finding it

difficult to take in what Samuel had just told him. On the one hand he was relieved, because he was apparently free to go and was not being charged with murdering Alice. But on the other, he was still distraught at the loss of his wife and felt he deserved to be imprisoned and punished for her death. It was his fault the cart went over and he knew it.

"Ah'll let ya know when the inquest is Dru," Jowett said. "Ah suggest ya go home now an' see that boy of yours. He's growin' up to be a fine lad. Ah can see yar father in him." Dru left the police house and quickly made his way to Anna's cottage. Eve was coming out of the front door. She was actually on her way to see him with a pie and some ale, and could not believe the sight of her brother walking towards her.

"Dru," she screamed and dropped the supper, running to him. He picked Eve up in his arms and spun her around. "Dru," she cried, and smothered his face with kisses. "Oh Dru," she said again. "He did it," she said.

"Who did what?" Dru asked her.

"Nothin'," Eve replied. It was a story for another day. Now it was time to welcome Dru back. As he walked into her cottage, Anna almost fainted. Even though she knew that James Barlow had been approached by Joseph and Eve to help secure Dru's release, she dared not hope it would be done.

"Oh, mi sweet boy," she said. Dru gave her a big hug.

"Where's Thomas?" he asked her.

"'E's playin' in t' garden," Anna told him. Dru went out and fetched his son. They all sat and talked about the last few days. Dru was in a very strange place however. He was happy to be out of the police cell but was dreading going home and found it hard to accept that Alice was dead. It was decided that he and Thomas should stay with Eve and Anna for the time being, just until Dru could cope better, perhaps they would stay until after the inquest. Eve went to tell Joseph about her brother's release and he soon came to the cottage. Dru and Joseph hugged each other, Joseph not quite believing that the Squire conceded and withdrew his accusations against his friend so easily. When Dru took his son into the garden to play for a while before supper, Joseph approached Eve.

"Ah can't believe that Addington changed his mind," Joseph said.

"Ah must admit, ah couldn't be sure that he would, but ah thought James would manage it somehow," Eve replied.

"What did Dru say about James bein' involved?" Joseph asked. Eve just looked at him without giving an answer.

"Ya haven't told him about our meetin' with James

Barlow, have ya Eve?" he asked her.

"Nay, ah haven't, not yet," she replied.

"So ya are goin' to tell him then?" Joseph questioned.

"Aye," Eve said. She was intending to tell her brother at some time that it was more than likely the intervention of James Barlow that had somehow persuaded Frederick Addington to change his testimony against him. However, Eve knew that this would be difficult for Dru to hear; he had hated the Barlows since long before Jonathan Barlow had played his part in taking his mother from their home and putting her in Paddow Asylum. It had been Jonas Barlow, James's grandfather, who had caused a great deal of hardship to Dru and Eve's grandmother, Elisa, and Mary, their mother, when she was very small. Elisa had attended the birth of one of Jonas Barlow's children, a sibling of Jonathan Barlow, but the baby died. Jonas held Elisa responsible for the death, even though the poor infant had been born with terrible deformities and showed few signs of life from the moment he was birthed. Dru remembered his mother telling him of the stigma that attached itself to Elisa for years after this event, which she, as her daughter, also suffered. Dru remembered stories of the hatred shown towards Elisa by the Barlow family and the accounts of how Jonas Barlow was fairly cruel to his grandmother, calling her a harridan and killer in public places. That cruelty continued down the Barlow line, as far as Dru was concerned, proven by the actions of Jonathan Barlow towards his mother. To now tell him that James Barlow actually did him a kindness, would be very hard for Dru to hear and accept. Eve needed to pick her moment carefully to let him know this, but before she did that, she wanted to talk to James and find out exactly what had passed between him and Frederick Addington.

Alice's funeral was held some days later, which was a horrendous affair for Dru. All sorts of stories had been spread around the village. It was now common knowledge that he had been arrested for murder at one point and some were suspicious of him still, even though he had clearly been released without being charged for anything. Some of Alice's family attended her funeral and were very cold towards Dru, but he was too distraught to notice. Little Thomas, thankfully, did not understand what was happening at all, except he missed his mother. It had been Eve who organised laying Alice to rest with Pastor Bell, which was not easy, given her dislike of the woman. She set that aside however, and gave her sister-in-law the best farewell she could manage and afford.

The inquest was held the following week in Ashton. Squire Frederick Addington presided over the proceedings. There were few people from Elmsley there, other than some of Alice's kinfolk, but not that many, considering she came from a large family. Anna, Eve and Joseph attended, as of course did Dru, who gave his testimony as best he could, breaking down occasionally when he spoke of his wife. Constable Jowett, who had been called as a witness, gave his evidence, as did the three men who went out to help fetch Dru home from the accident. None of those people who had been with Alice in Ashton just before the event were called to give witness nor was it mentioned that Dru had been arrested for his wife's murder. Altogether, it was a fairly short hearing, and after listening to the events of that night, the Squire directed the jury to pass a verdict of accidental death on Alice Jennus, which they did. It was a strange affair altogether and although safe from imprisonment or the gallows, Dru now had to find peace within his own conscience. The question was could he forgive himself for what he did?

Eve then asked Joseph to arrange a meeting between her and James Barlow. He felt sickened at the thought of her having contact with the man again, but agreed to do it. She told Joseph that she needed to find out exactly what was said between him and Frederick before she told Dru of James's intervention. Joseph did as Eve asked and she met

James at his bakery later that week; it was the safest place to meet, especially for James. Joseph let him in then went out to Anna's cottage, leaving the two to talk alone. James first told Eve how the old Squire had entrusted him with stories of the many unpleasant deeds that Frederick had committed over the years. He told her that he simply blackmailed Frederick with exposure if he did not withdraw his lies about Dru. They laughed together, especially when James mimicked the astonished face of Frederick when he realised he had to surrender to James's demands. Eve was so grateful to him, but she was not to thank him, he insisted. James told her that he enjoyed watching Frederick squirm; it was no more than he deserved. He also told Eve that he knew Frederick attacked her when she was found hurt outside Fellows Farm, but understood why she did not inform on him.

It felt so good to be laughing and talking together with James again. The years they had been estranged seemed to have made no effect on either of them. She asked after James's children, and he told her all about them. He asked after her life and if she was content. She lied and told him she was happy. He touched her face unexpectedly and she instinctively held his hand to her cheek. They stood looking at one another for some moments. He gently pulled her to his body; he just wanted to hold her, just for a few minutes. She did not resist, but slipped into his arms, resting her head on his chest. She could hear the beating of his heart. He could smell her hair, soft and fragrant near his face. He kissed her hair and then her cheek and then he found her mouth as she surrendered it to him. Years of denial were swept away in total and complete passion as James gently lay Eve down onto the floor. He unbuttoned her dress, exposing her naked body. He kissed her breasts and sucked her hardened nipples. Then James gently pushed his penis deep into her wet vagina and they were one. For some blissful moments the two enjoyed each other in complete love.

Eve should have felt regret at what she had done, but she did not. For so many years she had dreamed of taking James into her body, and now she had done it. She did not fool herself into believing that this could ever happen again, and she did not intend to allow it to. But Eve wanted to know the love of a man. Not just any man, but James. She had to know the love of James. After they had finished and lay in each other's arms, he told her that he wanted to be with her again. James wanted more of her; he loved her, and cared little of the consequences of that love. But Eve told him that this was the only time they would be together like this and that they would never make love again. She meant it. They argued

240

and James refused to accept what Eve was telling him, but she did not relent, and eventually he left, hoping that she did not really mean what she was saying and would change her mind.

Now Eve told Dru what James Barlow had done for him. On first hearing this, Dru was stunned. Why would the man want to do that for him he asked Eve? She told him that James, in spite of what Dru thought of the Barlows, was a good and fair man. She told her brother that she believed that James also did it for her. But for whatever reason, Squire Addington had withdrawn his accusation, and now he, Dru, was free to rebuild his life. Eve left her brother that day, knowing that it was going to be very difficult for him in the weeks and months ahead. She and Anna would care for Thomas whilst Dru worked, and Dru must try to build up his business and his life again. That would be hard, but he was now solely responsible for his child, and he needed to be courageous for his sake.

And so Eve's life settled down again, at least for some weeks. Her brother threw himself into his work and she and Anna delighted in looking after Thomas. He was a joy to have around and seemed to be coping very well without his mother. Then Eve began to feel ill and spent some time each morning being sick. She was with child. Anna was shocked and pleased at the same time, wanting to ask who the father was, but respecting Eve's privacy. Eve was not about to say who he was however, not even to Anna. Dru was less restrained and demanded to know who had done this to his sister; the man was to be made to take responsibility for the child. Joseph was deeply affected upon hearing this news, although not surprised. He guessed who the father was, but said nothing. Whenever they all sat down to eat together, the conversation always turned to how Eve was going to cope with a baby on her own, given that she would not declare who the father of her unborn child was. What was she to live on, how could she and Anna, and now a child, survive?

As if this was not a big enough problem for Eve, one evening, just before supper, Margaret, Eve's gossipy neighbour called at Anna's cottage with some very disturbing news. There had been an accident on a local farm that afternoon. It was the farm belonging to the Morley family. William Morley was helping his father remove some large tree trunks from their land, and was standing beside the heavily loaded cart full of logs. Something spooked the horse and it reared up, tipping the cart and its contents over and on top of William, who was crushed beneath the weight of it all. It was reported to Margaret that he died within minutes. Although somewhere in her mind Eve was not surprised to hear this report, she was still momentarily shocked and almost fainted in her condition. Margaret referred Eve back to what she had told Morley all those years ago, as if she would have forgotten.

"Ya said 'e would die in a terrible accident, didn't ya Eve?" Margaret remarked excitedly.

"Aye, ah remember," Eve replied dolefully.

"Well, 'e 'as! Yar tellin' came true," Margaret said, morbidly exercised by the whole event.

"Aye," Eve repeated. She was deeply unhappy at hearing this news. There was a knock at the door.

"That'll be Joseph come fer some supper," Anna said and went to answer it.

"Where is sh'?" a loud voice yelled. "Where's Eve Jennus?" The voice belonged to Henry Morley, the father of William.

"What do ya want wi' Eve?" Anna asked the man, but he did not answer. He pushed Anna out of the way aggressively and charged into the room, making his way towards Eve, who was sitting at the table with Margaret. Margaret screamed as she saw Morley rushing towards them. Eve stood and faced the man full on. He stopped before her, clenching his fists at his side, his eyes wild with grief, anger and fear.

"'E's dead!" he screamed at Eve. "Mi son, 'e's dead."

"Ah know Mr Morley, ah just heard it myself from Margaret," Eve said calmly. "Ah'm very sorry."

"Sorry?" Morley shouted again. "Ya 'ad sommit ti

243

do wi' this Eve Jennus. Ya're responsible fer William's death, ah know it." Anna came over to stand by Eve's side.

"Henry Morley!" she said firmly. "Ya're talkin' mad. How could Eve possibly 'ave 'ad owt ti do wi' yar son's death? Think about what yar sayin' man."

"Sh' told William 'ow 'e wor goin' ti die. Sh' told 'im!" Morley yelled again. He was shaking, and with every sentence he spoke, got closer to Eve, violence in his face.

"What's happenin' here?" Joseph said loudly from the door. He came in to see Henry Morley standing menacingly close to Eve and Anna. Margaret had scurried to the side of the room from where she would be out of danger, but still be able to see what was going in. Joseph summed up the situation instantly, having not long heard the tragic news about William Morley himself.

"What are ya doin' here Henry?" he asked.

"Mi son's dead an' sh' killed 'im," the man yelled. He now began to sob loudly. Joseph went over to the women and stood in between them and Morley, motioning that they withdraw behind him. Eve held on to Anna and they moved back. Joseph put his hands on Morley's arms.

"Ah'm right sorry fer yar loss Henry," he calmly told Morley. "But ya can't just come here and blame Eve fer this. It wor a terrible accident by all accounts, but it worn't Eve's doin'. Now sit down an' tell me what happened." Joseph managed to usher Henry into a chair. Eve fetched a bottle of brandy from the pantry and poured some in a cup for the man to drink. Henry told Joseph what had happened to William, crying inconsolably much of the way through the story. Eve looked at the man and felt very sorry for him. She understood his grief, but was careful not to say a single word. Joseph was very kind to Henry and offered to return with him to his farm. He was also concerned for Eve. William was one of four brothers and Joseph did not want any of them paying her further visits. He brought this up with Henry and elicited from him an undertaking that none of his other sons would be coming to Anna's home and that they would all stay away from Eve. Henry appeared to pull himself together a little and told Joseph he would manage to get home on his own, he was calmer now. Henry left without looking or speaking to Eve, but he did ask Anna if he hurt her when he pushed passed her at the door. She told him he had not, and Henry left.

Margaret, who had recorded every detail of the event so that she could spread it around the whole village, also left after proclaiming how shocked she was at Henry Morley's behaviour. When all was calm again, Joseph sat down.

"Ah'll have some of that brandy please," he asked

Eve. She poured him some and a little drop for Anna as well, who had turned quite pale with the commotion. "Are ya fine Anna?" Joseph asked.

"Aye, ah wor just shocked when Henry pushed mi out o' t' way," Anna replied. "But ah wor scared fer Eve. Ah thought 'e wor goin' ti 'urt 'er."

"Ah didn't," Eve said confidently. "Henry Morley is nay violent. He wor never goin' to hurt me."

"Eve," Joseph turned to her sharply. "Ya don't know that lass."

"Ah do," she protested. "None of the Morley family will hurt me."

"Ah just hope ya're right Eve," Joseph said. "But will ya at least be careful?" He was concerned for her even though she was confident about the Morley boys. It was not just that family alone who Eve needed to mind however. The news of William's death would be spread all over the village within hours and she had enemies in Elmsley. The whole sorrowful mess would be dragged up from the past and Eve would have to face the accusations all over again. However, at least Henry Morley was as good as his word and none of William's brothers bothered Eve. Of course, she had to face whispers behind hands and some people turning their backs to her as she passed them in the street, many had remembered her foreseeing William's death, and those who did not were soon told. Eve knew it was going to be difficult for her in the weeks ahead. The Morley family were well thought of in and around Elmsley. But she could not change what happened in the past, and what she said all those years ago. Eve just hoped that folks would believe she did not cause William's accident, even if she foresaw it.

Three weeks had passed since William's accident and when Eve visited her family's graves to put some flowers on them, as she did every Sunday, she was shocked to see what had been laid on top of her mother, grandmother and great grandmothers' graves. All had large, roughly-made wooden crosses laid over them. Eve stared at this sight for some moments, trying to make sense of what she was looking at. Then, out of the corner of her eye, she noticed someone over the other side of the churchyard. It was one of the Morley brothers, standing by William's grave. As Eve looked across to him, he turned and looked back at her.

"Eve Jennus?" he shouted. "That is you, isn't it?" he asked loudly. She had no option but to acknowledge the man.

"Aye," Eve called back. He lingered for a while, and then started to walk over to her. For some moments, Eve felt slightly apprehensive. The graveyard was empty but for the two of them, and she did not know what the man had in his mind. She scrutinised him as he came towards her, trying to remember which one of William's brothers he was; she had not seen any of them for years. As he came closer, she recognised him as William's older brother, Nathan.

"Mornin' Nathan," Eve greeted him. He nodded. "Ah'm sorry about William," she told him directly. He stared at her blankly, his face not showing any emotion and it was difficult for Eve to sense what he was feeling towards her.

"Aye," he said simply. "It wor a bad accident all right." Eve did not reply but shook her head in agreement. They both stood for a short while, not saying anything. "Ah heard about mi dad's visit to yar home. 'E wor out of 'is mind in grief," Nathan told her. "Ah think 'e wor sorry after."

"Tis fine," Eve said calmly. "There wor nay harm done." Nathan nodded again. He looked at Eve as if he was going to say something else, but then stopped himself. Nathan then noticed the wooden crosses on the graves. Eve was tempted to ask him if these were his doing, but she knew they were not. She bent down and casually picked the crosses up.

"They do that ti keep witches in their burial places," Nathan said matter-of-factly as he watched her perform the task.

"Who's they?" she asked.

"Whoever did that," Nathan replied.

"Ya don't know who did it, do ya?" Eve questioned him. "Ya didn't see anyone near my family's graves?"

"Nay. An' before ya ask, it worn't me," he said. "Ah don't believe in witches."

"Ah didn't think it wor you Nathan," Eve told him. He nodded again.

"Yar family's not well thought of in this village by some are they?" Nathan remarked.

"Nay, not by everyone," Eve said. "But there are certain folk around 'ere who owe their lives to my Nanna Elisa an' to my mam an' puttin' these crosses on their graves is evil. An' they think themselves to be good Christians?" She laughed mockingly.

"Aye," Nathan agreed. "Ah think tis shameful what they did. They should leave the dead to rest in peace." Eve studied Nathan. He was a good looking man, just two or three years older than she was. In their younger years, he had always been polite towards her, even when his brothers were taunting or bullying her in the street. Eve also knew Nathan liked her; she often caught him sneaking a glance at her when he did not think she would notice. Another time, another life, she thought to herself, and she may have been interested in him. As well as having a handsome face, Nathan was of the build and appearance that a woman could spend some pleasurable time bedding.

"Well, ah have to get back home," Eve said. "Ah'm sorry again fer yar brother, Nathan. Ah really am." He acknowledged her remark then stood and watched Eve as she left the churchyard and walked up the lane towards Anna's cottage. She was aware of his continued gaze, but did not look back, relieved that their meeting was civilised. When she got home, Eve told Anna that she had seen Nathan Morley at the churchyard and that they had spoken. Anna was pleased to hear that he was pleasant towards her, not that she was surprised. She remembered Nathan as a nice little boy, she told Eve. Joseph however, was not happy to hear that Eve had met any member of the Morley family whilst visiting the churchyard alone. He was constantly worried about Eve, especially in the condition she was now in.

It was the report of her bumping into Nathan Morley that instigated Joseph paying her a visit one evening with an important question. He had thought long and hard about what he wanted to ask Eve, and it now seemed the right time, and Joseph thought, the perfect solution. He was going to ask Eve to marry him, and he would offer to bring the child she was carrying up as his own. Before he went to speak to Eve however, Joseph wanted to talk to Dru. He needed to know that he would be happy for him to marry his sister. Dru was surprised at first to hear that Joseph loved Eve; the thought had never crossed his mind. But after considering what Joseph told him, Dru thought it would be a good thing for his sister, and he gave him his blessing.

"Ah want to ask ya sommit Eve," Joseph said nervously. He nearly lost all of his courage standing in Anna's cottage in front of Eve. She looked at him, waiting for the question. "Ah want to ask ya...will ya marry me?" he managed to get out. Eve did not respond in any way, she just continued to look steadily at Joseph. He took a breath and continued, before she could reply. "Ah know ya don't love me, an' ya never will, but ah'll be a good husband to ya. Ah'll not expect anythin' from ya but friendship...ah know ya love another man. Ah'm happy to bring up yar unborn bairn as my own. That'll stop the tongues waggin' around here an' give ya some peace an' protection."

"Joseph," Eve said. "Dear, kind Joseph. Why would ya want to marry me? Ya know ah'm trouble." Joseph looked at her and smiled. He had said what he never thought he could say and now felt free.

"Aye, ya're trouble," he told her, smiling, "but ah don't care. Ah can look after ya an' ah want to do that. Ah love ya Eve, an' ah allus will." Eve was suddenly overcome with emotion. It might just have been her pregnant hormones, but it was probably more to do with the total unselfishness and loyalty of her dearest friend.

"Aye," Eve said.

"Aye what?" Joseph asked her.

"Aye, I'll marry ya," she told him.

Chapter 19

The marriage between Eve Mary Jennus and Joseph Seb Locke was a very quiet affair. It was not held in Saint Guthlac Church; they had a civil marriage in Farnleydale, performed by a registering clerk. Anna, Dru and little Thomas were there to witness the union and the couple returned to Elmsley as man and wife. Joseph moved into Anna's cottage, as Eve would not leave Anna to live on her own. She was getting on in years now, and although reasonably healthy for her age, she needed looking after. Many people in the village were very surprised at Joseph marrying Eve, even though they knew he was loyal to the Jennus family. Some of his customers loudly voiced their disapproval of his marriage when collecting their bread and cakes from his bakery. How could he marry someone like Eve Jennus they asked? Did he not know what she was? Was he not concerned about what she has done? But they got a swift and discourteous response from Joseph. He was not going to put up with any nonsense from them nor would he hear their drivel about his new wife.

There was one person however, who was very distressed at hearing the news of Eve's marriage. James Barlow dismissed it as sheer gossip at first. It was only after some investigation that the truth of the rumour hit him. He was devastated. Having thought that he had just re-found and re-kindled his lost love, she was gone to him again. James had to find a way of speaking to Eve alone, but he could not send a message to her home. After spending some fruitless days trying to meet her accidently on one of her calls around the village or to a local farm, James realised that the only way he was going to speak to Eve was with the knowledge of Joseph, so he visited his bakery to ask permission. Joseph was not surprised to see James on his step early one morning.

"Ah would like to speak to Eve, Joseph," he said. "Ah know she's your wife now, but ah need to speak to her, with your permission that is."

"Ya have my permission to speak to Eve," Joseph told James, "but ah don't know if sh'll speak to you. Ah'll have to ask her."

"Of course," James replied, relieved that Joseph was not aggressive towards him.

"Ah'll ask her tonight an' tell ya what sh' says tomorrow," Joseph said. "If ya come back here in the mornin', ah can let ya know." James agreed, thanked Joseph for his kindness and left. It was not all kindness on Joseph's part, although he did feel some small measure of pity for James. However, James had the opportunity to be with Eve many years ago and had chosen Jayne Addington instead, for whatever reasons. So, as far as Joseph was concerned, James had made his bed and therefore should lie on it. His concern was for Eve. Joseph felt that, even though he was her husband now, he could not deny her the chance to speak with James. If she ever found out that he had turned the man away, then she might not forgive him, and Eve's trust was as important to Joseph as her friendship and possible future love. When supper was over and Anna had retired for the night, Joseph told Eve of James's visit and his request to speak to her. She thought it over for a time and then told Joseph that she would be there, at his bakery, when James went in the morning.

"Eve!" James said as Joseph let him in to his shop early the following day. He was surprised to see her there.

"Ah'll leave ya to talk," Joseph told Eve. "Ah'll be out back in the yard if ya need me, but ah won't come in until ya call." He then left James and Eve alone.

"Eve," James said again. He moved forward, as if he was going to embrace her, but she stepped back.

"Don't!" she told him and he did not move any nearer. He studied Eve, noticing that there was a change about her. She had a certain glow in her face and her breasts seemed fuller. James then realised that she was carrying a child; a slight bump beneath her skirt was just visible. He was shaken.

"You're with child?" he whispered. "The child...the child's mine!"

"Tis Joseph's," Eve said abruptly.

"Joseph is my bairn's father," she insisted. James nodded. He knew what she was telling him.

"Eve," he repeated, "Eve. Ah don't want to live without you. We can be together. We can go away. You do not have to do this. Ah'll look after you and our baby. Ah promise you Eve." She looked at James standing in front of her, almost begging. She loved him so much, but their fates were sealed.

"Ya have to go from here James, to yar wife an' family," Eve told him. "Ah'm married to Joseph now an' you and me are gone to each other. This will be the last time we speak like this. Ya have to leave now." James did not want to accept what Eve was telling him. He argued with her again, pleading with her, but Eve remained adamant. They were never going to be together and each must get on with their own lives. Their time and chance to be one had passed. James eventually left, despondent and telling himself that he was not going to accept Eve's rejection.

The months passed and Eve's bump grew bigger. Joseph made Mary's old room into a nursery for the new baby and Anna's cottage was prepared for the new arrival. There was much tittle tattle around the village and plenty of gossip about the date of Eve's coming birth; did she fall before the marriage, or did she fall afterwards? Margaret frequently popped in and told Eve all the latest rumours, mostly about her, but nothing was going to be allowed to spoil the happy event. Life was settled for the time being.

Dru was still working hard to re-build his business, with some success, and he had resolved himself to living a quiet life with his son. Dru remained very sad though, much to Eve and Anna's concern, but they hoped that eventually he would forgive himself and move on. Other than Thomas, Dru had no interest in anything much. He worked all day and sat in his home all evening, apart from the few days in the week that he could be persuaded to join Anna and Mr and Mrs Locke for supper with Thomas. Dru was something of a lost soul.

James had tried to come across Eve when she was out and about around Elmsley, but without success. As she increased in size, her midwifery duties became fewer and Joseph took on the job of delivering her remedies in the village and to the local farms. James had visited Joseph's bakery and spoke to him about Eve's birthing, and it was agreed, between Joseph and Eve that she would accept the help of Doctor Botheroyd, at James's expense, when her time came.

She began her labour one late evening in April, and

Joseph went to fetch the doctor while Anna sat with her. By three o'clock in the morning, Eve was holding her new baby girl. All went well with the birth and Doctor Botheroyd was satisfied to leave mother and infant in the hands of Anna and Joseph. The doctor was asked to report back to James on the birth and the well-being of mother and baby and he called early the next day at Stockley House, to tell him that both Eve and her daughter were fine. James was delighted to hear that they were safe and also pleased to hear that Eve had given birth to a little girl. Jayne had provided him with two boys, although they now had another child on the way.

"Ah'm goin' to call my babby Mary Elizabeth," Eve told Joseph. "That's if ya don't have any objections?"

"Nay, nay," Joseph said. "Ah think that's a perfect name fer such a beauty." He was as delighted with the little girl and was as happy as if she were his own. He held her, kissed her and loved her. Eve laughed at the way Joseph melted every time he went near the baby, and she was content. She was happy that she had married the good, kind and generous man sitting on the end of her bed, cooing over her baby's cot. Yes, Eve thought about James, but in her heart, she knew she had done the right thing in choosing Joseph.

Little Mary was a pretty baby and always had a smile. She had her grandmother's dark eyes and dark hair. James did get to see his daughter occasionally when he happened across Eve in Ashton or Farnleydale. She gave him some moments to look upon the baby, who had her father's soft curls and his broad smile. James may have wanted more from Eve, but he did not approach her again, not for them to be together. As Mary became a toddler, Eve resumed her midwifery duties, and her remedies and curing pastes became more popular than ever with the villagers and local farmers. She was very happy at this time. She felt safe and loved with Joseph and life was being kind to her, at least for the next few months.

It was the middle of May, just after little Mary's third birthday, when Anna closed her eyes to the world and went to sleep. She had been very busy that day, helping Eve tidy up the garden and clearing the vegetable patch ready for planting. Eve had told her not to overdo things, but Anna said she felt good and was glad to get out into the warm spring day after the long, cold and dull winter months. Anna went to bed early that evening as she said she was tired. She kissed Eve and Joseph good night and that was the last time they spoke to her. When Anna was not up early the next morning, like she always was, Eve went to her room and found her dead. She had passed away during the night. Eve stroked Anna's face and kissed her dearest Granny

Anna, who was as much family to her as her real Nanna, Elisa. She called to Joseph. He came in and checked Anna's pulse, but they both knew she was gone. Eve cried and asked to be alone with her and Joseph left the room and said he would make sure that Mary did not come in. After Eve had laid Anna out, she locked her bedroom door then went to tell Dru, and afterwards, speak to Samuel Jowett. The constable called a doctor in from Farnleydale to examine Anna's body, and, satisfied that she had died of old age, left Eve, Dru and Joseph, to their grieving.

As they laid Anna Rose Gledhill to rest next to her mother, father and two sisters, Eve's thoughts went back through her own life. She could just remember her Nanna Elisa's funeral, then her father and mother's. So many loved ones; she cried for them all. There were quite a number of people from the village who came to pay their last respects to Anna. She was well-liked and well thought of by many, and Eve felt that Anna would have been pleased that they were there. As she left the churchyard, Eve knew it would take her a long time to get used to not having her around. She realised how big a part in her life Anna had played and already missed her.

Joseph was his usual support in the days and weeks following Anna's death. The loneliness that Eve felt in losing her was partially filled with her noisy toddler Mary, and with caring for Joseph, who was her abiding strength and companion. Now Eve felt that her daughter was old enough to sleep alone in her own room, and one night, before they retired, Eve invited Joseph to her bed. He had never asked or even suggested that she allow him to make love to her. He had slept in a bed in the corner of Eve's mother's old room since their marriage. Joseph was completely surprised, and at first, did not know how to react. Of course, he had dreamed of this happening. To live in a home with a beautiful wife whom you loved and yet not be able to touch was very hard for him. But Joseph had told Eve he did not expect anything from her other than friendship and he was a man of his word.

"Are ya sure that's what ya want?" he asked Eve.

"Aye," she replied simply. "Ah want ya to be a husband to me Joseph. Ah want us to have a proper marriage." That night, Joseph lay with Eve and they made love for the first time. Eve gave herself to her husband completely and he fulfilled his duty to his wife to her great satisfaction. He did not ask Eve if she now loved him, and Eve did not tell him that she did. She could not lie to Joseph, but she cared deeply for him, respected him, and decided in her mind that she would do all that was within her power to make him happy.

A year passed in relative peace, but the following

bad winter caused some illness in the village. A particular outbreak of what was thought to be scarlet fever claimed two young lives. Eve was called upon to assist some of the stricken children, but knew she was almost helpless against such an infectious disease. When it was clear that there was an outbreak, Eve had urged everyone who would listen, to isolate themselves and their children as much possible until the disease passed. Eve herself did not let Mary leave the cottage and play with any other children and Joseph was kept at arm's length, given that he mixed with people in his bakery. Then one evening, Harriet Siddle called at their home begging for Eve's help. Eve was not feeling too well herself and turned down Harriet's request that she go and nurse her three children. She explained to Harriet however, in some great detail, how to treat the little ones herself, gave her some remedies, and told her not to worry because she knew that all three of her offspring would be fine. As she said this, Eve touched Harriet's arm, which the woman seemed to respond to.

"That wor a dangerous thing to say to Mrs Siddle," Joseph remarked as Eve returned to sit with him by the fire.

"Maybe," she replied, "but the woman wor beside herself wi' fear. If ah know that 'er bairns are goin' to be fine, shouldn't ah tell her that?"

"That's not the point Eve," he warned. "If anythin' happens to those bairns now, sh'll be sayin' ya had sommit to do wi' it. Ya should be more careful Eve. Ya don't owe these folks anythin'. Not many of them have helped you in the past."

Joseph was right of course, but that was of no consideration to Eve. She only saw the woman's pain and wanted to help her, as she believed it was her duty to do. Two full weeks went by and the outbreak in the village seemed to be abating, as no new cases were reported. Later that week, Harriet Siddle called again at Eve's home, looking much happier than the last time she was there.

"Ya wor right Mrs Locke," she told her. "All mi sick bairns got well. Thank ya fer what ya did an' thank ya fer t' remedies."

"Ah didn't do anythin'," Eve told the woman. "Ya must have nursed yar young'uns well." Harriet smiled and left. Eve was pleased for the woman and told Joseph when he returned home that evening. He was relieved. She also told him some other news. She was carrying his child. Joseph was at first speechless and then overwhelmed with joy. He kept asking Eve to repeat what she had just told him, just in case he heard wrongly. Such happiness he never thought he would experience again, not after losing his first wife when they were so young. Charlotte Locke had died from influenza not long after her and

Joseph had been married. The illness came suddenly upon her and took Charlotte away within days. After his wife's death, Joseph spent months in the deepest depression. It was Thomas, Eve's father, who helped him recover from his grief. He and Mary befriended Joseph and were always there for him, a debt that he had tried to repay to the Jennus family since then. Now he was sharing his life with a beautiful and lovely woman, who was going to give him the gift of a child. He was to be a father to his own flesh and blood as well as to little Mary. After the initial shock, Joseph called on Dru to come to their home with young Thomas and celebrate.

It was an easy confinement for Eve, much easier than when she carried Mary, and she was busy with midwifery duties and dispensing her remedies right up until her eighth month. However, it was not just her birthing and curing knowledge that people began to want from her. Harriet Siddle had told others in the village that Eve had predicted that all of her children would survive the scarlet fever, which of course they had. It was a slow trickle of people at first, but then the numbers calling on Eve to 'tell' them things increased. Harriet's story added fuel to the other 'story' of how Eve had predicted the death of William Morely, which had also sadly come to pass. Young women wanted to know about potential lovers and husbands, wives wanted to know how many children they would have and their life's prospects, and even the odd farmer wanted weather forecasts and warnings for cattle disease outbreaks to protect his crops and livestock. Eve was considered by many to have 'the sight', which of course, she did. However, the devoutly Christian folk in the village saw this as having the 'evil eye' and poured scorn on Eve and anyone seeking her advice. This made no difference to them of course, and they still kept coming to her, some even in secret. Folk also wanted Eve to 'touch' them and give them luck. The fact that she was with child only added to her 'potency' in the eyes of the needy.

Pastor Bell came to speak to Eve one evening and to find out was going on, because he had heard all sorts of rumours and needed to hear the truth of them. He was concerned because he felt there was some hysteria in the village. Apparently, a number of his flock had told him that Eve was performing miracles. When he told Eve this, she was stunned and spent some time putting the pastor's mind at rest that she had done no more than tell Harriet Siddle that she thought her children would get over the scarlet fever, if indeed that was what they had. She told Bell that all she did for those who called upon her for 'seeing' into their futures was to talk to them and give them some guidance, much the same as he would. Satisfied that Eve was not declaring herself to be a miracle worker or soothsayer, the pastor told her and Joseph that he would try and stop these rumours. Joseph expressed his gratitude to Bell that he was stepping in to help. Eve must be left alone now and be allowed to rest; she was very near her time. When the pastor had gone, Joseph once again pleaded with Eve to be careful. He pointed out how easy it was for anything she says and does to be misunderstood and how things can quickly get out of hand. She was about to have their second child and that was surely the most important thing that she must concentrate on at this time. Eve understood Joseph's concerns and promised him that she would not do anything to harm their family or herself. He had to be satisfied with that, whatever it meant.

Like their daughter Mary, the new addition to Eve and Joseph's family was a spring baby. Seb Joseph Locke came into the world late one night in the middle of May. He screamed his lungs out after he had slipped his way into life, whilst everyone else smiled. Doctor Botheroyd attended this second of Eve's births as well, on Joseph's insistence.

"You have a healthy little boy," Botheroyd told Joseph. "Mrs Locke is well and everything seems to be fine. Congratulations Sir." Joseph was so delighted that all he could do was stand before Eve with a silly smile on his face.

"So aren't ya goin' to hold yar son?" Eve asked him. He went over to the bed and peered down at the baby.

"Oh God, he's beautiful," Joseph finally managed to say. "Ah can't believe ah'm lookin' at my son. Thank ya fer givin' me this blessin,' he told Eve. Little Mary was still sound asleep in her room, totally unaware of the busy night that her mother and father had just had. She would have to wait until the morning to see her new baby brother.

Chapter 20

And so Eve now had two beautiful children and a loving husband. Life was being kind and she settled down to look after her family. She only had the odd few people coming to ask for her 'knowledge' now, so Pastor Bell's 'help' seemed to have worked. Of those that did, Eve was careful in her actions and words. She told Joseph she would be mindful of helping to create any damaging rumours about herself or her 'powers', and she kept to that promise. Eve saw nothing of James during this time. He never seemed to go to Ashton or Farnleydale anymore, and was not at Stockley House very much either, according to Eve's neighbour, Margaret. She visited with stories of how James Barlow rarely saw his wife these days. He had two boys away at boarding school and left his third son and wife alone much of the time on his estate. Apparently he could not bear to be at home with Jayne. Margaret's brother worked at James's stables and gave her the regular gossip on the Barlow family. If these reports were true, then Eve felt very sorry for James and his wife Jayne. She would not have wished so much unhappiness and loneliness on either one of them.

The truth of the matter was that James was very unhappy with his life. He only coped over the years because he saw Eve and his daughter Mary occasionally and harboured the belief that Eve had only married Joseph to give his child a name and to save her reputation, such as it was. But when James heard that Eve was carrying Joseph's child, he became very distressed, realising that both she and his little girl were gone to him forever. The thought of Eve making love with Joseph was unbearable to him. James threw himself into his business, opening other factories across Yorkshire and staying away from home for long periods of time. With his fast-growing wealth, James also began buying up land and property. It was all he could do to stop himself from thinking about Eve, and the life they could have shared, had he not been persuaded by his family and the old Squire to marry Jayne Addington instead of the woman he really loved.

Although Eve's life was fairly constant at this time, things were changing all around her. Elmsley was being transformed and so were the people in it. A new century had been heralded in the year earlier, and some of the old country ways were rapidly dying out; cottage industries being lost forever to a 'modern', mechanical era. Many villagers were leaving the land and going to work in the new industries that were mushrooming right across the county, including the factories owned by James Barlow. Whole families were being enticed away from a rural life to live in towns, so that the parents, and their children, could fill the burgeoning factories nearby, which were forever hungry for workers. The promises of greater wealth and increased comfort that were given as inducements to people to leave their homes and lives that their ancestors had followed for hundreds of years, did not, for the most part, materialise however. Stories came back to the village of people who had moved away, stories of how they were now living in just as much poverty and depravation in slum dwellings in the towns as the rural ones they had left behind. Those folk, women and young children, as well as men, were now trapped, often working cruelly long hours every day in awful conditions within noisy, dirty factories, and still unable to escape a wretched and poverty-stricken life. At least in Elmsley they were breathing fresh air in open spaces, not filthy fumes in dirty factories and living in overcrowded and unsanitary town slums.

On hearing these stories, Eve was reminded of how fortunate she was. She owned the cottage she lived in, having inherited it from Anna, and Joseph had a steady income. There were fewer people in the village, but he still earned a living for their family from the bakery. Eve was often paid some small amount of money to deliver babies and supply her remedies, and all together, that afforded the Locke family a reasonable existence. They grew some produce and kept poultry and Dru supplied them with pork meat occasionally, so they managed. The Locke children were growing up fast. Mary was a clever and inquisitive little seven year-old girl, although delicate, and Seb, a noisy, boisterous three year-old toddler. They got on well enough, in spite of their different characters, and Mary bossed her little brother around appropriately.

Life was settled for Eve's family and there was not much change, except for two big events that happened; one for the village, the other for Eve personally. The first was the marriage of Squire Frederick Addington to the daughter of Colonel Alfred Waterhouse Berkley, the Head of one of oldest military families in York. Elizabeth Berkley was not only very rich but was said to be beautiful as well, and far too good for the Squire, according to most of Elmsley and beyond. The second and more important event was that Dru met a lady from Farnleydale, a Lillian Metcalf, and they were married within a short time. Lillian was in service at a large house in the town, and Dru first met her when he delivered some repaired horse harnesses to her employers. The young lady was eighteen years Dru's junior, and when her brother first told her this, Eve was slightly concerned. However, once she met Lillian, that unease was mostly dispelled. She was a pretty, chatty, fun person, and Eve instantly liked her. If anyone could pull Dru from the sad place that he had inhabited since Alice's death, then Lillian could. Eve's only worry was that she was not just young in years, but she was, in some respects, quite childlike and fragile. Knowing how dominant Dru was, Eve only hoped that he would be gentle with his young bride, and to this aim Eve resolved to keep a look out for Lillian.

It was autumn now and the nights were drawing in fast. One late evening, an unexpected caller came to Eve's door, just before dark. It was Sarah Thresh, a young girl of seventeen that Eve knew of. She had been orphaned as a toddler and was taken in by the Streddlers, who ran a small, rented farm some miles outside Elmsley. Eve had known of Sarah, firstly from Margaret, who had given her regular accounts of the poor girl as she was growing up, which were not always comfortable to listen to. The Streddlers apparently treated the child quite severely, putting her to work on the farm from a very early age and treating the girl like a servant. Eve remembered her mother, Mary, calling on Pastor Bell a number of times to ask him to try and help the child, but it was never clear to Eve just how much help he was ever able to give her.

Eve invited Sarah into her home and she nervously came in. Looking at her dishevelled state, Eve offered the girl a warm drink and asked her to sit down.

Joseph, sensing their visitor needed to talk in private, said he had some chores to do and left the room. Sarah was a tiny little thing, all bones. She may have been seventeen, but she looked more like a twelve year-old. She was badly dressed in an ill-fitting skirt and a loose, sleeveless top, held together around her thin waist by a grubby apron. Even with her shawl, she was far too scantily dressed for such a late autumn night, and Eve was already thinking about the spare clothes she had that might fit her.

"What can ah do fer ya?" Eve asked as she set some hot tea and honey on the table for Sarah.

"Please Miss Eve, ah mean, sorry, Mrs Locke," she bumbled in her tiny frail voice. "Please, ah need yar help. Ah'm in some pain an' someone told me to come to you. They said as ya would help me."

"Of course ah'll help ya if ah can," Eve told her calmly. "Now tell me what the matter is." Sarah burst into tears. For some moments she could not speak. Eve went to the girl and put her arms around her. Sarah was so skinny it was uncomfortable to even hold her. "Now then lass," Eve said kindly. "Take yar time to tell me. Are ya in pain now?" Sarah nodded. "So where is the pain?"

Sarah pointed to her lower stomach. Eve kneeled down beside the girl. "Can ya tell me what sort of pain it is?" Sarah stopped herself from crying and looked at Eve.

"Please Mrs Locke, please help me," she begged.

"Ya have to tell me what's wrong," Eve insisted. "Ah can't help ya if ya don't tell me." Sarah then told Eve what had been happening to her and Eve listened in silence and with horror. Sarah was married to John Morley just over a month ago. He was nearly twenty years her senior and Sarah did not want to marry the man. But Mrs Streddler, the only mother she had ever known, insisted that she married him, or be put out into the street. Sarah thought the Steddlers may have sold her to Morley, but she could not be sure. At first, Sarah said, before they actually got married, John Morley was reasonably pleasant, but then he began to hurt her, especially when he took her to his bed. She had been a virgin and knew nothing of a man. The way Sarah described what Morley then did to her made Eve feel sick and outraged. The girl told her how she was in terrible pain, but that every night, sometimes two times a night, he wanted her sexually. She told Eve that she begged him to let her get well, but he would not listen, and now hits her if she does not let him do what he wants to with her. By the time Sarah had finished her account of the abuse she had received at the hands of her husband, Eve was so angry, she could barely speak.

"Ah need to look at ya," Eve told Sarah gently. "Ah won't touch ya, but ah need to see where ya're hurtin'." Sarah was told to go up to Anna's old room and lay on the bed. Eve then looked at Sarah's vagina and anus. The girl was so badly swollen and bruised Eve thought it a miracle she could sit down. The inside of her groin was also black and blue and she had a number of strange injuries about her buttocks and the tops of her legs, some of which looked like teeth marks.

"Did ya walk here from the Morley farm?" Eve asked her. Sarah nodded that she had. Eve was astonished. The farm was almost five miles away and in her condition, she must have been in pain with every step she took.

"Did ya tell his mother what he's been doin' to ya?" Eve questioned.

"Ah did try to tell Mrs Morley, but sh' told me to stop complainin' an' get on wi' bein' a good wife to her son," Sarah replied. Eve was sadly unsurprised. It was typical of many an attitude she had come across. She was still angry about Mrs Morley ignoring the girl's plight however; Sarah was not much more than a child and she should have cared about her daughter-in-law's safety.

"Does yar husband know ya're out?" Eve asked.

"Ah crept out whilst John wor asleep by the fire," Sarah said.

"Ah want ya to stay here an' rest Sarah," Eve told the girl. "Ah'm goin' to get somethin' fer yar pain. Ya just rest here now lass." Eve covered the girl with a warm blanket and went to fetch her some healing paste to put on her vagina and anus, and some tincture to drink for the pain. She also went to speak to Joseph.

"Sh's nay goin' back to that man," Eve told Joseph, after she had given him every grim detail of Sarah's abuse and injuries at the hands of John Morely.

"Eve," Joseph said. "Ya can't interfere between a man an' his wife. Ah know tis dreadful what he did ti t' poor lass, but tis not yar business."

"Sh's stayin' here wi' us," Eve stated. "Sh's got nay mother or father ti look out fer her. We can't let t' poor lass go back there. He's a beast. What kind of man does that ti his own wife?" Joseph did not reply. He was too shocked and disgusted that any man could treat a woman so badly. Eve left him to think it all over whilst she went back to Sarah and treated her injuries. Eve then told the girl that she could stay with them, but Sarah insisted that she had to go back to the Morley farm and to her husband. She was clearly terrified of him. Eve tried her best to persuade Sarah to stay, but she would not be dissuaded. After some time, Eve had no choice but to let Sarah go home, but she gave her a number of remedies to take back with her. There was more tincture for her pain, more paste to spread around her vagina and anus, and another bottle of Eve's 'special' tincture. This, Eve told Sarah, was to 'help' her husband sleep, and she was to put two drops into his drink every night before they retired. Sarah, now dressed in some of Eve's warm winter clothes, was then taken to just outside the Morley farm by Joseph in his cart, from where she walked the rest of the way back, so as not to be discovered. Eve was very concerned at her returning to her husband but had done all she could to help Sarah. However, early next morning, just after Joseph had left for his bakery, Sarah was standing on Eve's doorstep. She seemed terrified and begged Eve to help her again.

"Did the tincture not work?" Eve questioned her.

"Aye, it did," Sarah replied. "But when ah got home last night from seein' you, he punched me, 'cause ah'd gone out without his say so. Then he asked me ti get him some ale. Ah wor so afraid of what he wor goin' to do to me, ah put all o' that liquid ya gave me in his drink. Ah put it all in." Eve almost laughed aloud.

"Ya never did?" she asked Sarah.

"Ah did, an' ah think ah've killed him. Ah think ah've killed my husband," Sarah cried. "Ah don't know what ti do."

"Sarah," Eve said reassuringly. "There worn't enough in the bottle ah gave ya to kill him lass. He's just asleep. Where is he?"

"Ah left him in bed. Ah thought he wor dead,

'cause ah couldn't wake him up," Sarah told her.

"Nay, he'll just be asleep," Eve told her. Sarah looked relieved but still afraid.

"Last night ya said ah could stay here," she said to Eve. "Please let me stay now? If ah go back he's goin' to hurt me again an' ah can't take any more." Eve did not hesitate.

"Of course ya can stay wi' us," Eve said. Sarah managed a fragile smile. "Ya can have Anna's old room till Seb gets bigger an' needs it. But fer now that can be yar room." Eve gave Sarah a hug and she clung on to Eve for dear life. There was now much to be done and get prepared for. Joseph would accept Eve's decision, even if he did not agree fully with it. He would understand that she wanted to help the poor, abused Sarah. But there was John Morley and possibly his family to deal with, and that could be difficult, if not dangerous.

As expected, later that day, Eve had a visitor. However, it was not John Morley who came to her home; it was his brother, Nathan. Eve opened her door and invited him in.

"Eve," he greeted her solemnly. Sarah cowered in the corner of the room, terrified that Nathan would attack her and force her to return with him to John. Eve quickly went over and held her.

"Nathan," Eve replied in greeting.

"Ah've come to try an' find out what's goin' on," he

said in his normal expressionless voice. "John says that Sarah poisoned him last night. He's been right sick all day, an' thinks Sarah tried to kill him."

Sarah was shaking with fear by now and Eve told her to go upstairs to her room with Mary and Seb and lock the door. That would make her feel more secure, Eve thought. She also told her not to worry, because she would protect her.

"Sit down Nathan," Eve directed him and he sat. "Sarah was treated sommit dreadful by yar brother, an' now sh's stayin' wi' us," she told Nathan bluntly.

"Tis not yar place Eve," Nathan said. "Tis between husband an' wife to sort out their differences." Eve then described what John had done to Sarah in graphic detail. She left absolutely nothing out. Nathan looked extremely embarrassed, but also appalled at the report of the injuries sustained by the poor girl at the hands of his own brother. He sat in silence after Eve had finished.

"If ya think ah'm lettin' Sarah go back to that man, then you don't know me Nathan," Eve told him. "An' when ya get back to yar brother, ya can tell him that ah give him a warnin'. If he comes near Sarah again an' tries to hurt her, he'll have to deal wi' me. Make sure ya tell him Nathan, that if he does anythin'...an' ah mean anythin' to damage that girl any more than he has done already, ah'll let the whole village know what he did to her, an' ah'll make sure he never hurts another woman again." Nathan did not argue with Eve. He nodded that he understood her warning and left, without saying another word. When she had closed the door behind Nathan, Eve called to Sarah to come back with the children. As she came down the stairs, Sarah scanned the room for Nathan and was relieved to see him gone.

"John won't give up," Sarah told Eve. "He'll never leave me be."

"Well, ah've warned him Sarah," Eve said. "If he so much as comes near ya again, ah'll deal wi' him. Ya just have to be careful fer a while, till he gets the message." Joseph returned that evening to his new guest and the story of Nathan's visit. He offered to go and speak with the Morley family on Sarah's behalf, but Eve told him it was of no value. John Morley would do whatever he was going to do.

Sarah was a sweet soul to have around the home. Eve made sure she got plenty of rest and treated her injuries until they were healed. With some loving care, good food, and peace of mind, young Sarah blossomed. She was fortunately not left with child, something that concerned Eve for a few weeks, and with her growing confidence, Sarah's countenance took on a new glow. She loved the children and adored Eve and Joseph, who she began to look upon as something of parents.

"Ah know ah can't call ya mam," she said to Eve

one afternoon, "but can ah call ya Mother Eve?"

"Mother Eve?" Eve repeated. "Ah like that Sarah. Aye, ya can call me Mother Eve." And so, from then on she did. As well as helping Eve with the children, Sarah did some chores around the home and worked in the garden. She loved being a part of the Locke family. She was an intelligent girl and Eve was disturbed to find that she was illiterate, so she began to teach Sarah to read and write. She was an enthusiastic pupil and sat with Mary and Seb doing her learning. Joseph took Sarah with him to the bakery sometimes and showed her how he baked the bread and cakes.

It was on returning to Eve's cottage one late afternoon, having spent the day with Joseph, Sarah went missing. Eve was expecting her back before dark, the daylight in the winter months gone by four o'clock. When Joseph walked through the door at half past five without Sarah either, Eve became distressed.

"He's took Sarah!" she told Joseph. "Ah'm goin' to get her back."

"Ya can't go tonight," Joseph replied. "It's been snowin' fer the last hour. The roads will be too dangerous. Ah'll go at first light." Eve was extremely upset however and was not quietened by that offer.

"Ah can't leave Sarah there tonight," she cried. "Ah can't. What if he hurts her?"

"Eve!" Joseph almost shouted. "Ya can't risk yar life goin' out in this weather in the dark. Ya're not thinkin' straight. John Morley knows that you know what he did to Sarah. He'd be more than stupid to hurt 'er again." Eve calmed herself. Joseph was right, she knew that. Once her head was clearer, she asked him to see to the children and went into the garden. Eve had to do a few things to secure the safety of young Sarah until she could find and retrieve her.

Early the following morning, as soon as it was light, Eve set off on Joseph's cart to the Morley farm. She had persuaded her husband, after much argument, that she should go, not him. Eve was kept company by Constable Jowett however. She had gone to see Samuel last night, after putting out her protection for Sarah, and had told him the whole story, particularly why the poor lass had run away from her husband. Jowett, who had daughters of his own was mortified at hearing such a dreadful account, and gladly went with Eve.

The weather had not worsened overnight thankfully and the journey to the Morley's farm did not take very long. As she pulled the cart through the farm gates, Henry Morley came out of his house.

"What are ya doin' at mi home?" he shouted at Eve as soon as he recognised her.

"Is Sarah here?" she asked him.

"So what if sh' is? Sh' lives 'ere," Henry replied angrily.

"Ah want to see Sarah," Eve said. "Ah want to make sure that sh's safe. Ah want to speak to her."

"Well, ya can't," Henry shouted back. Samuel Jowett climbed down from the cart and walked over to Morley.

"Ah think it would be best Henry," he said calmly, "that ya go an' fetch Sarah. Just so that we can make sure that sh's here because sh' wants to be."

"Ya're on 'er side?" Henry protested. "Ya're 'ere ti do 'er biddin'?" Samuel Jowett stood his ground.

"Please go an' fetch Sarah," he repeated. Henry was furious.

"Ah'll not do that," he argued. "Sh's where sh' should be, wi'my son, 'er 'usband, an' ah don't see what it's got ti do wi' 'er or you fer that matter." Nathan came out of the house at this point.

"What's goin' on?" he asked.

"We've come to speak to Sarah," Jowett told him. "Ah've asked yar father to go fetch her an' he's refusin'. Tis not helpful Nathan." Nathan turned to his father. He looked surprised.

"Sarah's here?" he questioned him.

"Aye," Henry told him.

"When did sh' come back?" Nathan asked.

"John fetched 'er last night," Henry said.

"John?" Nathan asked loudly. He stared at his

283

father for some moments then looked back at Eve and Jowett. "Ah didn't know Sarah wor here," he told Eve.

"They want ti see 'er, but it ain't their business," Henry told Nathan. "Tis nowt ti do wi' them, what goes on between mi son an' is wife." Nathan did not reply to his father.

"Ah'll go fetch her," he told Jowett calmly.

"Ya'll do nay such thing!" Henry yelled at Nathan.

"Ah'm fetchin' Sarah," he yelled back at his father and quickly returned to the house. Five minutes later Nathan walked out of the front door with Sarah. Eve scrutinised the girl as she walked towards them. She looked terrified, then relieved to see Eve and ran to her. Eve got off of the cart and hugged Sarah tightly. She was crying and telling Eve how sorry she was for all the trouble she has caused. She told Eve how John had come into Elmsley last evening, just after she left Joseph's bakery, and forced her into his cart and back to the Morley farm with him. Eve consoled Sarah and told her that everything was fine. Constable Jowett then asked her if she had come back with John voluntarily. Sarah told him she had not. He then asked her if she wanted to stay with him. She told Jowett that she did not. He then asked her if John had hurt her. Sarah told him that John had not hurt her, other than when he grabbed her arm and forced her up into his cart. That was clear enough for Jowett, and he was happy to oversee the removal of Sarah from John Morley.

"Did he touch ya?" Eve asked Sarah. "Did John do anythin' to you?" Sarah shook her head that he had not. She told Eve that John had made her go with him but he had not hit her or forced himself upon her last night; he slept in another room. As they were speaking, John rushed from the house, screaming at the top of his voice.

"Sh's mi wife, ya harridan," he directed at Eve. "Leave us alone an' get out!"

Eve turned towards the man and stared straight at him.

"Ah warned ya John Morley," she said. "Ah warned ya not to hurt Sarah."

"Ya heard her," John shouted at Jowett. "Ya heard Eve Jennus threaten mi."

"Ah did not hear Mrs Locke say any such thing," Samuel told him angrily. "An' if ah wor you John Morley, ah'd make sure ya keep away from young Sarah or ya'll be answerin' to the law. Do ya understand?" John stood glaring at Jowett, but was careful not to say another word. Eve, Samuel and Sarah then left the Morley farm.

Chapter 21

With Sarah restored to the safety of their home, Eve and Joseph resumed their normal life. However, Eve did not assume that John Morley would leave Sarah alone and remained vigilant. Her concerns were justified. Some weeks after they had brought Sarah back from the Morley farm, John attacked the girl again. He became very drunk one afternoon at the Bull Inn and stumbled across the village over to Eve's home, where Sarah was in the garden, watching Seb and Mary for half an hour in the fresh air, whilst Eve took lunch to Joseph at the bakery. Morley went around to the back of the cottage, where Sarah was playing catch ball with the children. She screamed when she saw John and tried to protect herself as he lunged towards her and punched her face, shouting obscenities as he did so. Mary and Seb were terrified, and Mary ran out of the garden and up towards her father's bakery. Eve was on the way home and saw her hysterical daughter running along the side of the road, screaming. She picked the child up and ran back to the cottage. Eve charged into her garden, where she saw John shouting and threatening Sarah, who was hunched over against the wall of the house, desperately trying to protect her head with her arms. Eve put Mary down and picked up a shovel. John saw her and ran off.

"Are ya hurt much?" Eve asked Sarah. The girl looked up and nodded her head that she was not, although her lip was split wide open. Fortunately, being drunk, Morley's strength was depleted, so Sarah was spared the normal weight of his blows. Eve held the children and calmed them down, then took Sarah indoors to treat her mouth.

"Ah gave him some extra chances," Eve told Sarah, "fer yar sake, him bein' yar lawful husband an' all. But that's it now. He's got to be stopped. Are ya fine wi' that?" Sarah nodded that she was.

Joseph did not ask Eve for her permission or views on him going to the Morley farm later that night. He went there as soon as he heard of the incident that had occurred in his garden that afternoon. He called on Henry Morley with his own warning. He told him that if his son, John, stepped foot near his home again, where his children lived and played, then he himself would kill him. Henry knew Joseph well enough to know that he meant it. Joseph then demanded to speak to John, who was dragged from his bed, still in a drunken state. Joseph repeated his warning and added that if he ever went anywhere near his home, or indeed Sarah again, he would shoot him. Then he left the Morley farm. Eve was not surprised at Joseph's visit. She had come to realise, as she got to know her husband over the years that beneath the calm and gentle exterior, there was a strong and fearless man who would defend his family to the death. When she had told Joseph earlier in the evening what John had done that afternoon to Sarah in his garden, near to his children, she could not remember ever seeing him so enraged. He went totally silent and left the cottage. She knew where her husband was going and that she could not stop him.

Sarah was badly shaken by John's attack and it took her weeks to regain some confidence to leave the home. Eve slowly encouraged the girl to go out with her or Joseph and little by little she began to get stronger again. Eve gave enough information to Margaret about why Sarah was now living with her and Joseph so that the woman had a pretty good idea about the abuse John Morley had given his wife. Eve knew that the report would be all over the village in hours, which was exactly what happened. Within days, Margaret fed back to Eve and Joseph the disgust and abhorrence expressed by the decent folk of Elmsley. John Morley was now considered to be the scum-of-the-earth and beneath contempt in the community. He was ostracised and despised.

The following Christmas and Eve's birthday, came and went and the cold days of January took hold of Elmsley. With the awful weather, a certain peace fell over the village as people struggled to even get about. The local school had to be closed because of the cold, but Joseph remained forever busy, baking from flour stocks built up before the winter hit. As he always did in severe weather, Joseph let the poorer families in Elmsley use his large ovens at the bakery on Sundays after church to cook their own bread and meat. This saved them some fuel. Joseph had to keep the ovens hot anyway, but his help was still much appreciated by those in need.

It was one afternoon in the middle of January when Margaret called. She had a slightly frantic look on her face and hurried into Eve's cottage.

"Ah've got such a lot to tell you," she said excitedly. Margaret was so overwhelmed with the news she was carrying, that Eve made her sit down and take a breath. "First tis about Doctor Mason. He's run off wi' t' Squire's wife, Elizabeth," she managed to get out this information and stared expectantly at Eve and Sarah, waiting for their response. When they did not react, she continued. "Apparently, 'e's been givin' 'er a lot more than 'is medical attention!" Margaret laughed loudly at her own witticism. Eve and Sarah smiled, but at Margaret, not her news. "Ah spoke to mi sister, Ethel, who works in t' kitchen up at t' big house. Sh' said that Elizabeth Addington 'as never even been in t' Squire's bed. Sh' 'eard that 'e's got some bad rot disease on…ya know…on 'is tackle," she giggled again like a young schoolgirl. Margaret looked across at Eve seriously. "What's that disease they catch from whores?" she asked.

"Syphilis?" Eve replied. "But how would Ethel know that?"

"Ethel told me that t' Squire wor sick straight after 'is weddin' day. Then it all came out that 'e'd been in a Lock Hospital," Margaret explained. "One o t' Squire's man servants overheard 'im an' 'is doctor speakin' about it. It wor t' servant who told my Ethel. Lucky fer Elizabeth, they'd nay consummated their marriage. Course, 'er father went crazy when 'e 'eard, an' went straight ti see 'is daughter an' forbid 'er ti go ti t' Squire's bed. Bein' from t' military, Elizabeth's father 'ad seen what that disease did ti 'is soldiers. Ah reckon Doctor Mason guessed t' Squire wor sufferin' from that...syphilis, an' told Elizabeth. Mason's been after 'er right from t' start, accordin' ti mi sister."

Eve and Sarah had listened to this story with some fascination, especially Eve. She wanted to smile, remembering the entry of Frederick Addington's name in her mother's story, but refrained from doing so. The last thing Eve needed was for Margaret to spread around the village that she was laughing at the misfortunes of the Squire. No, she saved her jubilation until she was alone.

"An' then there's what's 'appened ti John Morley," Margaret stated. Eve and Sarah looked at one another. Margaret gathered from their faces that they had obviously not heard that bit of news either.

"What about Morley?" Eve asked calmly.

"He's right sick," Margaret paused, looking as if she had stumbled across a great secret. "He 'ad a slight accident when 'e were out fixin' fences wi' 'is brother, young 'Enry. He cut 'is leg, which 'e didn't think wor bad at the time. It wor only a small cut apparently, but now it's infected, badly infected they say." Eve listened to this report dispassionately, but Sarah was not so unmoved and looked quite shocked.

"Do they think he'll die?" she asked. Before answering, Margaret looked directly at Eve.

"Ah suppose that depends on whether or not tis God's will," she replied, still staring at Eve, "or if t' Devil 'as anythin' ti do wi' it."

"In John Morley's case," Eve said matter-of-factly, "ah'd say that he'll get whatever he deserves."

"Ah also 'eard that someone from the Morley family wor goin' ti ask you ti give 'im one o' yar curin' pastes," Margaret told her. "Would ya give 'im some remedy after what 'e did to Sarah?" she asked Eve.

"Nay, ah would not," Eve replied bluntly.

"What if 'e wor to die without it?" Margaret asked.

"John Morley's life is not my responsibility," Eve told her. Margaret did not seem surprised by Eve's attitude, but then wanted to move on to her next revelation.

"Well, the last bit o' news ah've got ti tell ya is

about James Barlow," Margaret said, looking at Eve. She believed that once upon a time they had been sweet on one another.

"What about him?" Eve asked casually, expecting Margaret to say he had come home to Stockley House or something like that. Instead, what she heard was quite upsetting, although she could not show any emotion.

"James Barlow wor attacked an' robbed," Margaret told her. "He's in York County Hospital. He wor leavin' one o' 'is factories an' got 'it over 'is 'ead. My sister told me that 'e wor near ti death when it 'appened, an' they worn't sure if 'e wor goin' ti make it at one point. Ethel said that sh' 'eard 'e's makin' some improvement now though. His wife's wi' 'im at t' hospital." Eve was horrified to hear James had been hurt, but then comforted to know he was now improving. What surprised her was why she had not had any sense of his being injured. Eve was also concerned at how upset she was, hearing about James. She had not thought about the man for some time and now suddenly she was overwhelmed with wanting to see him again.

Margaret had delivered all of her news and was now quite exhausted with the telling of it. Eve gave the woman some sweet tea to recover her. Sarah had sat mesmerised throughout the whole of her visit, listening to Margaret's tales. She had never experienced anything like them or the woman before. As Margaret went to leave, she stopped and studied Sarah for a few moments.

"What you need," she told her, "is a nice young man. We'll 'ave ti find ya one. A good lookin' lass like you should be out courtin', not sittin' in 'ere." Sarah blushed. "You leave it wi' me. Ah'll find ya a good un," she said and winked at her.

"Ah'm not sure what kind of man Margaret thinks sh's goin' to find fer ya Sarah," Eve said after she had left, "but it'll keep her 'appy fer a while doin' it." Sarah smiled, but she did not really want Margaret to find her anyone. She had been very sweet on a particular lad in the village ever since she was a small girl, and had always dreamed of being with him one day. His name was Ben Rackley, and he was the son of an out labourer on a local farm, but he went to work in one of the local wool mills when he was twelve. As a young girl, Sarah used to see Ben occasionally when she was allowed to attend church. There was also the odd time that she saw him in Ashton when she went with Mr Streddler to collect provisions. Sarah had a feeling that Ben looked at her favourably as well, but she never had the nerve to speak to him. Even when she was forced to marry John Morley, she often thought of Ben; her daydreaming about the lad kept her going through some very dark days. Sarah wondered if she should tell Eve about her secret love, then decided she would.

"Ah do have someone in the village that ah like...well...ah think ah've allus loved," she said shyly. Eve smiled.

"Do ya want to tell me who he is?" she asked. "Ya don't have to."

"Aye," Sarah replied. "his name's Ben Rackly."

"Little Ben?" Eve asked. "Well, of course, he's nay little any more. Ben's a nice lad Sarah. Has he asked ya to walk out wi' him?"

"Oh, nay," Sarah blushed. "Ah've never even spoke to him. Ah don't suppose he'd want me anyhow, not now."

"What do ya mean, not now?" Eve asked.

"Not now ah'm soiled," Sarah said sadly.

"If Ben Rackly's any kind of a decent lad, then he won't take a care that ya wor forced to marry that Morley beast," Eve told her. "We'll see about gettin' ya an opportunity to talk to Ben, but before we do all that, we have to get ya marriage to Morley finished." Eve knew that Sarah had to be rid of John for once and for all before she could make a new life and settle down with somebody else. But how to ensure this? Morley was clearly suffering from blood poisoning, from what Margaret had described, and could therefore die. That would release Sarah, but what if he got better? What would happen then? The answer to those questions would soon be clear.

Nobody from the Morley family approached Eve to help John, as she knew they would not. Henry Morley did however visit Joseph at his bakery, and begged him to ask Eve to take her 'curse' off of his son. Henry cried to Joseph that he and his wife had already lost one boy and begged him to plead with Eve to spare him the loss of another. Henry told Joseph that he knew John was no good, but to tell Eve, that if John was spared, he would make sure that his son never again interfered with Sarah, and that he would release her from their marriage. Joseph repudiated that Eve had not put any curse on John and told Henry that whilst he felt sorry for him, his son's life or death had nothing to do with his wife. Joseph still brought Henry's request back home to Eve that evening however.

"So Henry Morley thinks ah've put a curse on his loathsome son John does he?" Eve asked him.

"Aye, he does. If ya have Eve, ah'd like ya to take it off," Joseph replied simply. He had also learnt a fair bit about his wife over the years and knew enough of her knowledge not to discount anything. "It'll do ya nay good to see John Morley in his grave Eve," he told her sternly.

"There's probably nay cleanliness at the Morley farm," Eve argued. "Ah can't be held responsible fer their lack o' that or the way they are treatin' his wound."

"If ya give him some o' yar curin' paste ti put on his injury, he might get well," Joseph said. Eve stared at her husband. Did he know what he was asking her to do, she thought. Was he seriously suggesting to her that she helped the man after the way he treated poor Sarah?

"Aye," Joseph replied. "If he gets well because of somethin' ya give him, ya can't be accused of ever tryin' to kill the man can ya?" Eve stood thinking it all over for some time, and then told her husband that she was going to put the question to Sarah. It was she who had suffered at the hands of John Morley, therefore she, and only she, should make the decision of whether or not he gets remedies. Joseph could not argue with that and Eve went to Sarah's room to ask her. The girl was very upset at having to make that choice, but respected Eve's reasons for asking her to decide. Of course, the gentle lamb told Eve to help her despicable husband.

Later that evening, with Sarah minding the children, Joseph took his wife to the Morley farm to see John. Henry was at first very surprised to see Eve at his door, but then, realising she had come with some of her curing paste and tinctures, let her into his home. Mrs Morley stayed out of the way, but Nathan and young Henry, John's two brothers, were interested in what was going on and showed Eve to

John's room. He was lying on his bed soaked in sweat and he stank. Eve told the brothers to fetch boiling water in a bowl and some clean bedding. She had taken with her a bar of soap and strips of clean linen to bathe the wound with, which she had previously soaked in her own tincture. The brothers were ordered to take off all of John's dirty clothes and change his bedding. Once they had done that, Eve washed him and dressed his wound. She then poured some remedy down John's throat carefully and gave him something to make him sleep. Henry had been watching Eve from the side of the room, and was enthralled by what she had done for his son. He thanked her profusely.

"Ah don't want yar thanks," she told him. "Ah want ya to keep yar word an' make sure that John never comes near Sarah again, an' gives her leave to finish their marriage." Henry gave Eve his word. When she had finished with John, she spoke to the father. "Yar son's in a bad way Mr Morley, but ah think ah may have got to him just in time. Why didn't ya call in a doctor? John should've seen a doctor days ago. Ya nearly lost him Mr Morley, an' it wor nowt to do wi' me or me curses. If John had died, it would've been yar own fault." Henry nodded that he understood.

"But ah can't stand doctors," he mumbled. "Ah don't trust 'em an' so ah don't 'ave any chuck wi' 'em."

"Well that's maybe, but a doctor would've done fer him what ah just did," Eve told the man. "Anyways, ah'll leave ya wi' some remedies an' some paste." She called Nathan over to John's bed, he being the most intelligent person in the house, and told him what measure of tincture to give his brother and when to give it, and how to change the infected area and use the paste on his wound. That done, Joseph and Eve left the Morley farm. When they returned home, Sarah was eager to hear of John's condition and Eve was able to tell her that in her opinion, he would recover. She told Sarah of the promise Henry had made to her and how she hoped he would make John stick to it.

Some two weeks later, Nathan Morley called at Eve's home to tell her that his brother was well on the way to a recovery and thanked her on behalf of his family. She accepted his thanks. She also reminded Nathan to make sure that John settled his marriage with Sarah. Eve insisted that he do the deed as soon as possible, so he would know that he no longer had any claim on her. John would be glad to do this, Nathan told her, and intended to see to it as soon as he could walk; the wound was still tender. That was acceptable to Eve, but she assured Nathan that she would expect this to be soon.

During those weeks, Eve had tried to push the thoughts of James from her mind. She had hoped that Margaret would visit with some news of him, but she did not, which made Eve feel all the more frustrated. Joseph had also heard the story of James's attack by now and noticed some slight change in his wife's demeanour. He decided not to say anything about James to Eve however, and hoped she would be able to deal with whatever she was going through in her own way. Joseph suspected however, that she was struggling with it. Then, almost four weeks after Margaret had first brought the news into Eve's home about James, she came around with the latest report. Eve did her best to look calm and not too interested, but inside she was desperate for the information.

According to Margaret, James Barlow was now at home, much recovered from his ordeal. In fact, so recovered was he that he was seen out riding near Elmsley yesterday. Eve was relieved. Now she could put the man from her mind again and go on as before, she thought. That was difficult to do however, and after much trying Eve still found herself having to battle with a desire to see him, just to look at him; that would be enough. But as that was not possible, she threw herself into her children, her husband, her work, her home, and in helping Sarah. Eve was so busy that she went to bed exhausted every night, just so that she would not lie there hour after hour, thinking about James. Joseph knew her plight, but remained silent.

It was some six months later, when Eve was making her way back home from a birthing when she thought she saw James in the distance on horseback. Her heart began to pound and her legs felt quite weak. She so wanted to see him, and yet she dreaded the thought of it. As Eve stared in the rider's direction, he began to ride towards her. As he got nearer, she realised it was Frederick Addington, not James. She braced herself as he pulled his horse up near her.

"Well, it's Eve Jennus. No, I am wrong...it's Mrs Joseph Locke, the Baker's wife," he said in a slightly sarcastic tone. Eve just looked at the man. Ironically, she realised that she was standing in much the same place as when Frederick encountered her before his attack all those years earlier. She started walking away from him. "How dare you turn your back on me," he shouted to her. She ignored him and carried on her way. Frederick turned his horse and rode up to Eve, bringing the animal very close to her side. "Did you hear what I just said?" Eve looked up at him but did not speak. He nudged her with his horse, which was a full 17 hands high, almost pushing Eve over. She managed to steady herself from falling and then turned to face Frederick.

"What do ya want?" she asked him loudly.

"I want you to greet me with the courtesy and respect I deserve," he told her.

"Ah did," she replied bluntly.

"You ignorant whore," Frederick shouted at her and raised his riding crop as if to strike her face. She did not flinch and stared defiantly at him. He hesitated for a few seconds then withdrew his crop. After looking at Eve for some more silent moments, he pulled on his horse's reins and rode off. She stepped back as it thundered away from her. Eve stood for a few minutes watching after Frederick, and then smiled to herself. Imagine thinking that he was James she thought, and continued on her journey home. As she walked the lane back to Elmsley, her mind imagined the sight of Frederick's genitalia being eaten away with syphilitic lesions, and that made her feel quite content. Eve also decided not to tell Joseph of her meeting with the Squire. She knew it would worry him and although verbal, Frederick was actually no threat to her physically in any way at all.

Chapter 22

By the time Eve reached home, she felt strangely relieved of her desperate need to see James. It seemed to have lifted from her being, and she was able to look upon her husband with contentment once again, a feeling she was frightened would not return. Life reverted to normal for Eve over the following months, and she no longer feared hearing any news about James. That was just as well, because Margaret called one afternoon to tell her that James and his family were leaving Stockley House for good and moving to a large mansion in Swithindale, some fifty miles away. The estate he bought, known as Harlington Manor, was more in keeping with the Barlow family's new wealth and status, Margaret put forward as the reason for their departure from Elmsley. Eve was relieved in one sense, as she no longer had to be concerned that she might come across James unexpectedly when out walking, but felt sad also, knowing that she might never see him again. It took Eve some days to convince herself that she would be better off with him moving away however.

John Morley released Sarah from their marriage, and Eve set about helping her to get acquainted with Ben Rackley, her childhood love. Eve found out that he went to church regularly, so Sarah was packed off there the following Sunday and every Sunday after that, dressed in the finest clothes that Eve could put on her. Sarah looked the picture of prettiness as she left to attend her first morning service at Saint Guthlac, and Eve was happy to see her charge so full of joy and expectations, as a young woman should be. Sarah had also become friendly with Dru's wife, Lillian, and the pair often spent time together. It was Sarah who alerted Eve to some of the problems that Lillian and Dru were having. Eve was not happy to hear them, but listened all the same. Apparently, Dru had taken to drinking alcohol more frequently and in greater quantities than he used to, and with the drink, was becoming difficult for young Lillian to handle. He was often angry with her, and Thomas, who was almost a man now, at times felt the need to stand up for Lillian against his father's verbal abuse towards her. On one occasion, when Dru was worse for drink, and came home shouting for his supper, Thomas told him off, and Dru slapped his face hard. Eve was very distressed to hear this report. Sarah begged her not to tell Dru where she heard the story from. If he thought that she had told her, Sarah said, she feared he would stop Lillian from being her friend. Sarah told Eve about her brother's increasingly awful behaviour because Lillian was carrying Dru's child, but was too scared to tell him. Eve understood Sarah's concerns but was not going to sit idly by whilst her own brother bullied and harmed his family, especially his now pregnant wife. It was not going to be allowed.

"Ah've been hearin' stories that ya're treatin' yar wife an' yar son badly," Eve put to her brother directly. She had invited herself into Dru's home one evening.

"Who told ya that?" Dru snapped, staring across the room to Lillian, who was mortified at what Eve had just said.

"Never ya mind who told me," she replied. "Is it true?" Dru looked guilty, then angry, but Eve maintained her stance.

"Ah only slapped the boy once," he admitted. "He wasn't hurt. An' ah've never hit mi wife, have ah?" he put to Lillian. She nodded a no.

"So ya say," Eve replied. "An' why are ya drinkin'?"

"Ah don't know," Dru answered honestly. "Ah just seem to need a drink before ah come home." Eve looked hard at her brother.

"Ah tell ya what ya're goin' to do," she told Dru. "Tomorrow night when ya've finished at the smithy, ya're goin' to come straight around to us to talk to Joseph and me. Ya're not goin' to go to the Bull Inn first. Do you agree?"

"Aye," Dru said. "All right."

"Yar husband's goin' to be late home tomorrow Lillian," Eve told her, "but he'll not be at the Bull, he'll be at our place talkin'." Lillian nodded again. When Joseph and Eve had Dru's full attention the following night, they tried to find out why he was drinking heavier. There was clearly something wrong and they tried to uncover what that was. Dru found it hard to explain, but he did say a number of times that he missed Alice. Eve was surprised to hear this and reminded Dru of the times he complained about Alice to her and Anna, saying that he could not cope with her spending, her laziness around the home, and how badly she cared for their son. Dru agreed that it sounded strange, but still maintained that he missed his first wife. He declared that he had loved Alice like he could never love Lillian. Eve expressed how sad she was to hear that, given that Lillian was now carrying his baby. Dru was stunned. Why had she not told him he asked? Eve explained that Lillian was afraid to, she was frightened of his reaction and, under the circumstances, Eve told her brother that she would have felt and acted the same way. Dru left Joseph and Eve's home with plenty to think about. After he had gone, they sat and talked about Dru and how they could help him. Eve believed that her brother still felt guilty about Alice's death and that was probably what was going on in his mind. Perhaps the new baby might help them, she hoped.

Sarah reported back over the following weeks that Lillian and Dru seemed to be getting on much better, and that he was pleased to be a father again. Dru was not angry about her speaking out either. He apparently had reduced his drinking and was much more pleasant to be with. Young Thomas was also relieved that his father had changed his behaviour. Eve made sure that she regularly spoke to Lillian from then on however, just to make sure that her brother did not revert back to his heavy drinking and bullying.

It took some months, but Sarah came home one day and told Eve and Joseph that Ben Rackley had asked if he could walk out with her. Eve was very happy for Sarah and looked forward to seeing her fulfilling her dreams. And so, the months that followed were full of expectation. There was a new baby Jennus arriving and a hope that Sarah might finally find a decent husband to share her life with. The children were well and growing up fast. There was relative peace in the village and no major outbreaks or contagious illnesses for Eve to busy herself with. Even the birth rate seemed to be dropping, so Eve's midwifery duties were called upon less often.

As she did quite regularly, Margaret brought the latest items of Elmsley news to Eve. James had finally moved his family to Harlington Manor, which Eve felt a little upset about when she heard, and there was a new doctor in Ashton, a Doctor Edward

Cheetham. Margaret told Eve that Agnes Little had called him out to treat her youngest boy, and found him to be a brusque and unpleasant man. When Eve heard the name of this person, a cold feeling went through her; she knew that Doctor Cheetham was going to be a formidable man to deal with and that she needed to be careful of him. Eve resolved however, that she would not allow him to stop her from helping neighbours if asked to do so. That proclamation was soon to be put to the test though.

It all began with Betty Hallot, a woman who had called at Eve's home one morning asking for her help. Betty was forty-two years old and had given birth to eight children, six of whom had survived. She thought she was with child again and begged Eve to help her. Betty's husband seemed to have run off, leaving her with the six hungry mouths to feed and a possible further child on the way. Could Eve abort this unwanted baby, was the question the woman put to her. But Eve could not help Betty in any way with an abortion; she could face a long prison sentence if she did. All she could do was talk to her and try to find a way of helping her cope with another baby. A week after speaking to Eve however, Betty returned with the news that she had 'seen bleeding', and was therefore sure she was no longer carrying a child. Before long, Eve was being approached by numbers of women, all asking for her help to either prevent a pregnancy or to end one. Joseph became anxious for his wife and begged her not to get involved with any of these women. Eve assured him that she was being careful but said that she would not turn away any woman who wanted to prevent a pregnancy. She promised him however, that she did not assist terminations. Although slightly reassured, this also frustrated Joseph, but he knew his wife well and could only hope that whatever help she gave, she would do it discreetly.

However, events over the following week would test Eve's resolve to help others and worry Joseph further. Constable Jowett called to see Eve at her home one evening in an official capacity. There had been a complaint made against her from Doctor Cheetham, accusing her of aiding women to abort their babies. This was an extremely serious accusation and Jowett came to warn Eve about it. He told her that if Cheetham obtained any evidence that she had performed abortions, then he would have no choice but to arrest and charge her for that offense. Joseph was beside himself hearing this and protested to Samuel that the allegation was utter nonsense, and that Cheetham had no right to accuse his wife of anything so dreadful. Samuel told him that he might personally agree with him, but he could not ignore the doctor and warned Eve to mind him. He told her that Cheetham had already spoken to the Squire, who would like nothing better than to see trouble at her door. Eve thanked the constable for coming and warning her, and assured him that Cheetham would not get evidence of her having performed any abortions, because she had not done so. However, on the orders of the Squire, Jowett visited a number of women in Elmsley, investigating the allegations made by Doctor Cheetham. Not one of the women that the constable interviewed supported the man's accusations though, and through Margaret, they all told Eve of Jowett's visit. Eve now had the full measure of Cheetham, and knew she had to be more vigilant in the future if she wanted to help any woman with preventing a pregnancy. Jowett reported back at the next meeting of the newly elected village council, Cheetham now being one of them, that he could gather no evidence that Eve Locke had been administering assistance to women to abort their babies. The doctor was furious. He had decided, as soon as he heard about Eve and her supplying of the old remedies, that he would put a stop to her doing this in any way he could. Cheetham had been successful in the town where he lived previously in getting a woman convicted of carrying out abortions, with very little evidence, and she was sent to jail for many years. He also congratulated himself on removing two other women from the town who practised the old ways, and what he considered to be 'superstitious nonsense', and 'quack medicine'. He had managed to destroy the women's' reputations little by little by having some spurious accusations against them for administering poison in their so-called medicines, upheld by the law. One woman disappeared from the town as soon as she realised she faced being arrested, and the other one was sent to prison for six months, largely on Cheetham's say so. With such victories behind him, the good doctor thought he was invincible.

Walking in the village with her children one morning, returning home from a visit to see Lillian, her sister-in-law, Eve passed Cheetham's carriage. He was just climbing up on to it when he saw her and stepped back down.

"Mrs Locke?" he called to her. She turned to face a rotund, middle-aged man with a red complexion. He looked more like an Inn keeper than a doctor, she thought. He was short in height with a thick neck and a double chin that spilled over his high collar. He had very small eyes and sported a thick black moustache. Eve particularly noted his short, stubby fingers on the end of fat hands. He was altogether unpleasant to look at.

"Aye," Eve replied simply.

"I am Doctor Cheetham," he told her expectantly. She knew who he was. He did not take his hat off, which would have been the courteous thing to do.

Eve nodded a greeting to him in the same manner. "I would like a word with you please," he added.

"Aye," she repeated, and stood looking blankly at the man.

"As the local, qualified physician, I do not intend to put up with your medieval tinkering with the health of the people in Elmsley," he told her sharply.

"Has there been complaints made against me?" she asked. "If there has, who made um?" Cheetham glared at her.

"I am making a complaint against you," he stated.

"About what exactly are ya complainin'?" Eve asked bluntly.

"I want you to stop giving out your quack remedies," Cheetham sneered at her. "And," he continued, "if I ever find you helping any woman to abort her child, I will see you in jail."

"Firstly, Doctor Cheetham," Eve squared up to the man. "Ah'm nay breakin' any law wi' my remedies. If folks want me to help them, then they have the right to ask me. Ah don't demand any payment, so ya can't make anythin' of that. Secondly, Doctor Cheetham, ah've never performed an abortion, so ya can stop makin' yar lies an' accusations. Now, if ya'll excuse me, ah have to get my children home to be fed…unless ya have sommit else to say to me?" She stood defiantly glaring at the man, waiting for his further response. Cheetham was incensed, his face

311

getting redder by the second. After waiting for a further few moments for the doctor to reply, Eve turned her back on him and walked away. When she saw Joseph later that evening, she told him about her meeting with Cheetham. Although she did not seem unduly concerned, Joseph was, and again, begged her to be careful. It was obvious that the doctor was not about to let her alone and clearly had her set in his sights as a target.

The weeks and months past by and Eve was proud and delighted to help Lillian birth her first child, another son for Dru. The whole delivery went well and mother and baby came through it fine. The new member of the Jennus family was to be named Edward Dru Jennus, Edward being Lillian's father's name. Dru was totally smitten with his new baby boy and Thomas with his tiny baby sibling. The Jennus home felt warm and full of love and Eve was happy to see her brother looking so well, content and happy. Dru's smithy and forge were doing good business again, and young Thomas was now working with him as an apprentice to the trade and doing well, by all accounts. Thomas looked like his father more and more as he matured, and seen from a certain angle, her nephew reminded Eve very much of her own dear father, who he was named after. Further good news arrived with the announcement by Sarah and Ben that they were getting married. It was late summer now and the wedding was to be held where Eve and Joseph wed in Farnleydale; it was going to be a civil marriage. Eve and Sarah set about making new dresses for each of them and one for young Mary, who was turning into a real beauty.

She was now years of age. Mary had Eve's long legs and eleven thick, dark brown hair, which curled, just like her fathers' and she also had James's eyes and wonderfully long eyelashes. Everyone said Mary looked just like her father, meaning Joseph. It made little difference however, because to Joseph, Mary was a gift to him from God and he adored her. Apart from three freckles across the bridge of her nose, Mary had also inherited her mother's porcelain complexion and rosy red lips. The girl looked physically strong, but Eve had sensed, ever since she was quite small, that her daughter was not very spiritually robust. Mary found it hard to cope with things at times and got easily upset.

As Seb grew older and stronger-willed, Eve often witnessed Mary giving in to his demands, however unfair or unjust they were. Eve had to interfere and stop him from taking advantage of his big sister on many occasions. Seb slapped Mary around her face one day quite hard, when she did not do as he demanded her to, and Mary did not retaliate, just stood in shock, looking fragile and hurt. Of course Seb received a number of very hard slaps from his mother for doing this. Eve was not going to have any son of hers abusing a female, and that lesson would begin at home. It was the first and the last time Seb ever lifted his hand to Mary. Eve tried to build some strength into her daughter, as did Joseph. They spent hours trying to instil into Mary a sense of herself and her own power, but it was almost as if she did not want to be strong. Eve was anguished at times over her daughter's lack of courage and fortitude, and she was concerned for her future. Joseph comforted his wife by saying that Mary was still very young and would grow tougher as she matured more.

Sarah's wedding day came and it was a lovely occasion. She looked beautiful in the dress that Eve and she had made for the occasion, and was so happy that even Eve cried…a very rare sight indeed these days. It was so rare that Joseph could not take his eyes off of her as she dabbed the tears away.

"Ah don't think ah've ever seen ya cry over somethin' like this," he told Eve.

"Well, aren't ya lucky?" she joked with him. "Ya could've married one of them women who grizzle all the time."

"Ah know how lucky ah am," he told her and squeezed Eve's hand as they watched Sarah and Ben embrace with the words 'you are now husband and wife'.

The next celebration was the christening of Edward Dru Jennus at Saint Guthlac church, not altogether the most comfortable place for Eve to be. She had not been inside the church since the funeral of Granny Anna, and was saddened as the memories of all of her family who were buried there intruded into the service for Edward. It was also slightly strange for Eve to watch her brother soak up the whole religious service. Dru had 'found' Christianity when he got married to Alice, not having been brought up particularly as a Christian by Mary and Thomas. He began to worship at the church with her when she was alive. Alice had been quite religious and Dru was pressured to go with her to church. But he had carried on going after her death, and remained doing so to that day. Pastor Bell, now getting on in years, was still taking the services at Saint Guthlac, and looked genuinely pleased to see Eve and Joseph sitting in the stalls. As Eve listened to the pastor's Christening sermon and watched him perform the rituals, she remembered how hard he had tried over the years to turn her into a true convert. He was kind to her though, and for his sake, she pretended to be in awe of the religion and its beliefs. Of course, Bell had no idea that she really practised her own faith, but then there was no reason for him to know. Eve's religious convictions lay in a different direction from Christianity, but she respected all other belief systems, even if they did not respect hers. Sarah and Ben were the chosen godparents to Edward and the day ended with a special meal at Eve's home, with everyone content that the ceremony went well. Even Pastor Bell and his wife joined the festivities briefly for a toast to the baby, the first time either had ever entered the home of Eve, the woman with the 'evil' eye.

Chapter 23

So, with Sarah's wedding and Edward's christening out of the way, Eve and Joseph set about preparing for the coming winter. Sarah and Ben moved into the spare rooms above Joseph's bakery. Ben was earning a liveable wage at the factory and Sarah would clean the shop and baking area for Joseph, as part payment for the living accommodation. The situation suited everyone and it was hoped that the young couple would soon settle down to a happy married life. Ben was a good man and Eve felt no apprehension whatsoever for Sarah to leave her cottage and go to share a life with him. He was a quiet and thoughtful young man, which afforded Sarah the peace and tranquillity she needed. She had had some tearful weeks prior to her wedding in anguish over whether or not she would be able to let Ben have sex with her. Eve spent some hours talking to Sarah, trying to reassure her that with time, she would be able to be intimate with him. Joseph spent some hours talking to Ben, trying to help him understand how the traumatic experiences that Sarah had gone through with John Morely would affect her, and to make him fully realise that he needed to show her a great deal of love and patience in their marital bed. Both Eve and Joseph thought they had done a fairly good job in helping the couple to cope with what was possibly going to be a difficult time.

However, a week after Sarah was married and had moved away, she arrived back on Eve's doorstep, asking if she could 'come home'.

"Ah can't let Ben near me," Sarah told her in floods of tears. "Ah can't let him touch me, ah just feel sick to my stomach every time we go to bed." Eve was not surprised to hear Sarah say that or to see her return, but she was disappointed. Eve had hoped that the young couple could find their way through the difficulties of sex, given Sarah's dreadful abuse, but that obviously was not the case.

"There's nowt to worry about lass," Eve calmed Sarah. "It wor never goin' to be easy." She took in the distressed girl and put her to bed with some tincture to calm her down. Joseph was in Ashton buying provisions and Eve expected him home in an hour or so, and would talk to him about Sarah then. However, not long after Sarah had arrived, Ben called at Eve's cottage. He looked very unhappy and asked if his wife was there. Eve told him Sarah was, but that she was asleep upstairs, having arrived in an upset state. Ben was clearly distressed. Eve sat him down. She felt very sorry for the young man, and was not sure what she could say to him other than things would be fine if he would give Sarah time. But Ben seemed to be angry with her.

"Ah don't understand why Sarah should come here," he complained. "Sh's not yar daughter is sh'? Ah mean, sh' only lived wi' ya fer a while."

"Ben," Eve said calmly. "Sarah has been through dreadful abuse. Joseph told ya all of that didn't he? An' Sarah's like one of ours. Sh's got nowhere else to go. Of course sh's goin' to come to us. Sh's upset, sh's frightened an' sh' needed to be quiet fer a little while. Ah suggest ya go home. Let Sarah stay here wi' us tonight an' ah'll speak to her in the mornin' when sh' feels better." Ben was agitated and reluctant to go, and for a moment or two, Eve thought he was going to argue with her, but he did not. Just after he left, Joseph arrived home and Eve told him what had happened. He was also sad to hear this news but understood Sarah's problems. He took a quick drink of tea then left to go and speak with Ben.

Sarah stayed with Eve for a few days in the end. She would not speak about her problems and every time Eve broached the subject, Sarah would say she felt ill, or went to her old room. By the fifth day, Ben came to Eve's cottage and asked to speak to Sarah. Eve left them alone, once she thought that Sarah was happy to be on her own with her husband. She remained close by however, collecting holly from the tree in the garden with the children for the Christmas wreaths. When she returned indoors, both Sarah and Ben were smiling. Eve did not ask what had been said between them and Sarah did not tell her. She just told Eve that she was going home, kissed her and the children goodbye, thanked her, and left with Ben. Both Joseph and Eve were relieved that she happily went back with her husband, and just hoped that they would now work it all out.

The weeks were rapidly falling into winter. The weather, which had so far been relatively mild, turned sharply for the worse. The previous four winters had been reasonably fair, and had lulled the community into a false sense of security; Elmsley folk had gotten used to the ease that a not-so-bad winter afforded them. Very heavy snow hit the whole region late in December and Christmas was spent locked away in relative safety at home. It remained unremittingly cold for a solid three months however, with significant snow falls weekly. Everything froze beneath two feet of ice and even the carriageways, such as they were, became impassable. Horses could not cope with the depth of the snow, let alone the ice beneath it, so anything needing to be carted around, could not be. The local farmers' winter animal feed began to run out by the end of February, due to their cattle having to be kept indoors for many weeks. They could not let their livestock outside onto the land, firstly for fear of them freezing to death in the bitterly cold conditions, and secondly because they could not graze for food anywhere, anyway. The outlook became increasingly grim and the only solution was to slaughter some of the animals. This was always done with trepidation as, although it provided instant nutritious food to eat, once killed, it would be hard for farmers to build up their herd numbers again. It was also very near the breeding season, the worst possible time to destroy livestock. No one living in Elmsley and its surrounding farms was immune. Work coming into Dru's smithy and forge was much reduced and after many weeks of bad weather, his income began to suffer. Along with everyone else in the community, the Locke and the Jennus family lived off the harvested food from the previous summer and autumn and from what their animals produced. However, they too were struggling to feed their own livestock, few as they were, as the duration of the freeze continued. Joseph managed to keep the bakery going, but people living in the outlying farms simply could not get into the village, so even his living suffered.

Then further dreadful news was brought by Margaret to Eve's home. Diphtheria was suspected to have caused the death of an infant boy in the village; the symptoms suffered by the child were reportedly those of this much dreaded infection. Within hours of the baby's death, fear for their own young gripped the whole community, but there was nothing to be done except wait and see if anyone else contracted it. Eve knew however, that the continuing bad weather, with its freezing, damp conditions, would only help to weaken the resistance of the small infants and vulnerable elderly in the village to the disease. As best as they could, Joseph and Eve tried to make sure that they helped any of their elderly neighbours in need and the parish council stepped up to give some food aid and wood for cooking and heating to the poorest in the community.

It was at times like this that Eve was called upon, as were her mother and grandmothers before her, by some local folk, to use her 'powers' to protect their homes and children from infection and death. She was asked to do such things by those considered to be the most ignorant in the village, because they still believed in the power of charms and spells. It was very difficult for Eve. Out of pity for those neighbours, she would sometimes pander to their old superstitions and beliefs, simply to help alleviate their dreadful fears, knowing she would be condemned yet again by the religious and pious in the community for doing so. Of course, Eve knew that her remedies could not stop the spread of diphtheria, nor could any charm or ritual prevent this deadly disease from claiming the lives of her neighbours or their children, and she would tell them this also. But people only hear and believe what they want to when faced with a feared killer such as diphtheria.

What Eve had learned from studying her grandmother Elisa's 'story' in her book was something of the spread of diseases like diphtheria; Elisa had experienced an outbreak in the village many years ago. Eve did her best to advise people to keep away from the infected households and to have no contact with anyone in them, as she had done when the scarlet fever hit the village. However, in giving this guidance to her neighbours, she brought scorn upon herself from Doctor Cheetham, who took great offence to her saying anything to anyone about how to deal with the outbreak. He considered Eve's advice to be interfering by an ignorant woman and castigated her for doing so. After all, what would a simple peasant like her know about such diseases? He, on the other hand, was learned and educated, even though his more 'modern' medical treatments were not effective against such a ferocious disease as diphtheria either. Doctor Cheetham however, still condemned Eve's herbs and plants to the dark ages, and did not want her administering any of her remedies to the people in 'his' care. From a medical point of view, the doctor was defending a professional position, but it could be said that the opposition to Eve was also to do with the fact that his livelihood depended on the treatments he supplied to the community, and Eve, virtually giving her mixtures and preparations away, damaged his pocket as well as undermined his authority.

Meanwhile, the dreaded diphtheria claimed six more young lives, a nursing mother, and two elderly folk. When Eve was asked by Ada Emmet for her help with her remaining three children; she was the mother of the first boy that died in the village, Eve was torn. She knew in her heart that she could not do very much for the stricken family, and if she entered the infected house, she would then have to stay away from her own family for some time. Eve eventually decided not to go to the Emmet's home. Within days of her doing that however, two of the poor dead boy's siblings looked as if they had gone down with the diphtheria as well. Their lives could have been in danger. Ada, distraught and heartbroken, took herself to Eve's cottage again to condemn her for not coming and helping her family through the crisis. Inconsolable, Ada Emmet accused Eve of abandoning her neighbours and not caring. Eve was more than upset by this and tried to make Ada understand that she could do nothing more than give some remedies to help with the children's' symptoms and discomfort. But Ada began to cry hysterically and collapsed into Eve's arms, begging for help. She held the sobbing woman and heard herself promising to go and nurse the children through the disease.

Indifferent to her own safety, but with Joseph's agreement, Eve went to the infected home and spent the next days and nights caring for the sick youngsters. Doctor Cheetham, who had tried to treat the first Emmet boy who died, made a point of visiting the family again, even though he was not called upon to do so. He argued vigorously with Ada Emmet, that whatever help Eve might be giving her children, it was wrong and useless. But Ada refused to send Eve away. In fact, Ada Emmet sent the doctor away. This infuriated him. Cheetham was now more determined than ever to rid himself of Eve Locke. However, if the doctor thought he would do that by discrediting her, he needed to think again. Within three days, both of the Emmet youngsters were out of danger and seemed to be making a recovery.

With no more children contracting diphtheria over the following weeks and no other cases reported, the whole of Elmsley breathed a sigh of relief. Prayers were offered up to God in Saint Guthlac to thank him for his blessing. The community had tragically lost seven infants and three adults, but everyone knew they had still escaped the worst ravages of a disease such as diphtheria, which could have easily taken half of the entire population in the village and outlying farms, particularly their infants and the old and infirm. So, in spite of their terrible losses, there was cause for some small celebration in Elmsley. The bitterly cold weather was also abating and with that, the mood of black despair in the community began to lift.

One man however, remained angry; the focus of his fury was of course Eve. She, exhausted from her vigil and engrossed in seeing Joseph and her children again, was largely unaware of the extent to which she had upset Doctor Cheetham. Eve had little idea that in helping nurse the Emmet children back to health she had made a vicious enemy of the doctor.

As the darkness of the winter months began to turn to lighter and warmer days, the people of Elmsley and the local farmers took stock of the damage that the prolonged freeze had done to their herds and livelihoods. Some farmers had lost significant numbers of their animals. Both Dru and Joseph had managed to keep theirs alive and Dru was once again beginning to be busy in his smithy and forge. Everyone hoped they had seen the worst of the winter and its destruction and Eve and her brother were deeply relieved that neither family had lost their young; Mary, Seb, and baby Edward and Thomas were all safe. Lillian and Eve had taken every precaution for their family's safety by not having contact with others in the village, and although Dru and Joseph had to go about their jobs, contact was kept at a minimum with their customers. It was only when Eve believed that the danger had passed that she resumed her normal activities and let the children go outside and mix with other youngsters.

As well as the villagers and local farmers counting the cost of the harsh winter and the diphtheria epidemic, which it was now known had swept through all of the local towns and villages in the county, the members of the parish council met to discuss what needed to be done to help those effected worse by the hard winter months, and of course, the bereaved families. Their discussions were soon guided in a certain direction however. The council consisted of Pastor Bell, Doctor Cheetham, who had now moved to a large villa on the outskirts of Elmsley, two owner farmers, Cuthbert Lamb and George Hopkinson, and of course, Squire Frederick Addington.

"I don't believe the other Emmet children had diphtheria," Doctor Cheetham pronounced to his colleagues at the meeting. "I went to the house myself and those children did not have diphtheria symptoms, I am quite sure of it. The woman, Eve Locke, fooled poor Mrs Emmet into believing that she was curing the diphtheria. Locke is a liar, a quack and a fraud," he stated loudly and with total conviction. The other men in the room looked at one another.

"That is a serious allegation doctor," Cuthbert Lamb remarked.

"Yes, it is Mr Lamb," the doctor replied. "It is a serious allegation, but it is true." He had the full attention of the men in the room and now he was set to do his worst by Eve.

"The woman is a know-nothing. She is a pitiful stock of knowledge. She has no training, no certificates, no diplomas or a medical degree. She has never been to university or been trained in medical matters, and yet she is being allowed to treat the people in this village as if she were." He looked across the faces of those present for their reactions. Cuthbert Lamb and George Hopkinson looked uneasy at his strong attack on Eve. Both knew Joseph quite well and Dru even better, they regularly gave him their business. George, the eldest of the two men, even knew Dru and Eve's father, Thomas Jennus before his untimely death. Both men did not want to agree with Doctor Cheetham, nor did they want to be seen to disagree with him. Cheetham continued, being fired on by the fact that no one had actually spoken up for Eve.

"The Locke woman pretended that the Emmet children were very sick and then miraculously cured them. I am telling you, Locke is a charlatan and a quack and she is dangerous to this community. She has to be stopped!"

The room was silent for some moments then Squire Addington spoke.

"Eve Locke has always been trouble for this village," he said. "Is she not the one who cursed Morley when he was a boy and then he died? His death was recent, was it not?"

Pastor Bell spoke up. "Eve was a child herself Squire when she said those silly things to Morley," Bell told him. "Your father did not charge her with any offence. Eve Locke does much good in this community. She saved the life of John Morley," he pointed out. "And John is the brother of William Morley."

"That is utter nonsense!" Cheetham snapped. "I heard about that case. All Locke did was clean the man's wound. She did not cure anything. And as for her doing good in the community...well. She has no medical training Bell. She should not even be delivering babies." The pastor was silenced.

"I agree with Doctor Cheetham," the Squire stated. "I agree that Locke is committing the offence of fraud and quackery." Lamb and Hopkinson looked even more uncomfortable but still said nothing. "She is also considered to be a witch by some in the village, is she not?" the Squire added mockingly.

"A witch?" Cheetham almost choked on the ale he was drinking. "She calls herself a witch? Well that explains a great deal."

"I really think we need to be careful Squire," Pastor Bell said very respectfully, having found some bravery from somewhere. "Eve Locke is well thought of by some folk in Elmsley. I know her past is a bit, well, strange to say the least, but she does do a lot of good work in the village. And Mrs Locke has never called herself a witch Sir, that really is just superstitious nonsense and gossip put about by the ignorant folk in Elmsley." Bell felt the need to put his views forward. He had gotten to know Eve over the years and considered her to be well-meaning and honest, even if she did live at the edge of what he would preach as being 'the Christian way of life'. Although Bell was aware that some in Elmsley believed Eve was a witch and had done some witch-like things in her life, the pastor firmly believed that she was harmless. If the truth were known, Eve had actually helped his family in the past as well. Mrs Bell would not be one of the voices in the village to condemn Eve, and Pastor Bell knew that.

"Come, come man," the doctor railed on the pastor harshly. "By letting those that do not know any better think she is a witch with some sort of power over them, Locke is praying on the minds and beliefs of those fools. That is why they flock to her when something happens to them or they get sick. These idiots believe this nonsense and she encourages them to."

"Wi' all due respect Doctor Cheetham," Lamb spoke up, "that is hardly the same as Eve Locke sayin' that sh's a witch, an' that sh' can cure 'em when they is sick."

"Yes, and I do think we should be careful what we are accusing Mrs Locke of," the pastor repeated.

"She's breaking the law Bell," the doctor almost shouted back at him. "Good God man, you of all people should want her stopped. Eve Locke has got no respect for me, or the law, or your church, and she clearly has not got any Christian decency."

"The doctor is right Bell," the Squire spoke in his authoritative voice. "If the woman is committing a crime then she should be answerable to the law."

"Aye, but has sh' committed a crime Squire?" Lamb argued. The Squire did not reply to Lamb, just looked into the distance and mumbled something. He looked pale and unwell and was sipping water throughout the meeting. Doctor Cheetham stared at Cuthbert in disgust for arguing with him. He secretly held both Lamb and Hopkinson in contempt. Cheetham had not foreseen having to sit on a council with two farmers who were clearly below his social class. It was Pastor Bell who was instrumental in getting them voted on to the parish council before

Cheetham's move to Elmsley. Bell wanted to make sure that some ordinary folk had a presence on it. Doctor Cheetham turned to the Squire.

"We can use the 1735 Witches Act," he stated calmly. Pastor Bell rose from his chair.

"The Witches Act?" he shouted. "This is madness Sir," he addressed the Squire. "Cheetham, what are you thinking?"

"Aye, tis a bit harsh doctor?" Lamb said. "Ah'm not disagreeing wi' ya sayin' that Eve Locke is a nuisance ti yarself, but ya surely can't have 'er punished fer bein' a witch. We stopped doin' that years ago."

"The Witches Act?" the Squire mused, thinking aloud. He was not sure himself how to react to Cheetham's suggestion either and looked across to him to check that he was serious. The doctor did not flinch. "How could that be done?" he asked him.

"It is one way to stop her," Cheetham said. "Of course we cannot have Locke arrested for being a witch Cuthbert," he said to Lamb sarcastically. "But we can have her tried for being a charlatan and a fraud. That carries a prison sentence. We just use the 1735 Act."

"This is not acceptable," the pastor protested loudly, "and I'll have nothing to do with it." Bell glared at the doctor and stormed out of the room. Hopkinson called after him, but Cheetham told him to let the pastor go.

"I think he has got a little too close to the Locke family," he said.

"Ah don't want to be a part o' this either," Lamb told the Squire and rose from his chair also. Hopkinson, who had said nothing during the meeting, simply stood up and walked out of the door. Lamb followed behind him.

"What is wrong with the people in this village?" Cheetham asked. He was surprised that his plan had not been accepted by the other men on the council. "I can understand Bell. He does not have the courage to do anything like this, but Lamb and Hopkinson..." The doctor paused for a moment. "I suppose that is what happens when you are dealing with the lower classes." The Squire laughed.

"My dear doctor," he said. "You are more arrogant than I am. But do not be fooled into thinking that Cuthbert Lamb and George Hopkinson are mere peasants. They are both very wealthy men. They own almost as much land and livestock as I do." The Squire sat back in his chair and smirked at Cheetham. He thought the whole episode was extremely amusing. Cheetham did not!

"Well," the Squire said as he took another drink of his water, "I'll look into the matter. If I think Eve Locke is indeed a danger to this community then I will certainly act and report her to the authorities in

Farnleydale. I will let you know my decision Cheetham," he concluded.

Chapter 24

Doctor Cheetham thought his plan to remove Eve by having her charged as a fraud and charlatan was an excellent one, and that all he needed to do now was convince the Squire to report her to the police. He did not care much for the opinion of Pastor Bell or Lamb and Hopkinson. He had little respect for Bell and still regarded the two owner farmers as low in class, even if they were wealthy. What Cheetham did not know was that Eve had done Cuthbert Lamb and his family a service some two years earlier. Cuthbert's wife, Ellen, had fallen badly at their home and hurt her arm. When called upon to help, Eve not only strapped her arm up very well and gave her remedies for the pain but, because Ellen could hardly do anything with an injured arm, Eve tidied their house, dressed their three children and even cooked a meal for the family and had it on the table when Cuthbert arrived home from his day's work. Lamb was not about to forget that. The day after the council meeting, he paid Eve a visit to inform her of Cheetham's intentions. Lamb was so disturbed by the doctor's vindictiveness towards her that he did not care that he was breaking parish council rules by disclosing what he said at the meeting. Lamb also told Eve that Pastor Bell and George Hopkinson objected to the doctor's plans, just so that she would know that none of them wanted anything to do with his plotting. Lamb did not, nor did he ever, like Cheetham. He suffered him because the Squire had more or less insisted that he sit on the council, Cheetham now being his personal doctor and confidant. Botheroyd had recently retired from medical practice and from being the Squire's physician.

Eve was not surprised to hear of the doctor's plan but she was disturbed to learn of the lengths the man would go to in order to remove her from his society. Her mother's warnings about doctors came to mind. She smiled to herself. Mary thought it was Doctor Mason whom she must be careful of, but it was more likely to be Cheetham that generated her mother's future 'sight' and concern all those years ago. Eve thanked Cuthbert Lamb for calling on her with his report. Whilst he was there, he collected some paste for his bad feet, which had been playing him up recently.

Eve did not tell Joseph of Cheetham's plan to have her charged with being a fraud, because she knew he would be very upset to hear this. But whilst Lamb was talking to Eve about the threat to her from Cheetham, George Hopkinson was calling on Dru at his smithy and telling him what had gone on at the parish council meeting as well. Dru was incensed when he was told what the doctor was planning. Like

Lamb, Hopkinson was very worried with what he heard Cheetham suggest they do to Eve and told Dru so that he could warn his sister. Dru took this information directly to Joseph at his bakery. Joseph immediately shut his doors for the day and rode over to Doctor Cheetham's villa. Fortunately for the doctor, he was out making calls on patients in Farnleydale, according to his elderly housekeeper. Joseph left a message with the woman to tell Cheetham that he, Joseph Locke called to see him, and he would be back.

Frustrated not to see the doctor and confront him with the accusations he was making against his wife, Joseph rode home in a strange mood. He was tired from his day's work, but he was also annoyed with Eve. By the time he reached home, Joseph was short tempered and ready for an argument.

"Why did ya not come to tell me about Cheetham an' his threats?" he confronted Eve not long after walking through the front door. "Ya should've come to tell me straight away," he said angrily.

"Ah didn't want to get ya upset," Eve replied quietly. She could see Joseph was distressed now anyway and wished she had. "How did ya find out?"

"George Hopkinson told Dru an' he called at the shop an' told me," Joseph said. "Then ah went to see Cheetham." Eve looked at him expectantly, waiting for his report on what happened next. "He wasn't

337

there, which wor just as well, 'cause ah think ah would have done him some harm if he had of been. Ah wor that angry!"

"Ya shouldn't have gone there," Eve told him.

"Ah shouldn't have gone there?" Joseph asked incredulously. "What should ah do Eve?" he said angrily. "Should ah just let ya be arrested an' put in jail fer years? Is that what ah should do?"

"Nay, but..." Eve began to say.

"Nay!" Joseph repeated loudly. "Ah'm nay goin' to do nowt any more. An' ah want you, as my wife to stop doin' some of the things ya do that put yarself in danger. Ya help folks around here an' some of them'll never stand by you if ya get into trouble. Slightest trouble at their door Eve an' they'll turn their backs on ya. Ah want ya ti stop it, 'cause ah can't take much more of this. Ya never think about me an' the children. What would happen to us if ya wor sent to jail? Who would look after our children?"

Eve was shaken. She never thought she would hear Joseph say those things to her. After some moments of staring at her husband, Eve sat down. She was trying to decide how to respond. After some uncomfortable minutes, she did.

"Joseph, first of all, ah want to say that ah love ya." She spoke very calmly. "Ah know that what ah do is difficult fer ya to understand, an' ah've allus appreciated ya acceptin' who ah am. Ya're a good

338

man an' a good husband. As fer what ah do...well. Elmsley's got a trained midwife comin' to live here, Margaret told me. She found this out from her friend who works fer Cheetham at his villa. That means soon ah won't be doin' any more birthin'. The authorities have set up these trainin' schools an' this lady, or rather nurse, went to one of them. As fer my remedies...as long as someone wants them an' tis not against the law, then ah'll carry on makin' them. Even if ah stopped givin' 'em out right now, Cheetham will still try an' do me some damage; that's the nature of the man. All ah can say to you is that he can't hurt me. Ya have to trust me Joseph. An' there's nowt that ah'll ever do that'll damage my family. Fate's in control of that, not me." Joseph looked wearily across the table to his wife. He knew she would not stop being who she was, no matter what he said. It then dawned on Joseph that Eve had just told him that she loved him.

"Did ya mean what ya just said?" he asked her. "Do ya love me?"

"Aye," Eve replied, smiling. Joseph went to his wife and kissed her and hugged her.

"Ah can live wi' what ya do ah suppose, but please be careful Eve," he begged her, not for the first time. "Cheetham's a dangerous man."

"Nay," Eve replied confidently, "He's not...he just thinks he is."

As correctly reported by Margaret, a middle-aged widow woman by the name of Mrs Ann Hubbard moved into Elmsley a few weeks later and took over the midwifery duties in the village and local area. Although subordinate to Cheetham, she was an educated and fairly tough sort, and Eve felt she would not be pushed around too much by the man. Nurse Ann was a pleasant soul and sought Eve out to chat with her about her future 'charges', unbeknown to the doctor of course. Eve liked the woman and was happy to hand over the role of midwife to her. Ann expressed a hope that she might be able to call on Eve if she ever needed an extra pair of hands, although that was not very realistic with Cheetham around. However, the women parted company on good terms, both respecting the other's knowledge and experience.

With that part of her life probably over, Eve concentrated on teaching Mary to find the right plants, flowers, berries, herbs and fungi for her tinctures and curing remedies. Mary was now a blossoming thirteen year-old and, although of a fairly delicate nature, she was becoming quite adult in her ways. Mary loved learning, so teaching her was a pleasure for Eve, who, from her own experience of school, never sent her daughter there. Mary was happy not to go and have to mix with the local children anyway. She had experienced bullying outside on occasions and was not robust enough really to cope with it. Of course, she had a small number of children in the village that would play with her, but by and large, she did not mix well. Mary was a very good artist though, and would spend hours doing watercolour paintings of wild flowers from the meadows, dissecting them and exploring the inner world of the plant kingdom. Joseph had bought her some paint cakes when she was quite young and over the years her natural talent with a brush had grown. Her pictures were beautiful. This solitary pursuit matched the quiet and introverted Mary, who liked nothing more than sitting at her little desk underneath her bedroom window, lost in another world; a world of colour, and the magic of nature. Although Eve would have liked her daughter to be a little more outgoing, she knew that her character was what it was and could not be changed.

Seb, on the other hand was completely different to his older sister. Now a noisy ten year old, he was quite a handful for Eve. Unlike Mary, Seb hated lessons and because he was such a livewire and exhausting, Eve sent him to the local school for some peace. She had no concerns for him being bullied. In fact, Eve was more worried for the other children there. Seb had a wild and unpredictable side to his nature and wanderlust; he was always off somewhere, roaming the fields and hills and woods. Joseph tried to interest his son in the bakery, but in his heart he knew that Seb was not going to follow him into his profession. Seb's very few attempts at baking anything resulted in badly cooked loaves being launched across the bakery floor when they did not turn out properly. No, Seb was far more interested in hunting and catching prey, and would come home, even at his young age, with fare he had trapped and killed from the fields. He was particularly adept at catching rabbits, but brought home the odd pheasant and duck. Eve was worried about Seb, and Joseph was forever trying to instil in him that he must not go on to anyone's land or risk getting into trouble for poaching. Poachers were treated more harshly than any other person accused of other types of theft.

After a warning from the new Police Constable Matthew Webster that Seb had been seen on the Squire's land, Joseph finally put his foot down and threatened his son with a beating if he strayed too far from home again. Webster, a young and friendly man, had recently replaced the retired Samuel Jowett, who had vacated the police house and was now living in nearby Ashton with his family.

Webster came with his warning to Joseph, having told the boy off himself on a previous occasion when it was reported to him that Seb had been seen meandering in the woods on the Addington estate, suspected of snaring rabbits there. It was hoped that between the constable's warning and his father's threat, Seb would behave himself and do as he was told. Joseph meanwhile would try to encourage his son again to get interested in the bakery. Seb did stop his hunting expeditions, at least temporarily, which gave Eve and Joseph some peace of mind for a while.

Although he was busy placing Nurse Hubbard into the community as its new midwife, Cheetham had only temporarily postponed his plan to damage Eve with his charges of fraud and quackery. As soon as he felt that he had replaced her with Mrs Hubbard and dispensed with Eve helping the pregnant woman of Elmsley and outlying farms, Cheetham managed to engineer a luncheon meeting with the Squire so that he could put pressure on him to report Eve Locke to the authorities. Also joining them was James Barlow. He was visiting his brother-in-law on some business. Frederick always needed money and wanted to sell yet more of his land to James, who had been steadily buying up parts of the Addington estate for years. Not realising that the doctor intended to discuss his plan to have Eve charged with fraud, the Squire thought nothing of the two men meeting at his table. The first hour went well enough and the meal was washed down with some good local ale. As James had already finished his business with Frederick before lunch much of the discussion around the table was general chat. Then Doctor Cheetham launched into his scheme of how to deal with Eve Locke. Frederick was caught by surprise and squirmed when the doctor brought her name up, and looked straight across the table at James.

James stared at Cheetham in astonishment and did not take his eyes off the man whilst he set out his plan to have Eve arrested and charged with fraud and quackery, listing the false evidence that he would bring to the court against her. The doctor then boasted of how he did that to a woman in the town he came from and that she was jailed for seven years. The Squire had tried several times to silence Cheetham and veer him away from the subject of Eve Locke, but he had gorged himself on strong ale and was in full intoxicated voice. James did not say anything to the doctor; just let him finish setting out his plan. He then turned to Frederick.

"And you have agreed to do this?" he asked him pointedly. James appeared outwardly calm, but Frederick knew him well enough to know that he was seething inside with anger.

"No, no, we were just considering the idea," Frederick mumbled in response.

"I thought you were thinking it over. I thought you

liked the plan Sir?" Cheetham noisily piped up. James ignored him and continued to stare at Frederick.

"You were actually considering having Eve Locke charged with this offence?" he put to his brother-in-law again.

"No, as I told you, it was just an idea," he answered nervously.

"Yes, and it is a dammed good idea too!" the drunken doctor laughed as he lit up a cigar. "All you have to do Squire is tell the authorities, they will do the rest." Cheetham was of course totally unaware of James's building fury, but Frederick was fully aware of his brother-in-law's ire.

"Be quiet man!" he shouted at the doctor and slammed his hand down hard on the table. "I only said to Cheetham that I would think about doing it," he told James defensively. "I would not have done it." The doctor looked confused. He could not understand Frederick's obvious concern to tell James that he was not going to carry out his plan. Cheetham went to say something else, but Frederick held up his hand and silenced him. "I think you should leave," he ordered the doctor. Cheetham struggled from his chair and straightened himself up. He was completely mystified by Frederick's behaviour towards him.

"Cheetham," James addressed him abruptly. The

doctor turned and faced him.

"Yes Sir," he replied.

"I had better not hear of this nonsense again about having Eve Locke charged with any offence. Do you understand?" he told the doctor icily. Cheetham looked over to the Squire for some kind of support, but Frederick just waved him gone with his hand.

"He will not Sir," Frederick told James firmly. The doctor took himself from the room noiselessly and left Addington House in a bewildered state. He had no idea as to why he had upset the Squire so, or James Barlow for that matter. As soon as Cheetham had left, James turned on Frederick venomously.

"Ah warned you once Frederick that if you did anything to hurt the Jennus family or Eve Locke's family then ah will do you great harm."

"I have not done anything to hurt anyone," Frederick argued amiably. He knew he had to placate James and not make him any more upset than he already was. James controlled his rising anger and lit a cigar. After taking a number of draws from it and calming down, he spoke.

"Ah'm going to tell you something now Frederick and ah want you to listen very, very carefully," James said menacingly. "As well as all the information your father told me about your little 'indiscretions' ah also hold some knowledge that ah will make very public if you so much as look at Eve

346

Locke the wrong way in the future." James walked over to the large window and looked across the neat lawns and shrubberies that bordered the long, stoned drive up to the house. In the distance he could see the tail end of Cheetham's carriage leaving the estate. James stood there for some moments, trying to further calm his temper so that he would deliver his communication clearly. With his composure returned, and speaking slowly and clearly, he continued.

"Your grandfather, Squire Edmond Addington was the father of Mary Shetcliffe, Eve Locke and Dru Jennus's mother." He paused and turned to study Frederick's face, which showed no change after this revelation, but his eyes gave away some shock. He did not say anything however. "Edmond told me this before he died. He told me that as a young man, he had an affair with Elisa Shetcliffe, whose father, Jabez Bowlin, worked on the Addington estate as an out labourer. Edmond said that he loved Elisa very much and their affair resulted in the birth of Mary Shetcliffe, who, of course, later married Thomas Jennus. Elisa's father worked for your great grandfather, Squire Harold Addington. It was he who settled on Elisa's father and mother, their cottage and land, which was part of the Addington estate back then. Not only did Harold have the greatest respect for Jabez and his family, he was embarrassed for his son's total lack of it. The settlement was by way of giving Elisa, who would inherit the cottage and land, some security in her life for herself and her child. Elisa, along with her parents, vowed never to say who the father of Mary was and they never did. They kept their word. It would have ruined the Addington family if that had ever become known. So you see my dear Frederick, Eve Locke and Dru Jennus have the same blood running through their veins as yours. You share the same grandfather and the same ancestors."

"Why should I believe you?" Frederick said crossly. "For all I know you have made this whole story up."

"My dear brother-in-law. Ah have all the legal papers that were drawn up by your great grandfather, of his settlement on Jabez Bowlin and Maria Shetclifffe," he told Frederick. "Your grandfather also gave me a signed and sealed envelope containing the lawful declaration that he was Mary Shetcliffe's father. He entrusted these documents to me because he had no faith in you. Edmond wanted to protect his daughter Mary and his grandchildren, Eve and Dru, after his death, even though they would never know who he was.

"I want to see these documents," Frederick demanded.

"You cannot see them," James replied. "However, you can speak to my lawyer, who has had sight of them and ah'm sure he will confirm their authenticity to you."

"I will speak to him," Frederick spat out.

"Then ah will instruct him to pay you a visit," James said. "Regarding Doctor Cheetham," he added. "You had better make sure that the insidious little man has no contact with Eve Locke and minds his business. If ah hear that he has done Eve any harm or injustice then ah will hold you responsible for his actions and ah'll make everything ah know public. Is that understood Frederick?"

"Yes," Frederick answered angrily. He hated James, but he had borrowed so much money from him over the years and now relied on his buying pieces of land from him whenever he needed to pay his gambling debts, that he dare not ignore or upset him.

Content to know that he had put an end to the plans of Doctor Cheetham, James left Addington House. He no longer rode his horse there and back to his own estate, instead, riding in a splendid black carriage that was not only warm and comfortable, but also had window blinds so that he could see out, but nobody could see in. That way, he could travel in and out of Elmsley, on the occasions when he came to do business with Frederick, without the worry of coming across Eve and her knowing it was him. He could also study her and his daughter if he passed them.

James had seen Eve walking the fields with Mary, a year or so earlier, and had strained to look at the face of his daughter as he sped past in his cocooned brougham. He so desperately wanted to call to his driver to stop so that he could speak to Eve and the girl, but they were gone from his sight as quickly as he had come upon them. And what would he have said to them, James thought? What would Eve have said to him? No, it was better that they did not see him or know he had even passed. He would still imagine Eve running across the fields though, every time he went to Addington House, just as he remembered she had done when they were youngsters.

Chapter 25

Squire Addington heeded the warning from James and ordered Cheetham to call on him, whereupon he told the doctor to relinquish his plan to accuse Eve of fraud and have her arrested. The doctor was loath to do this however and even attempted to argue with the Squire. Frederick was furious and screamed at him to do as he was told. Cheetham left Addington House with the Squire believing that he would do as he had instructed. But the doctor was too conceited to be averted from performing what he felt was his moral and medical duty. As he left Frederick, Cheetham decided that he would have to speak to the authorities himself and call upon them to deal with Eve Locke. The Squire Frederick did not have the sort of powers in the community as his predecessors held. Although he remained Justice of the Peace in the local court, the legal system had been slowly evolving over the previous few decades and was now centrally controlled by Her Majesty's Government.

Cheetham planned to go in to Farnleydale some days later to consult with the Chief Constable, now responsible for safeguarding and administering local law and order. It would be to him that the doctor would take his accusations and 'evidence' against Eve. However, the day before his planned visit, the doctor went down with what seemed like a bad cold. He felt so poorly that he would have to abandon his visit until he felt better. For the next two days, Cheetham had a raging temperature and his chest became painful when he breathed. Then a red rash covered his face and soon spread all over his whole body. He reasoned that he had contracted measles. Cheetham had visited a child in Ashton whom he suspected of having the disease, and seeing his symptoms, he surmised that he probably caught it from her. It took the doctor three weeks to get over the measles, and he was quite ill. A week into the disease he was so sick he sent one of his house servants to Farnleydale to fetch a doctor colleague from there to see him. Before he left on his errand however, his servant suggested to him that he call in Mother Eve from the village; apparently her remedies were very successful with treating the measles. The servant did not get a favourable response.

Even after he recovered, Doctor Cheetham remained weak. It would take him some time to get around to considering his campaign against Eve again. He firstly had to attend to his patients, some of whom, whilst he was incapacitated, had been calling on Eve for her remedies. Hearing these reports did not aid his recuperation. By the following month however, Cheetham decided it was time to think about riding into Farnleydale with his case against Eve. But, just before he set off that Monday morning, the doctor began to vomit. It progressively became worse and he spent the next week laid up in bed again, retching violently throughout most of the days. Once more Cheetham's doctor friend from Farnleydale was called out to him. The doctor's colleague was concerned that he could barely keep anything down except a few sips of water, and suggested he go into York Infirmary. Cheetham did not want to leave his home however, so a nurse was hired to care for him. The sickness slowly eased off and had left the man by the third week. After days of hardly keeping anything down, save a few sips of tepid water, the once rotund figure of Doctor Cheetham was much thinner. This at least made him slightly more pleasant to look at. However, the dark circles under his eyes, and the pallid, slightly green-shaded skin on his face began to give him a corpse-like appearance. He just did not look well at all, which concerned the patients he was now visiting, who expressed their worry that he might be contagious with something.

A full two months passed before Cheetham managed to regain some of his strength and a slightly normal colour to his face. Now he really was intending to speak to the Chief Constable about Eve Locke and ordered his carriage to be ready for the following morning at ten o'clock. The doctor told his servant that he would have his breakfast and then leave afterwards, getting back to see any patients in the village after lunch. That morning, Cheetham arose from his bed feeling fine. He had a good breakfast and was being helped on with his day coat by his servant, when he had a hot sensation around his genital area. Looking down, the doctor realised that he had pissed himself. The servant was shocked and embarrassed, and did not know whether to leave the doctor or try to help him. Cheetham was so surprised himself, that he just stood there staring at his crutch, watching the urine make a bigger and bigger dark patch as it soaked through his undergarments and then his light grey trousers. He sent his servant away and went to his dressing room and changed into a completely new outfit, putting his 'accident' down to perhaps a slight chill in his bladder. Having dispensed with the soiled clothes, he once again put on his day coat and made his way to the front door. Then a noisy explosion occurred from his anus. Cheetham was mortified as he tried to control the diarrhoea gushing from him and filling up his newly changed undergarments and then running down both legs. He held his trouser bottom full of excrement and carefully walked back to his dressing room. The stench of his faeces, even for him, was overwhelmingly grotesque. His visit to Farnleydale had to be postponed yet again.

It was not until Cheetham was riding to see one of his patients some two weeks later that it struck him that every time he tried to go to speak to the Chief Constable to carry out his 'duty', he fell ill or suffered a mishap. After musing for a few moments on a thought that Eve Locke might have something to do with these phenomena, he dismissed the idea as ridiculous. 'How could she?' he thought. Then a faint glimpse of a consideration passed through his mind, remembering that some people in the village thought she was a witch. 'No', he argued with himself. He was a man of science. He could not possibly believe that someone could have that sort of power. Belief in witches and their curses was just old wives' tales and superstition. 'No', he thought again. Locke could not have anything to do with his being unwell; it was coincidence and just one of those periods that one goes through. His next attempt to see the Chief Constable in town would be successful, he assured himself.

To that end, Cheetham organised his carriage to be ready again the next day. The weather was fine and dry, so that would not prevent him from going to Farnleydale. He felt quite well and had done his full toiletry, so that should not encumber him either. The doctor put on his day coat, left his house and climbed into his barouche. He smiled smugly, having made it thus far without incident, the thought of Eve and her witchery slowly banishing. He raised his stick and tapped it on the side of the carriage to signal his driver to go. His driver whipped the horses lightly and the carriage moved off. As the barouche went through the gates to his villa, Cheetham's confidence grew and he settled in his seat to think about the conversation he would have with the Chief Constable. As he gazed out of the window at the passing countryside, the doctor felt his nose running and took out his handkerchief to wipe it. Examining what had just left his nostrils, Cheetham noted spots of blood. He then blew his nose and it suddenly began to pour with thick, red, hot blood. He held his head back to stem the flow, but it only got worse and started pouring down the back of his throat, making him want to gag. He yelled out to his driver, as best he could, for him to stop, which eventually he did. Cheetham climbed out of his carriage and held his face over the grass verge, away from his body, blood still gushing from his nose. A wind blew up and Cheetham's attempts to limit the damage that the blood would make to his clothing became futile. His handkerchief was soaked and no longer of any use and he called to his driver to give him his scarf or shirt, or something that he could hold to his nose. The doctor's day coat was now heavily splattered with blood, as were his trousers and shoes. He could not possible go to Farnleydale in that state and ordered his driver to return him to his villa.

"I am telling you that I cannot believe my being prevented from going to speak with the Chief Constable in Farnleydale is purely coincidental," Cheetham was reporting to his fellow members of the parish council at their next meeting. The Squire was not there that evening, as he was said to be feeling unwell again. A message had been sent to Doctor Cheetham to attend to him after the meeting had finished.

"So what are you saying?" Pastor Bell asked the doctor. He was very angry that Cheetham was still pursuing his vendetta against Eve Locke, and told him so.

"If I was not a man of medicine and science," he replied, "I might well think that Eve Locke, Mother Eve as she now is being called in the village, is using some sort of witchery on me." Cuthbert Lamb and George Hopkinson, who were both in attendance, looked at one another. Cuthbert laughed out loud.

"But ya are a medical man an' a man o' science," he goaded the doctor. "Don't tell us that ya believe in witches?" he laughed again.

"No, of course I am not," Cheetham replied. Cuthbert went to continue with his baiting of the doctor, but George winked at him, messaging that he wanted a turn.

"Now then Cuthbert, ah wouldn't dismiss what t'

357

good doctor 'ere is sayin'," he told him. "We all know t' truth about Eve, don't we?" he added with a serious face.

"What do you mean by that?" Cheetham asked.

"Tis common knowledge," George paused tantalisingly.

"What is?" Cheetham asked again.

"Well…Eve, sh' comes from Shetcliffe stock. There's plenty o' stories about that family," Cuthbert joined in. Pastor Bell huffed. He knew what the men were doing and almost put a stop to it, but having heard Cheetham declare earlier that he was still trying get Eve charged with fraud and quackery, even the pastor felt he deserved to hear what Cuthbert and George were planning to tell him.

"Aye," George said. "All o' t' Shetcliffe females 'ave allus been known fer their witchery. Do ya remember when t' Devil 'imself came to t' village?" he asked Cuthbert.

"Aye, it wor t' night Eve wor born. T' devil wor s'posed ti 'ave been watchin' over 'er birth, wasn't 'e?" George replied.

"The Devil? Eve Locke's birth? What are you talking about Hopkinson?" Cheetham yelled at him.

"T' night when Eve Jennus, as sh' was then, wor bein' born, t' Devil came ti Elmsley an' left 'is footmarks around t' Jennus cottage. 'E wor there ti see 'is own comin' int' t' world." Cuthbert explained in an unnerving voice. "Pastor Bell remembers that night, don't ya Bell?" The pastor nodded.

"Yes, I remember," he confirmed.

"You are telling me, that the Devil came to this village to watch Eve Locke being born?" the doctor asked incredulously.

"Aye," both men said at the same time. Cheetham stared at them. He wanted to pour scorn on their reports, but, for a few moments he half believed what they had said. Then his logical mind returned again.

"This is nonsense!" he spat out, but all three men stared blankly at him, none were going to give their joke away, at least, not yet. "I am sorry gentlemen, but this is all just blind superstition." He studied his colleague's faces again. As he continued to do so, Cuthbert was the first to break down and begin to laugh, followed by George and then Pastor Bell.

"How dare you find sport with me," Cheetham shouted at the men, realising they were playing with him, but that just made them laugh even louder. "How dare you, I say," the doctor repeated.

"Ya deserved it man," George told him. "Now leave t' woman alone. Sh's nay doin' you any 'arm."

"Eve Locke is harming this community," Cheetham argued back.

"Ya mean sh's harmin' yar pocket more like," Cuthbert replied.

"So, you are all against me are you?" Cheetham snarled. "And you Bell, I am surprised that you should take a stand against me with these men."

"I am afraid, Doctor Cheetham," the pastor told him, "that you will get no support or sympathy from any of us here for your plans to destroy Mrs Locke."

"Very well," Cheetham said angrily. "I see I am completely on my own in this matter. Even the Squire seems to be afraid to do anything about the woman. But I am not."

"On yar own 'ead be it then," Cuthbert warned him loudly. Cheetham snatched up some papers from the table and stormed out of the meeting, making his way to attend to the Squire Frederick, as instructed.

"Have you been attempting to go to Farnleydale to see the Chief Constable there?" Frederick asked Cheetham pointedly, after he had finished examining him and recommending a medicine.

"Yes Sir," the doctor replied, surprised at the question. He had not mentioned to anyone what his plans were, apart from earlier that evening at the council meeting, and no one there could have had time to tell the Squire.

"May I ask why doctor?" Frederick asked calmly. Cheetham hesitated and fumbled around for his reply.

"Erm...well, I thought I might discuss the Locke case with him," the doctor said. He looked at

Frederick's face, which looked like an impending thunder storm. "Just to discuss it, nothing else you understand," he lied.

"Cheetham," Frederick addressed the doctor sternly. "Did I, or did I not give you strict instructions not to pursue this business with Eve Locke?" Cheetham nodded a yes. "Then please tell me why you ignored me?" he added. The doctor squirmed.

"Squire," Cheetham replied apologetically, "This really is a medical matter Sir." Frederick stared at him in disbelief.

"I do not care what it is," Frederick screamed at him. "I gave you an instruction and you ignored me, you bloody fool." He was so angry, saliva was pouring from his mouth. "I will ruin you. Do you hear me?" he continued to scream. "I will make sure that you never practise medicine again, anywhere." The doctor was stunned. He did not expect such a venomous attack from the Squire. All sorts of arguments lined up in his brain to put to Frederick in his defence as to why he should continue with his persecution of Eve Locke, but just as soon as they came to him, the fear of making the Squire his enemy, overrode all such arguments. He stood without a word to say.

"Well?" Frederick screamed at him again. "What say you man?"

"I will of course do as you have instructed me Sir," he mumbled. The Squire, still livid, screamed at Cheetham again.

"And what have I instructed you to do?" he yelled.

"You have told me to stop taking action against Eve Locke," the doctor mumbled again.

"So you have heard me this time?" Frederick said in a slightly, but not much of a lower voice.

"Yes Sir," Cheetham replied.

"Good," Frederick said. "And if I hear that you have gone to speak with the Chief Constable about any of the Locke family, or the Jennus family, I will destroy you. Do you understand?" Cheetham nodded that he did and after the Squire waved him gone, he left, his tail firmly stuck between his legs. All the way home, the doctor sat in silent shock. He could not understand the Squire's adamant stand in his defence of Locke. It made no sense to him at all and he could not comprehend how the man could have even found out about his plan to go to the Chief Constable. Clearly, he was going to have to find another way to destroy Eve Locke. He would certainly not give up, his sort very rarely do. Cheetham was a fanatic, and fanatics, who unquestionably have right on their side, do not give up.

Frederick sat in his room after the doctor had left, very angry at Cheetham. He instinctively knew that the man was a loose cannon. The doctor had ignored him once and therefore could ignore him again. Frederick was very frightened of James hearing about Cheetham's attempts to see the Chief Constable in Farnleydale with his accusations and so-called evidence against Eve. If James found out, he would think that he put him up to it, or at least agreed to the doctor doing it. Frederick needed to speak to James directly and therefore sent one of his servants to ride overnight, the fifty miles to James's estate, to bid him visit Addington House as soon as he could. Later the following day, James called on Frederick. They sat and discussed Cheetham and Frederick vowed to James that he had nothing to do with the doctor's plan or attempted visits to Farnleydale to bring trouble down on Eve Locke. James was not wholly convinced by Frederick's protestations of innocence but, considering his call to him and frankness about Cheetham's acts, he was willing to acknowledge an attempt on his side to stop him from taking his planned action against Eve. However, James was not about to let Frederick off of the hook that easily.

"Ah'll hold you responsible for Cheetham then," James told Frederick.

"But I have been honest with you James, I cannot stop the man," Frederick bleated. "I have threatened him, but I just do not think he will listen to me."

"Well then you had better get rid of him. My warning still stands Frederick," James reiterated. "Any harm comes to Eve or Dru, or any member of their families through the actions of that man, or you, and ah will carry out my threat." Frederick was horrified. He knew James meant what he said, but he also believed that Cheetham would continue with his plots; he knew enough of the man to know he was a dangerous fool. James left Frederick with much to think about. Getting rid of Doctor Cheetham, as suggested by James, might be his safest option.

On his return back to his own estate, James directed his driver to take a detour and go through Elmsley. He had the notion that he wanted to pass Eve's cottage. Safe behind his screened windows, nobody would see him, whilst he could clearly see the village and all its activities. James had to remember which end of the village her cottage was and almost thought he had passed it, when he saw a young lady come out of the front of what he now realised was Eve's home. The youngster was unmistakably his daughter Mary, her long dark hair blowing gently about her face in the light autumn breeze. She was beautiful, James thought, just like her mother. In fact, for a second or two, she reminded him of Eve, the first day he saw her walking towards him on the lane out of Elmsley, all those years ago. James's carriage soon passed the girl, but he stared at her out of the back window until she could no longer be seen. His heart sank and he sat back into his lonely silence, yearning once again to see Eve. Even a glance would suffice he thought...just a glance.

Chapter 26

With the immediate threat of Doctor Cheetham removed, Eve was relatively safe for the while. When next she saw Cuthbert Lamb in Elmsley, she asked him to convey her gratitude to George Hopkinson and Pastor Bell for their humanity in not supporting Cheetham in his accusations against her. Cuthbert warned her however, that in his opinion, having some knowledge of the man and his manner, the doctor would not give up trying to remove her from his society. Eve heard his warning.

But life settled down to some calm for the time being. Joseph relaxed a little as far as Cheetham was concerned and never paid him the visit he threatened; Eve talked her husband out of doing that. Mary was maturing and filling out in all the places a young woman should and soon began to menstruate, leaving behind the little girl. Eve was now training her daughter in the ways of her ancestors and Mary was a quick and eager learner. She began her own story early with her beautiful drawings and paintings.

Seb was also growing up fast and although Eve and Joseph had managed to curb his poaching activities, he was still always off somewhere, anywhere, as long as it was away from home. Dru and Lillian seemed happy enough, much to the relief of everyone. Young Thomas was turning into a quiet, handsome man, and an honest, good and true soul, as Eve would describe him. He was a great help to Dru in his smithy and forge and was popular with the village and beyond. His future looked set. The baby Edward was now a strong and healthy child, running around and getting up to every mischief, just as he should. Sarah and Ben announced they were having a baby and the whole family gathered together that following Christmas to feast and celebrate their blessings as well as Eve's birthday.

Sometime mid-January, in the New Year, Margaret visited with the news that Doctor Cheetham had suddenly moved away, somewhere up in Scotland she was told by one of the servants who used to work for him at his villa. Joseph was more than relieved to hear this news but Eve was a little surprised; this was none of her doing. Maybe he just got frustrated in trying to find enough 'evidence' on her she thought, but for whatever reason he was gone from Elmsley, Eve was glad. It would be interesting to see what the new doctor was like, whenever he arrived.

That winter saw another spread of influenza in the village. Concerned that it could be a killer infection, Nurse Hubbard called upon Eve to help in any way she could. With Cheetham gone and nobody local having filled his post yet, the nurse was grateful for

Eve's tinctures, once she satisfied herself that they were safe. However, this particular influenza outbreak did not appear to be as devastating as some of those that had passed through Elmsley before. But caution is always the best policy with something so contagious, so between Nurse Hubbard and Eve, they managed to quarantine and treat the sick, thus reducing the spread of the virus. It did unfortunately take in its wake some elderly, weak folk, but thankfully a very few.

One afternoon, as she was returning from a visit to a farm just outside Ashton in Joseph's cart, Eve noticed a carriage coming towards her in the distance. She had seen this particular barouche regularly being driven through the village. On two occasions, she had also seen it on the lane going out of Elmsley. Eve was curious as to its occupants, who she had never been able to see, the blinds on the windows preventing anyone looking into the carriage itself. Then she suddenly knew who was in it. James, she thought. It was him inside the carriage. Realising this, Eve did not know quite what to do, whether to ride off quickly or remain stationary whilst the carriage passed her. Neither option was appealing, but before she could decide, the barouche was upon her. Eve sat still and focussed her eyes on the carriage windows, letting its occupant know that she knew who he was. As it drew alongside Eve's cart, the barouche stopped. After a few moments, James opened the door and stepped out on to the gravelled road. Eve also climbed down from her cart.

"Mrs Locke," James said, taking off his hat and bowing his head.

"Mr Barlow," she replied, trying to appear calm and casual.

"Are you well?" he asked, barely able to look Eve in the eye.

"Aye, ah am," she said, staring into James's face. He had changed very little, she thought. He was still the most handsome man she had ever seen and her heart was racing at the sight of him. There was some greyness of hair about his temples and he had lost his boyish looks, but they were only replaced with a maturity of the face that was sexually appealing to her. Eve wanted him. Once he had gotten over his initial embarrassment, James looked at Eve. She was still lovely, he thought. Like him, she had some strands of grey hair in amongst her long brown locks, but to James, she was as beautiful as ever. Her noted her body, which was still slim, although more shapely, her breasts were fuller, but still pert. After he had examined her body, James studied Eve's face, her eyes, her lips, and her milky complexion. He still loved her.

"And your family, they are all well?" he enquired.

"Aye, they are thank you. An' yours?" she returned

the asking.

"Yes, my sons are all grown up," James replied. "My eldest, James, he is at military school now. My second son, Harry is with him, and my youngest, Charles, is still at boarding school, but he will be joining his brothers soon." Eve nodded.

"And your children?" James asked. He wanted to tell her that he had seen Mary once from a distance, and how lovely he thought she was, but he could not be that candid in front of his driver.

"Aye, Mary is growing up fast, almost a young lady now. Sh's well. Sh's becomin' a fine artist," Eve knew he wanted to know something about his daughter. "Seb, my son, he's a typical lad an' he'll soon be a man." They stood wanting to say so much more to one another, but neither could think of any other small talk and anything more than that was out of the question.

"It was good to see you again Mrs Locke," James said, conscious of his driver's presence. He knew only too well what servants hear and gossip about, he paid one who worked on the Addington estate quite handsomely to keep him informed of what went on behind the walls of Frederick's house.

"Aye," Eve replied casually. "It wor good to see you too." James bowed his head again, climbed into his carriage and his driver drove him off. Eve watched until she could no longer see James's barouche and then made her own way home. It had felt good to see him again, and Eve thought about James the whole journey back to Elmsley. She collected her children from Lillian's house, who was giving them lunch that day. As she walked through her door, she saw Joseph sitting there; he had closed his bakery up and gone home. Eve was surprised to see him so early in the day, but he looked pale and shivery. She made Joseph some tonic and sent him to bed. Eve did not mention to her husband that she had seen James, there did not seem to be any reason to. Whilst she had enjoyed seeing him, Eve could now control her emotions much more, something the years had taught her to do. Back with her family, James was returned to the compartment in her heart where he was kept under lock and key.

Joseph was ill for almost a week. During that time, Eve took on some of his baking work. She had learned how to produce most of what he sold and actually enjoyed doing it. Mary, Seb and even the heavily pregnant Sarah helped out as well. Eve would bake all morning, then nurse Joseph in the afternoon, cook a meal for the family, then return to the bakery in the evening to set up the trays for the following day's baking. Dru helped Eve out with the logs and keeping the ovens going. It was hard work, but Eve was more than capable of doing it. It was not the work that she found difficult, but the response of a few customers who came in to the shop. Once they realised that it was Eve who had made the bread and cakes, some would not buy them, proclaiming that they would not eat anything that she had touched. So, at the end of the morning's baking, there was some produce seemingly wasted. Eve would not allow this to upset her though and just gave the bread and cakes away to the very poorest families in the village, who gratefully received her gift.

Joseph felt slightly better after a few days, but Eve would not let him back to do his work until his colour had fully returned. She made no mention to him of the hostile customers she had dealt with. Joseph went back to his baking and seemed to be much recovered, but he fell ill again some ten days later and then had to rest up at home and return to his bed. Eve could not think what could be wrong with her husband and decided to call in a doctor from Ashton to examine him. Doctor Brent visited the cottage and attended Joseph two days later. He examined him, but could not immediately give any particular diagnosis either. Joseph's heart appeared to be sound and his pulse strong, but he was clearly listless and getting progressively weak and had a yellow look about his skin. He did not have pain anywhere, but his urine was strong in colour and in odour. The doctor concluded his examination with a diagnosis of a kidney infection and offered Joseph a herbal mixture to help shift the infection. But Eve had already tried the remedy that Doctor Brent prescribed and it had not made any difference to Joseph's symptoms. She said nothing to the doctor however, and it was decided that he would return in a few days' time to check up on his patient's recovery. Eve then tried various tinctures on her husband, but none seemed to make him feel any better. Then Joseph began to complain about some severe discomfort in his groin and lower back. Again, Doctor Brent was called out, but all he could offer was more of the previous herbal mixture he had already advised. Again, he left. Eve was now becoming very concerned for Joseph. Other than some pain remedy and the usual mixtures she would give for bladder or kidney problems, she had nothing to give to her husband.

All of the family rallied around to help Eve, but as Joseph's illness became more severe, she had to close the bakery and look after him. As the days passed and he continued to show no sign of return to his normal health, Eve became afraid. It came to her that she had to face the prospect of losing Joseph and she dreaded the thought of it. After what was now weeks of illness, he suddenly took a turn for the worse. Eve was frantic. It was just midnight, and she had been sitting with Joseph all of that day and evening. When she heard her husband fighting to breath, she sat him up and tried to get some air to him. This seemed to calm him and help his breathing and Joseph settled back down to sleep. But at one o'clock on that Sunday morning, he died, quickly and quietly. Eve sat holding Joseph's hand, shocked and distressed. For some minutes she could not believe her husband had passed away and kept feeling for a pulse and checking for any breath leaving him. But when it was clear that Joseph had gone, Eve became wretched and heartbroken. Why could she not save her husband? Why could she not have stopped the infection, if that was what was wrong with him? How could she have lost him so easily? Why did she have to lose him? The questions crowded her brain until she ran out of them, and then Eve cried bitter tears.

She sat with Joseph for the rest of the night. She did not wake her children from their sleep, but would ask Mary to fetch her uncle to the cottage in the morning. Mary became hysterical when she heard her father had died and insisted on seeing him. The sight of Joseph however, so pale and cold, brought on more hysteria and she was inconsolable. Seb threw a tantrum when he heard his father was dead and ran from the cottage. Eve had to fetch Dru herself in the end, who then went to call on the constable. He would send a message to Ashton for

Doctor Brent to come out to examine Joseph's body.

It was an extremely sad time for Eve. She took Joseph's death very badly. He was some years older than her, that was true, but he was fit and very rarely ever ill. In fact Eve could not think of any time, in all of the years that she had known him, when he was really sick. Of course, he had the usual tooth ache occasionally and the odd cold, but nothing of any note. Doctor Brent, after his examination, was satisfied that Joseph had died of natural causes and issued a death certificate stating kidney failure, possibly brought on by kidney disease. Why Joseph should have had this happen to him however, would always remain a mystery. The doctor gave Eve what he thought could be the reason as to why he developed this disease, telling her that it can be inherited and passed down through the generations. Brent had learned this new medical knowledge only recently from his journals. Whatever caused kidney failure however, Eve was further distressed to hear that Joseph may have been suffering from the symptoms of this for some time, without telling her. This upset Eve greatly. She also felt dreadfully guilty remembering how much James was on her mind that day when Joseph came home ill.

Joseph's funeral took place later that week. Eve decided to lay him to rest next to his first wife,

Charlotte. Over the years, Joseph had never failed to lovingly attend to her grave and Eve did not think it fitting to bury him next to her family in the north end of the churchyard, where she herself planned to be interred. Burying Joseph with Charlotte raised a few eyebrows, but she cared little for the opinions of the owners of them. Quite a few villagers attended Joseph's funeral. He was extremely well thought of in the community. Even the elderly, retired Samuel Jowett came from Ashton to pay his respects 'to an old friend', he told Eve. She held up quite well on the day, supported by her brother Dru and his wife Lillian. Ben attended, but Sarah was so heavy now with child, it was unadvisable for her to be there, but she sent a message of sympathy and love to Eve. It did not need to be said how upset Sarah was at the sudden death of her 'dearest Joseph'.

"What's he doin' here?" Dru asked. The burial had just finished and he had his arm around his sister, helping her as they left the graveside. Eve looked up, wondering who her brother was referring to. James was standing a short distance away from the funeral party, over by a large yew tree that stood in the corner of the churchyard, at the front of the church. "Why's he here?" Dru repeated, stopping to look at the man questioningly. Eve did not know how to react. She could not quite understand why James was there herself and she was partly angry and partly puzzled.

"Ah don't know," Eve finally replied. "Take Mary and Seb back home with you Dru," she told her brother. "Ah want to talk to James Barlow." Dru ushered the children out of the churchyard gently and he and Lillian left with all of them.

"What are ya doin' here James?" she asked him.

"Ah wanted to pay my last respects to Joseph," he replied. "Ah also wanted to tell you how sorry ah am for your loss."

"Ya should not be here," she told him.

"What will people think?"

"Ah don't care what people think and neither do you," James said bluntly.

"Ya're right, ah don't care," she agreed. "But ah don't understand why ya should be payin' yar respects to my husband?"

"Eve," James replied. "Joseph was a good man. He's looked after the woman ah love and brought my child up as his own in a loving and safe home. Do you not think that ah should pay this man my deepest respect for what he did?" Eve stared at James. She understood what he was telling her, and she could find no argument with that. Before she could say anything else, James said what he also went there to ask her.

"Ah'm a wealthy man Eve, and ah intend to give you an allowance for the rest of your life and ah will

377

be leaving some money for Mary. Ah offered Joseph a yearly sum, but he refused it. Ah understood that, but he's not here now and he cannot provide a living for you and your children." James looked at Eve and knew she was preparing herself to refuse his offer. "Before you turn me down, ah just want to say that ah will never expect anything from you. If you want me to, ah will not speak to you or see you again, but please do not refuse my help. You and your family need to survive." Eve was taken aback. Joseph had never mentioned to her that James offered him money. But what should she say to James now? How should she respond? How would Joseph have felt about her taking his money? What would he think? But Joseph was gone. Eve knew she could not earn a living from the bakery. Most of Joseph's customers had deserted his shop and now bought their bread from Ashton. No, she would have to sell the bakery, but the small income she received from her remedies and curing pastes would not keep her, Mary and Seb. As Eve stood and looked upon the concerned face of James Barlow, the alternative to his allowance loomed strong and clearly across her mind. She did not want to see her daughter go into service, nor Seb be a farm labourer. With James's money she could give them a better future.

"Ah'll nay turn yar offer down James," she told him. He was surprised. He thought Eve would certainly refuse any help from him. After his initial amazement, James was so pleased he could not hide his feelings and smiled. At last he could do something for Eve and his daughter, he thought. This mood lasted for a very few seconds however, as she then told James that she would accept his money only on the condition that she would not speak or meet with him ever again. He had no choice but to agree, and Eve left him soon afterwards in Saint Guthlac's churchyard to return home to her grieving children.

"So what did Barlow say to ya? Dru asked Eve later in the day. She had given Mary a tincture to make her sleep as she had been crying since early that morning and was exhausted with the upset. Seb had gone out to walk with Dru's son Thomas, so that he could be kept an eye on.

"He told me he wanted to make a regular allowance fer me an' the children," she replied. "An' ah accepted it."

"Ya accepted Barlow's money?" Dru almost shouted. "Ya agreed to take his money? An' why would he want to give ya an allowance anyway?" Eve looked at her brother. Could she trust him with her secret? She was tempted to tell him that Mary was James's child, but did she dare?

"Because he still thinks a lot of me an' wants to help," Eve replied. She did not think she could trust

Dru to remain silent. "He can afford it Dru. James is one of the richest men in Yorkshire, an' ah have to think about Mary and Seb now. Ah need to be able to provide fer them. Maybe ah can send Mary to one of those nursin' schools an' pay fer an apprenticeship fer Seb." Dru was confused. He still could not quite understand why James Barlow, a man his sister had not seen for many years, should even contemplate giving her anything, let alone an allowance.

"Ya don't have to accept his money Eve," Dru told her. "Ya know ah'll take care of you and yar bairns." Eve smiled gratefully at her brother.

"Ah know ya'd try Dru, but ya struggle at times yarself. Ya've got ya own family to look after. Ya don't need to be keepin' us as well. Nay, ah've made up my mind. Ah'm goin' to take James Barlow's money."

Chapter 27

James Barlow was true to his word and set up a monthly allowance for Eve. Each four weeks, without fail, a messenger from his solicitor's office in Farnleydale called at her cottage with a small package of money. Mary and Seb, although inquisitive, did not ask their mother what the package contained or where it came from. Eve had sold Joseph's bakery shop recently and they thought it was something to do with that. She put some money she raised from the sale into the bank in Ashton. The rest, Eve used to do repairs to her cottage, particularly to the roof, which needed re-thatching.

Sarah and Ben had a little girl, who they named Annie, brought into the world by Nurse Hubbard and Eve. Mother and baby were fine and Eve could not have been happier to see her sweet Sarah safe, loved, and settled. After the cruelty the poor girl had suffered most of her life, at last she had found love, contentment and peace. Ben was an excellent husband and promised to be a wonderful and doting father. Eve felt she no longer had to worry for Sarah, although now she was the nearest thing to a grandmother to little Annie, a part she was overjoyed to play.

The rest of the Locke family remained well, and Eve

settled down into a quiet life without her dear Joseph. She could never have imagined just how much she would miss him though, and not a day went by when she did not think about him, talk to him, or look at his photograph; the one they had taken years earlier in Farnleydale with Mary and Seb, not long after he was born. But Eve was now alone and determined to do her best for her daughter and son. With the allowance from James, the three of them lived in reasonable comfort and with careful budgeting Eve managed to put some money away for Mary and Seb's futures. Without the worry to earn a living, she was also able to continue giving help to people with her remedies, especially those with little or no income who could not afford a doctor's fees.

A new doctor did finally arrive in the village, a Doctor Melbry. He seemed pleasant enough and did not appear to feel threatened by Eve and her 'potions' and 'curing pastes'. Nurse Hubbard had something to do with that, she thought. But Melbry acted as if he was content to leave those who wanted to be treated by Eve to their own decisions. When she first came across the doctor in Elmsley, he was polite and friendly. Melbry seemed to know who she was and introduced himself. He was very young, Eve thought, or perhaps it was her that was getting older. He was well-dressed and smiled a great deal. Those features would make him popular with the ladies of the village, Eve thought. He also had a slight flirtatiousness about him, even towards her; further adding to his attractiveness for the lasses, she surmised. But Eve was content to know that Doctor Melbry would not be causing her any problems.

And so the years passed. Eve saw nothing of James. She glimpsed his carriage occasionally on its way to and from Addington House, but it passed without stopping and although she missed seeing him, she was glad James never tried to see or speak with her. Eve did not know if James was in the carriage or if he saw her or not. But she chose to believe that even if he was, he had not seen her.

The Squire Frederick Addington was reported to be virtually an invalid now and rarely left his rooms. Gossip circulated around the village, largely spread by Margaret of course, that he would die without a direct heir to his estate and title, which looked increasingly likely. The eldest son of his sister Jayne, James Addington-Barlow, would be the next Squire, by all accounts.

Mary was now a lovely-looking young woman, with her mother's long burnished, dark brown hair, which hung in curls down her back, and her father's eyes and eyelashes and broad smile. She was petite and graceful, very much like Eve's mother, Mary's namesake. There had been much interest in her from a number of young lads in the area, but she was very shy and timid and would not consent to walk out with any of them. Eve was heartened to think that her own history and that of the Shetcliffe family, was not causing Mary too many problems as far as suitors were concerned. One young lad in particular seemed very keen on her and was more persistent than the others. His name was George Wade. Eve knew the family and was somewhat surprised at George's attraction to her daughter, given that he came from that home. The Wades were devout Christians and were very much against her and everything she and her ancestors had stood for. Old Florence Wade, George's grandmother, had been an arch enemy of Elisa, Eve's own grandmother, and had accused her of some dreadful deeds over the years. Things had settled down a little with the following generations, but George's mother, Martha, was always ready to point a finger at Elisa and Mary Shetcliffe. Eve's mother told her quite a few stories about the Wade family and their allegations of causing them bad luck. Every time something unpleasant happened to any Wade, they blamed the Shetcliffes for it.

But thoughts of love, marriage and the immediate future, for all the young lads and lasses in the village, would soon have to be suspended. A dark cloud was hanging over Europe that whole summer and there was constant talk of war. Reports soon began to pour into the village from Farnleydale that a country called Serbia had been invaded by Austria-Hungary, and then another country, Germany, had invaded Belgium, Luxembourg and then France. It was all happening so far away, but suddenly Elmsley, as small a village as it was, along with the rest of the country, seemed to be getting caught up in the frenzy of the whole business. Eve's heart sank when Margaret rushed into her cottage one evening with the dreadful news that Britain had also joined the war. It was the beginning of August, 1914.

The harvesting had just begun in earnest across the farms surrounding the village and after a perfect summer, it promised to yield an abundance of crops. Seb was working on Cuthbert Lamb's farm. In spite of all of Eve's best efforts, her son wanted to work on the land. He balked at any suggestion of learning a trade or getting some kind of formal education at a university. However, in spite of not being 'bookish', Eve had made sure that Seb could read and write well and had numbers and also knew some knowledge of the world. He was no scholar, but he was bright, intelligent and articulate, and Cuthbert Lamb wanted him to work by his side. He spoke to Eve about taking her son under his wing and training him up to manage his farm one day, which was one of the largest in the county. Cuthbert had four daughters of his own, but no son. He liked Seb very much and, if he had his own way, would see one of his daughters married off to him. Eve eventually relented, having given up on the idea of Seb ever becoming a master tradesman or graduate, and agreed that her son could be in the employ of Cuthbert Lamb. After her initial disappointment of wanting her son to do more with his life than work on a farm, she was persuaded by Dru that given Seb's character, a life outdoors was the best thing for him. And, Dru pointed out to his sister, Seb could not be in better hands than those of Cuthbert Lamb.

However, late one evening, Seb came home after a long day working in the fields, fired up with the excitement of war and action in far-off places, and bursting with enthusiasm to go and fight for his King and country. A number of young labourers who had been working around the local farms for the harvest time had gone to Flanders already and many lads in the village were talking about joining up as well. Eve was mortified. She told Seb that he was not going anywhere. He was only seventeen and this was not their war. Seb did his usual shouting and arguing with his mother, furious because Eve did not understand how he felt and would not listen to him. He was a man, Seb told her loudly, not a little boy any more. Why could she not see that, he screamed at her before he stormed out of the cottage. Eve sat holding her head in her hands, terrified at the knowledge that her son wanted to go and fight in a war that she knew could kill him. But what could she do to stop him? Seb was a stubborn and headstrong lad and could not be told anything.

Mary suggested to her mother that she ask for the help of Cuthbert Lamb to persuade Seb to be sensible and stay at home, and somehow get it through to him that what he was contemplating was dangerous and that there was no glory in death. This tactic worked, and with Cuthbert's intervention, Seb seemed to settle down and get on with his job, much to Eve's relief.

Then, not four weeks later, during the first week of September, Seb came home with some news. He had, along with three other lads working on Cuthbert's farm, volunteered and enlisted in the 4th Battalion Yorkshire Regiment. Eve was shocked to her core when she heard Seb say this. Her whole body froze in silent panic. She wanted to scream at her son, shake him and lash out at him. Eve felt as if a knife had just been plunged into her heart and then twisted until she could no longer breathe. How could he do that to her? How could he wound her like that? How could he be so stupid, so naïve? Eve was distraught. She could not bring herself to speak to her son or even look at him. Seb was sitting at the table, smiling a silly smile. He knew full well that he had damaged his mother but was telling himself that she would get over it and be fine. Of course Seb had no idea what level of pain he had just inflicted on Eve. Mary sat opposite her brother, also shocked at what he had done, especially since their mother had forbidden him to do it only weeks ago.

Mary watched her mother nervously. Eve had not seemed to react when Seb told her he had joined up; she just carried on cooking the evening meal. When she had finished, she put two plates of food on to the table, one for Mary, the other for Seb then she walked out of her cottage without looking at or saying a single word to her son.

"Have ya any idea what ya've just done to our mam?" Mary asked her brother. She had gotten over her shock and was now angry with Seb. "Do ya know how much ya've hurt her?"

"Don't start on me Mary," Seb retaliated. "Ah can't just carry on as if there's nay war on. Ah should go an' fight, like the others. Mam'll be fine. Sh' seemed all right to me."

"Don't be a fool," Mary told him, "Mam's in a dreadful state. She begged ya not to join up an' ya ignored her. How could ya do that to our mam?"

"Ah want to go," Seb replied loudly. "Ah want to fight fer my country. There's a lot of us from the village and farms around here who've volunteered.

We're all goin' together. Ah want to go an' see some action Mary. There's nothin' in Elmsley fer me. Ah want to get away, just fer a while."

"Seb, ya're only seventeen," Mary said. "They shouldn't have let ya join up."

"Ah told 'em ah was eighteen...ah will be soon," he replied argumentatively.

"Oh Seb, what are ya thinkin'? This is a war. Tis not some kind of fancy trip to another country. People are dyin' over there in Belgium and France, hundreds of them." Seb was silent. He really had not intended to hurt his mother, but it had all happened so quickly. His friend Jon came to the field where Seb and the other lads were working and told them that a recruitment officer from the army was in Ashton, and was calling for volunteers. They finished their work early and just thought they would ride into town and hear what the man was there to say. Apparently, the British army had just had to retreat from what the officer called the 'Battle of Mons'. He told the crowd of people that had now gathered around him, that any man of fighting age should volunteer to defend their home, their loved ones and their country. The Germans outnumbered the regular British soldiers, and unless their country fights them with every able-bodied man, the Germans would defeat the French and then invade Britain. Seb described how everyone was shouting at

389

the tops of their voices, and when any man stepped forward to volunteer, the crowd roared and cheered and clapped. His best friend Jon stepped up, then the two lads that he worked with. They all looked back at him, standing alone, and before he could think, he had stepped up as well.

Eve was kneeling by Joseph's grave. She was tidying it up, in between sobbing and talking to him. She was lost and afraid, and at that moment in time, felt totally helpless and alone.

"Eve?" a voice behind her said. She looked up to see Nathan Morely standing there. She could not make out his features clearly, as he stood with the setting sun behind him, but Eve knew it was him.

"Nathan," she replied, controlling her tears.

"Are ya upset, can ah help ya?" he asked. Eve dare not speak a word in reply, because if she attempted to say anything, she would cry again. She nodded her head as if to say there was nothing wrong. "Ya must miss Joseph?" he said kindly, surmising that her upset was for her late husband. Nathan had been quietly attending to his brother William's grave, which was not too far away from where Joseph was laid to rest and had heard some of Eve's anguished conversation with him.

"Tis my son," she finally managed to say. "Tis Seb, he's volunteered to go an' fight." At this, Eve broke down and wept into her hands. "He's only seventeen an' he's joined up. Ah don't know what to do?" Nathan looked down at Eve sympathetically.

"Ah've heard there's quite a few youngsters in the village that've joined up," Nathan said. "My brother Henry; his eldest 'as volunteered as well. Henry told me he weren't happy about it, but 'e reckons that those who don't sign up'll only get conscripted later on anyway."

"But my lad's only seventeen Nathan," Eve cried.

"Aye, so is Timothy, Henry's boy," Nathan replied. "He lied an' said 'e wor eighteen. Ah just don't know what to think. Tis all very worryin'. Ah'm sorry to hear about Seb joinin' up though. Try not to worry Eve. It won't do ya any good to fret." Eve stopped herself crying. She appreciated Nathan speaking so pleasantly to her. In fact, she could not remember him ever saying so much. He had always been a man of few words. She stood up from Joseph's grave, shook down her skirt and looked directly at Nathan.

"Ah didn't kill William," she told him. "An' ah didn't curse him neither." Nathan was taken aback. He had not expected Eve to say that to him, and she had not expected to say it. The thought had suddenly come to her mind that she had never told Nathan that, and she felt the need to say it.

"Ah know ya didn't," he replied simply. He paused, studying Eve's face. She explored his also. For some brief moments she thought she saw something in his gaze, something in his eyes. Then he looked away, before Eve could read anything more from him.

"Ah only saw what wor goin' to happen to William," she continued.

"Ah know," he repeated. Eve felt relieved, even forgiven. "Ah never thought ya killed him. What made ya say this to me now, after all this time?" he asked her.

"Ah don't know," Eve replied. "Ah just felt bad seein' ya here at ya brother's grave, ah suppose."

"Tis William's birthday today," Nathan told her. "Mi mam allus asks me to come an' put somethin' here. Sh' can't walk now an' so ah do it fer her. Mi dad, well, he can't bring himself to come to William's grave. If truth wor known, he wor mi dad's favourite." Eve was saddened to hear Nathan tell her that.

"Ah'm so sorry fer William dyin'" Eve said.

"Ah know ya are," Nathan told her. Again they stood in silence for some moments, he seemingly fidgeting with embarrassment. Eve realised at that precise moment that Nathan Morely was sweet on her. He realised that she now knew that, and became nervous.

"Well, ah best be goin'," Eve told him, and gathered up the pulled weeds from Joseph and Catherine's graves. "It wor good to see ya again Nathan."

"It wor good to see you as well," he replied, and Eve

left the churchyard and made her way home. She was calmer now and felt better-minded to talk to Seb. When she got indoors, Dru was standing by the wood burner, warming himself. It had turned cool outside and he had been out walking the village, and decided to call on his sister on the way home. Eve was pleased to see him. She looked around the room for Seb, but he was gone and so was his coat from the hook behind the door. Mary was sitting quietly at the table, reading her book.

"Mary just told me about Seb," Dru said directly. "Thomas has volunteered to go an' fight as well," he told his sister, before she could even greet him.

"Thomas as well?" Eve gasped. She looked at her brother's face to see how he might be coping with that. Dru did not look any different, but it was always hard to tell what he might be thinking if he did not want you to know.

"Aye," he replied.

"When did he do that?" Eve asked.

"Ah think it wor the same time as Seb," Dru told her. "They wor all at the meetin' in Ashton."

"Oh Dru," Eve sighed. She was now upset about Thomas also. She loved him as if he were her own son. "What are we to do?"

"There's nowt we can do," Dru replied. "Tis already done." Now Eve could see the fear spreading over Dru's face and she knew he felt exactly the same as her. "Ah've been speakin' to quite a few friends down the Bull Inn an' there's loads of their youngsters signed up too. It's a tragedy. Thomas told me that he'll look out fer Seb." At this, Eve began to sob again. She was heartbroken. Mary came over and held her mother.

"Mam, Seb'll be fine," she told her. "'Tis nay good ya worryin' like this. Ya'll make yarself ill." Mary looked across to her uncle for support.

"Aye," he spoke up. "They reckon that the war won't last long. An' our Thomas'll look after Seb. Ah know he will." Eve tried to control her crying but she was finding it very hard. Every time she thought about Seb, a surge of fear welled up in her and all she could think about was losing her son.

Seb came home shortly afterwards and Eve and he spoke quietly. He told his mother that he was sorry to have caused her so much heartache and did not join up to deliberately hurt her. He explained how it happened that he stepped up alongside all of his friends, although there was no hint of regret in his countenance. If anything, she had not seen Seb so animated and enthusiastic about anything before. As she examined her son, Eve could see nothing but excitement and expectation in his face. She argued that he was still only seventeen and that she could tell the enlisting officer and he would be turned out. Seb told her that if she did that, he would only join up again in a few months' time, when he was eighteen. At least if he goes now, he will be with everyone he knows and grew up with and they can all look out for one another. He argued that Thomas was going with him now as well.

Eve felt helpless. She could give him some protection if he stayed near, but so far away, she knew Seb would be on his own. Facing that, Eve quickly understood she must not show him any of her fear or trepidation for what lay ahead of him. It would not help Seb in any way. Whatever fate had in store for her son, Eve knew in her heart that the clock had been set and was now on its countdown.

There were sixteen lads in all from the village and local farms going off together. They were to report to Farnleydale Town Hall the following Monday morning at 7 o'clock sharp to collect their uniforms and kit bags. They would then be transported up to a barracks near Danberry, a large town just outside of York. Here, they were to join all of the other soldiers who had volunteered from the North of Yorkshire and be trained for battle. Four months later, the 4th Battalion Yorkshire Regiment was to be moved to the coast in readiness to leave Britain for Belgium or France. And so, by the middle of the following winter, both Seb and Thomas were trained and ready to go off to fight for their country.

Eve, Mary, Dru and Lillian journeyed to Danberry

Station to say their goodbyes to the lads as they left the barracks with their regiment for Dover. Dru's youngest lad was being looked after by Sarah for the day. Danberry Station, when they got there, was chaotic. There were people everywhere and Dru told all the ladies to stay in the waiting room until he could find out the information on the platform and train's departure time that was to take Seb and Thomas to the coast. Eve felt sick with apprehension. She had only seen her son twice in the four months he was in the Danberry barracks.

It was now a cold and bleak January morning. That past Christmas was the first one that both Seb and Thomas had ever been apart from the family. Eve had hardly eaten for days, knowing this time was approaching. Mary had been as supportive to her mother as she could be, but Eve closed herself off emotionally and was only holding herself together by blocking all demonstrations of care or affection from anybody, even from her daughter. It was not deliberate, just Eve's way of coping with having to say goodbye to her son. Dru returned with the platform number and the time that their sons' train was leaving for Dover. As the clock ticked on, so Eve's panic began to take hold. Dru could see her stress rising.

"Ya must not let the lads see ya upset," he told his sister harshly. "Tis hard enough that they're goin'.

They don't need to see yar tears as well." Eve nodded that she understood, and took some deep breaths. Supported by Mary, along with Lillian and Dru, she went to platform 3. The train was in the station, the steam billowing from the engine and engulfing the carriages at its front end. The noise of the engine, which was being stoked up ready to leave, and from the crowd of people who were now arriving to see off their husbands, sons, brothers and loved ones, was becoming overwhelming for Eve. Then suddenly they appeared. Seb and Thomas came up behind them. Eve turned to see her son, dressed in his full uniform, with a rifle and kit back thrown over his shoulder. He looked so grown up, yet his face was that of a boy, her boy. She desperately fought back her fear and her tears, and fixed a painful smile on her face. Seb's eyes were bright with excitement and he kissed Mary and hugged her tightly, then caught hold of his mother, and they held each other for some moments, she never wanting to let go of him. Thomas was kissing Lillian and then embracing Dru, who was grey with emotion. Eve then held her nephew and kissed him repeatedly.

"Look after Seb fer me," Eve begged Thomas, "an' bring yarself back to us safely." He smiled.

"Aye, ah'll do my best," Thomas told her. With that, orders were passing along the platform for the soldiers to climb aboard. Doors slammed shut and the engine seemed to get louder, steam now gushing from the train and billowing out along the platform. It was at this point that Mary caught sight of George Wade. He was leaning out of one of the windows saying goodbye to a young lass that Mary recognised as one of his sisters. George noticed Mary and smiled at her. He was a good looking young lad and she suddenly wanted to speak to him. Mary ran along the platform and returned George's smile, just as the train began to move off.

"Ah'll be back to marry ya," he called out to Mary. She smiled broadly.

"Ah'll be waitin' here fer ya," she called back. Mary then searched for her brother and managed to see him at the window of two carriages further down the train. Seb waved and smiled as he went past her. Minutes later, the train and all the young soldiers were gone.

Chapter 28

A month later, Eve received a letter from Seb telling her that his battalion had arrived in Belgium. They had not seen any action yet and were waiting for orders to come through telling them where they were going to be sent next. His letter was quite cheerful and told her how everyone's spirits were high and how they were going to kick the Hun all the way back to Germany. Seb did not tell his mother about the rumours that were reaching him and his friends of the huge losses that the British Army were sustaining.

Every two weeks, much to Eve's surprise, she received a letter from Seb telling her that all was well and that she must not worry for his safety. Reading these helped Eve with the missing of her son. Dru was hearing from Thomas regularly also, and both lads seemed to be coping with being away from home and their health was holding up. Having fought in a number of battles in Belgium, Seb and Thomas's battalion were then moved to France. Of course, neither son mentioned in their letters home of the terrible conditions they now found themselves fighting in, or the misery and death of their fellow soldiers that they increasingly faced daily. But Margaret was constantly bringing to Eve's cottage news about sons, husbands and brothers belonging to families in and around Elmsley who had been killed and of the terrible conditions they died in, so she knew the reality of the situation in France for Seb and Thomas.

Every time she heard of another life lost, it would take Eve weeks to get over the shock of hearing such dreadful accounts. Every day she cried for Seb. She desperately looked forward to receiving a letter from her son, but feared what it might say; Thomas and Seb having agreed to write to each other's family in the event of anything happening to them. Then there were stories of the Germans using gas on the British soldiers and their allies, and the terrible toll this was inflicting. Thousands were said to be dying a horrible death. Eve and Dru had to wait an agonising wait to hear that their lads were not amongst these casualties.

And so it went on. With each report that trickled into the village of a horrific battle, Eve and Dru had to wait for good or bad news. Each time there was a major offensive and encounter, Seb and Thomas survived the fighting. As the months, and then the first year passed, it became clear that this ghastly war was not going to be over as quickly as everyone had hoped. The war had now raged for two long years and it was 1916. Eve knew that the longer it went on, the more lives it would take. Her days were filled with worry for Seb and Thomas; her nights were full of terrors. The stress was taking its toll on her health, and many mornings Eve struggled to get out of her bed and face the day. Few things helped her to cope with missing Seb and Thomas, but with Doctor Melbry having enlisted as well, Nurse Hubbard called on Eve to help her with patients, which was a blessing, as it at least took Eve's mind off of her worries for a few hours.

It was on the afternoon of the 5th of July that a letter arrived from France. It was not Seb's handwriting on the envelope, neither was it Thomas's. Mary took it, as Eve was assisting the nurse with the birth of Sarah and Ben's second child, a baby boy. Ben had been turned down for the army. He tried to volunteer twice, but because he had a deformed foot; something that Eve never knew about, Ben was deemed to be unfit to fight as he could not walk any great distance, and certainly could not run. His work at the mill was also considered to be important for the war effort, as the factory had turned itself over to making army uniforms and equipment, such as blankets. Ben had been made a manager at the mill, owing to the now shortage of men, so for him and Sarah, the war was not proving to be devastating.

Eve returned home from the birthing and immediately saw the letter lying on the table where Mary had set it down. She went over and picked it up, the blood rushing from her head, making her sit down before she keeled over. Mary instinctively poured some brandy into a cup and put it on the table in front of her mother. Eve stared at the envelope, not recognising the handwriting. Her only ray of hope in those few seconds was that the letter had not been sent to her by Thomas. Everything in her body screamed out telling her not to open it, but she had to.

Dear Mrs Locke,

I am sorry to have to write to and inform you that your son was killed in action last Saturday (July 1st) and wish to express my sincere sympathy with you. He died instantly and did not suffer. Your son was buried on the 3rd July. Everyone in the company liked him. He was always so cheery and willing to do anything that was necessary. We shall miss his pleasant face. It seems very hard for a mere boy to die so young, but it may be some consolation to you to know that he died in one of the most magnificent advances ever made by the British troops.

My greatest sympathy for you at this time.

Captain R G Stodden, 4th Battalion Yorkshire Regiment.

Eve barely read the words, she had no need to. She sat in total shock, unable to speak or move. Mary took the letter from her mother's hand and read it.

She screamed.

"Mammy!" she cried out in fear, and falling to the floor, buried her head in her mother's lap. Eve clutched at her daughter, and that was how they remained for some time; Mary crying hysterically and Eve sitting bolt upright in absolute silence. "Seb," Mary repeated, over and over again.

Seb had been mowed down by German machine guns at what was to be known as the Battle of the Somme. The British offensive had begun on the 1st July, and was fought on either side of the river Somme, in France. This battle was to be one of the largest of the war, and by the time the fighting paused in late autumn of that year, there were more than 1 million casualties. The volunteers of the British army were destined to fight at the Somme, and it was to be one of the bloodiest military operations ever recorded. Seb was killed on the first day of this offensive, along with twelve other lads who had joined up with him that evening in Ashton. Only three of his comrades from Elmsley survived the battle. Two were injured, one seriously, the other not. One of those injured was Thomas. There was one uninjured man, and he was George Wade.

Dru came to Eve that evening with the news that Thomas had been wounded at the Somme. His commanding officer had written to tell him that his son was injured, but that his wounds were not considered life-threatening. The worry was for infection however, and the officer had evacuated Thomas to a Base Hospital in Le Touquet as quickly as he possibly could. Dru did not know until he arrived at Eve's cottage that Seb had been killed. Mary let her uncle in and told him the dreadful news. He was shocked, and stood before Eve, unable to say anything. She had not spoken a word since reading the letter, and still sat staring directly ahead. Dru knelt down and touched his sister's face. She was ice cold and trembling. He picked her up from the chair and pulled her close, one of his hands supporting her head gently to his chest. It was then that Eve broke down and Dru stood and held her in silence.

It was almost six months before Eve could even begin to pick up her life again after Seb's death. Some villagers were very kind to her and Mary, and had it not been for the support of Dru and Lillian and Sarah and Ben, Eve might not have coped at all. She received messages of condolence from those that her family had helped over the years. Others visited, such as Cuthbert Lamb, who was so upset at Seb's death, he openly wept. One of the letters she got was from James Barlow. He was very compassionate in his words and offered any amount of help to Eve that she might want or need. But there was nothing he could do for her. James told Eve in his letter that all of his sons were serving officers in France and all fought at the Somme also. His eldest, James, had been seriously wounded in one of his legs, and was being treated in a hospital in Le Havre. They expected him to be transported back to England soon. His second eldest and youngest sons were both unharmed, and remained fighting in France. At the end of his letter, James asked Eve if he could see her. Perhaps they could meet somewhere? If she agreed, would she tell him in her reply?

Eve was comforted to read James's letter and it helped her not to feel so alone. But could she see him? They had not spoken with each other now for some years and after much thought, even though tempted to meet with him, Eve decided not to see James. It would only drag up all of her old feelings for him and she was so emotionally insecure, she could not cope with that at all. The last thing Eve wanted to do was to lean on James and she knew she might do that should they meet again. So James never received the kind of reply he had hoped for from Eve, just one thanking him for his kind thoughts towards her family.

Thomas returned home during this time, still weak and suffering somewhat from his wounds, but it brought some light back into Eve's life momentarily. She was overjoyed to see her nephew and when he walked through her door, she could not speak for some moments. After hugging Mary, Thomas held Eve and they both cried. He felt so bad that he could not prevent Seb from being killed and spent some time telling her what had happened to him and how he had made sure that her son was buried properly and decently. Thomas told Eve that George Wade had helped with the burial and marked the grave so that they would know where Seb was after the war had finished. Mary had been listening to this story and she asked Thomas to tell her more about George. Thomas had nothing but praise for the man. As far as he knew, George was well and had already written to him. He had asked Thomas, before he left for the hospital at Le Touquet, if he would speak to his cousin Mary to see if she would write to him. This caused Mary to be wholly embarrassed, which made Thomas smile.

"Can ah take it that ya like this fellow?" he asked her. Mary blushed again. "George certainly likes you. He never stopped talkin' about ya." Eve looked at her daughter.

"Do ya like him Mary?" she questioned. Mary nodded a yes. Eve felt a mixture of happiness for her daughter, tinged with some apprehension. She was unsure of George Wade. However, Eve was grateful for the care that he had shown her son and for that she liked the man. Mary would thank George on behalf of Eve in her letter to him, one that would be the first of many.

Upon hearing of the death of Seb, the new pastor at Saint Guthlac Church had visited Eve a number of times to apparently offer her solace, but she would not speak to him. Pastor Ramsdon had replaced Pastor Bell, who retired a year earlier. Eve did not like Ramsdon. She thought he was stupid and arrogant. He persistently called at her cottage though, clearly determined to speak with her. That opportunity came a week or so later when Eve came across the pastor when she was tending to her family graves in the churchyard. Ramsdon walked over and spoke to her. Eve did not want to be rude to the man, but ended up telling him what she thought about God and his mercy and how he moves in so-called mysterious ways. She told Ramsdon that she did not want to hear it and would he please leave her alone. It was in the pastor's reply that Eve realised he had an added agenda, other than to help her with her grieving. Ramsdon had obviously heard the stories about her, and seemed to be intrigued as to why she was known as Mother Eve. He also referred to her 'visions', as he called them, and tried to press her into telling him something of them and where she thought they 'came from'. Eve lost patience after some of the man's questioning and ended up turning her back on the pastor and walking away from him.

"Aye," Cuthbert Lamb said to Eve one evening

when he called to see how she was. He also brought her some mutton and fruit from his farm. "Pastor Ramsdon is a strange one. Ah'm not sure about t' man. Ah have ti deal wi' him ont' parish council. He took Bell's place when 'e retired, but 'e is an odd 'un." Lamb looked at Eve with a surprised expression on his face. "He's fascinated about you though. He's allus asking us sommit about ya. So is t' new doctor that's just come on t' council; Doctor Finnan. Ah met 'im last week. He's ti be t' new doctor around 'ere."

"What do ya think of him?" Eve asked. She had not seen Margaret for over a week, so was not kept up with the gossip. Margaret would surely know about the new doctor.

"Seems ti be a reasonable man," Cuthbert replied casually. "But 'e wor very interested in you an' yar history as well. Ah didn't say much an' neither did old George. Ya know what 'e's like, ya'd be lucky ti get two words from 'im." Cuthbert laughed, thinking back on the last council meeting where Pastor Ramsdon spent over half an hour trying to prise information out of George Hopkinson on Eve. George just sat there, smoking his pipe. He had nothing to say about her and therefore he said nothing.

"George just said nowt, every time 'e asked 'im a question about you," Cuthbert relayed to Eve. "He just kept sayin' that 'e 'ad nowt ti say about ya an' what wor 'e askin' 'im such questions fer? Ah didn't understand miself. Pastor Bell wouldn't 'ave told Ramsdon anythin' about ya before 'e retired. Ah know fer a fact that 'e liked you an' yar family. An' t' last doctor 'ardly 'ad time ti know ya before 'e left, so what's it all about?" Eve was surprised to know that she still caused such interest. Things had been very quiet in her life over the last few years. She had deliberately been careful in her predictions; the few she did make were to very secure people whom she knew would say nothing. Nobody had accused her of any wrong or evil doing for some time, and Nurse Hubbard would not have said anything detrimental against her to the new doctor. Ann had become a friend over the years since she first moved to Elmsley and even used some of Eve's remedies herself.

"Well," Eve said to Cuthbert. "Thank ya fer tellin' me. Ah don't know why the pastor is so interested in me either, but no doubt ah'll find out." Cuthbert left with a jar of his usual foot cream.

A few days later, Margaret scurried in to Eve's cottage with her latest round of gossip. The first thing she mentioned was the new Doctor Finnan. He had come down from Edinburgh, she informed Eve. He was reportedly a brusque man with a stern face and a loud voice, which apparently had scared a number of children he treated in the village. Finnan had bought Doctor Cheetham's villa, which had stood empty for some time. Margaret told her that the new doctor planned to turn part of the villa into a surgery from where he could see patients, instead of him having to visit them at their home. Finnan was nothing like Melbry, Margaret complained, who she hoped would come back to Elmsley when he returned from the war. The next piece of news related to Squire Addington. Apparently he was very weak and could be dying. Margaret had been informed by her relative working at Addington House that the Squire Frederick was on his last legs and was not expected to see out the week. She questioned what would happen to his title and estate, with no descendant able to take his place. Eve was able to give Margaret some news for once and told her that James Addington-Barlow was returning to England, having been wounded at the Somme. No doubt, once he recovered, the young man would be taking on his inheritance. Margaret was intrigued as to how Eve knew this and Eve had to think quickly with her answer. Margaret must never know that the elder James had written to her, and she was angry with herself for nearly giving the woman more gossip to spread around the village about her.

"They reckon 'e's dyin' of that disease ya spoke about years ago. Apparently, it don't go away proper, even after treatment. It wor syflis or sommit?" Margaret stated.

"Syphilis," Eve corrected her. Yes, it might well be, Eve thought to herself. He had been suffering with something for years. She felt little pity for the man though, and reminded herself of the date in her mother's story.

"Ah'll let ya know if ah hear anythin' else about t' Squire," Margaret told her. She then went on to mention two other men, both husbands and fathers, who had been killed in France. Margaret used to be more descriptive about these deaths, but after Seb dying, she kept the reports short. Eve was always sad to hear this news, as she knew of most of the men and their families who lived in the area. She wanted to know about them however, so that she could be sure to send her sympathy to those families suffering their terrible loss. Eve also did what she could for some of the impoverished widows left with children to bring up. She and Mary called upon the better-off families in the village and local farms to donate provisions, and they made up food parcels and delivered them to the neediest. Eve also found herself helping other mothers, wives and sisters to cope with their bereavements. She knew exactly how they were suffering and could therefore empathise with them. Sometimes Eve would sit for hours talking with the bereaved. To the wives she could draw on the loss of her own husband and to the mothers she spoke about the loss of her dearest Seb. To Eve's horror, one couple in the village, Mr. and Mrs. Bale, lost four sons within weeks of one another. They were desperately praying for Jack, their fifth and youngest lad, to survive. In Eve's heart she felt that he would, but was careful not to say that exactly to Mr. or Mrs. Bale, even though she knew that was what Mrs. Bale wanted from her. In fact, the woman asked Eve outright. The way she gave the woman hope without actually saying anything was through a smile as she left the home.

So, in a strange way, Eve was finding solace in helping to heal other people's desperate feelings of loss, as well as heal her own. Nothing was going to bring her son back, but by doing something useful, she could lessen her own tragedy. Eve's bereavement 'counselling' around the village did not go down very well with Pastor Ramsdon however. He felt it was his job to help the families who had suffered loss. He considered Eve's visits to those whose menfolk had been killed, as pure meddling. Eve was preventing him from giving religious instruction to his flock during their bereavement, and Ramsdon resented her for that. It even sent him a little mad. The man tried to make Eve's visits redundant by dashing around to the homes as fast as he could after they had received the terrible news. He often intruded when he was not called upon and insisted the families kneel in prayer, when all they wanted to do was be allowed to cry or scream, or talk or just sit in silence. If the bereaved had spoken to Eve, Ramsdon demanded to hear what she had said to them. The pastor was indeed a stupid man and his egotism became more evident with every visit to a tragic home he made. In desperation, he began to call Eve unchristian to those he visited, saying that she was not quite 'wholesome'.

However, some of those he spoke to respected Eve and argued with him over his denigration of her. With his extreme behaviour, Ramsdon was rapidly losing the goodwill of many folk in and around Elmsley. For once in her life, Eve actually was getting some support from her fellow villagers. When Cuthbert Lamb heard about the way Pastor Ramsdon was acting, he rounded on him at the next council meeting and more or less told him to keep his mouth shut, pastor or no pastor. He even challenged the man to exercise what he preached and act like a Christian towards Eve, who was only trying to help fellow sufferers. Ramsdon did not take kindly to being told off and instead of humbly accepting the criticism, went the opposite way and increased his activities. But Eve had been in that position many times before, so paid little heed to the man and his antics, until a visit from Sarah late one morning.

Sarah and Ben had finally decided to have both Annie and their little boy, Josh, baptised. Their delay in doing so was not an irreligious act, it just had not happened. Now, with the atmosphere of war pervading every part of the village and affecting countless lives, their thoughts had turned to God and they felt it time to baptise their children. Sarah took her children to visit Ramsdon one afternoon with that request. The first comment he made was that neither Ben nor her attended his church regularly, which was a fair comment, because they did not. However, he then accused Sarah of being a friend of Eve Locke, as if there was something sinister in having that relationship, and of somehow being 'in league' with her. Sarah was mortified. She did not have the wherewithal to argue with the pastor and with such a sweet nature, was incapable of defending herself. Sarah simply did not understand why Ramsdon was being so hostile towards her. Distressed by the conversation, she took hold of both children and ran out of his office. Sarah went straight to Eve and was in quite a state by the time she got there.

"What's wrong?" Eve said, opening her door to a weeping Sarah and two upset children. Eve took Annie's hand and led her indoors and then took little Josh out of Sarah's arms. Sarah then told her what had happened with Ramsdon. Eve was sorry but not surprised and spent the next half an hour calming her down. When Sarah had gotten over her ordeal, Eve packed her off home and made her way to the pastor's house, which stood behind the church.

Ramsdon was rather shocked to see Eve Locke standing at his door and for a few moments was not sure how to greet her. Eventually, he invited her into his house. Ramsdon offered Eve a seat, which she declined. She then faced the man and asked him directly what he thought he was doing to Sarah Rackley, and why he did it? He acted surprised and said he did not know to what she was referring. Eve more or less called the man a liar and told him to stop his campaign against her and anyone associated with her. There was no justification for his behaviour and certainly no good reason why he should be cruel to Sarah. She added that if he continued, she would report him to his superiors...she knew how to. Ramsdon was furious. How dare the likes of her challenge him like this he told her? Eve did not reply, but simply turned and left. The pastor stood in his front room thinking over Eve's visit. He was angry and shaken. After a few minutes of thought he persuaded himself that he had just been in the presence of evil and he must act against it. Pastor Ramsdon, although a man of the cloth, was deeply superstitious and was a firm believer in Satan and hell. It was his lack of intelligence that made him gullible and such an enthusiastic supporter for notions of wicked and sinful goings-on. Eve was a perfect person to fire up the pastor's imagination. However, he was also terrified of his soul being 'taken' by the Devil, so after some consideration, Ramsdon decided that he would not do anything else to upset Eve. The pastor was genuinely afraid of her and her 'evil' powers.

The man was certainly stupid. After trying to succeed in three different professions and failing miserably, Ramsdon chose the church. He scraped by in his theological studies and had worked in two other parishes before being sent to Elmsley. As it was such a small village with only a few hundred parishioners, his bosses thought he might manage not to make too many mistakes there. He was recognised as being odd and none too bright, but deemed harmless by the hierarchy of his church. Ramsdon had moved to Elmsley with an elderly mother, whom he shouted at quite a lot. She was a frail old dear and harmless enough, and anyone who overheard the way her son spoke to her, had sympathy for the woman. Pastor Ramsdon was not only stupid, arrogant, unintelligent, and, as it became apparent to many, also cruel. He should never have been accepted into the church as one of its representatives. Eve did not have to do anything to discredit the man; he was doing that all by himself.

However, having spoken to Sarah and Ben some days after his meeting with Eve, Ramsdon gave them some sort of an apology, and their two children were baptised the following spring. Eve attended the ceremony, much to the discomfort of the pastor, and it was a fine christening. Not long after he performed this ceremony however, Pastor Ramsdon suddenly left Saint Guthlac Church, taking his poor old mother with him. Nobody, not even Margaret, knew why or where he went to, and not many people actually cared. Within a week of his leaving, a new vicar, Reverend Arnold, arrived at Elmsley. Arnold was a rather large and jolly sort of man. He was loud and friendly and Eve instantly liked him.

The christening of Annie and Josh had been a pleasant day for Eve, but now she had to face the ordeal of Seb's first birthday after his death. She spent much of that day at the graveside of Joseph, crying and talking to him of their wild but beautiful son. Eve's heart was so heavy with grief that she could not think how she would ever get over the loss of Seb.

Chapter 29

A difficult and painful year passed for Eve but finally some good news arrived in Elmsley; the war was over. Those men and boys who had left their homesteads to fight for their country began to return, some wounded, some not. Jack Bale was amongst those who had survived the war intact. He would go home to his parents and tell them how his four older brothers died bravely and selflessly, along with his best friend and two cousins.

Mary had been writing to George Wade regularly, and in his last letter to her, he said he would soon be coming home. Mary went to Danberry Station with some others in an open carriage to meet the train he would be on. It was an emotional reunion and Mary was very shy to see George again. They had been writing to one another for the past year, but had only ever exchanged those few words they shared when he left for the war that day three years ago. George clearly felt a great deal for Mary and she certainly looked upon him favourably. After he had seen his family and they had celebrated his return home, he paid a visit to Eve at her cottage. He seemed slightly uncomfortable in her presence, but Eve put that down to him being nervous because of his feelings towards Mary. If the truth were known, this was not really the case.

George had grown up being told all sorts of fanciful stories about Eve, her mother Mary, and her grandmother Elisa; in fact all of the history of the Shetcliffe family, who had always been deemed, by the Wades, to be their enemies. George himself was a fiercely religious man, having had it drummed into him since childhood that the Christian way was the only way; all other beliefs were heathen and ungodly. So, when he stood in Eve's cottage and told her that he would like to marry Mary, George did not reveal his predisposition to disliking her and everything that she stood for. No, he smiled pleasantly and was the perfect suitor for her daughter, espousing his love for Mary and his great plans for their future. Eve was so caught up in her daughter's obvious happiness she did not sense the future misery that the man would cause both her and Mary in years to come, not then anyway. It would have made little difference if she had. Mary was totally smitten with George Wade. She was getting older and was feeling almost desperate to find a husband and have children. There was also a dreadful shortage of young men in the area; at least ten females for every eligible male. The war had almost wiped out an entire generation of men in Elmsley and the local vicinity. And George was handsome, strong, attentive and very good with words. He was also a local hero, having won a medal for bravery in the field. It was no wonder he swept the shy, retiring, gentle and fragile Mary off of her feet.

When George told Eve that he wanted her daughter for his wife, Eve's heart sank, but she shook off all of her trepidation, believing it was just the thought of another child leaving the home that was making her feel so fearful. Eve had to smile when she looked at the face of Mary, flushed and so full of love and expectations. Eve could hardly say anything to her and George, except that she blessed a union between them and wished them every joy.

Mary Elizabeth Locke and George Alfred Wade were married in Saint Guthlac Church three months later. It was a simple and sombre ceremony; the Wades preferring an austere service for their son. Mary looked beautiful in her grandmother's wedding gown, which George had argued vehemently against her wearing. But Mary had always dreamed of getting married in that dress and veil, and George had to relent or look to be uncaring and unkind. Eve and her brother and his family sat on one side of the church along with Sarah, Ben and their children. Pastor Bell and his wife also attended the day, as did the Lambs, Hopkinsons, their neighbour Margaret, and a small handful of other people. On the other side of the church sat the Wades and a number of their friends from the village and local farms. The Wades were a large, serious family, and even the children looked dour. There was a barely a smile between the adults and Eve could feel their frostiness seeping across the stone floor of the church towards her. She tried not to look over at them, and they did the same for her.

The small reception after the wedding was held in the village school hall, which although not very large, managed to accommodate the wedding gathering, because some guests left directly after the service. As Eve made her way through the churchyard to go to the school hall ahead of the party, she caught sight of James. He was standing over the far side, looking as if he was attending a grave, but Eve knew he had come to see something of his daughter's wedding. She barely acknowledged him and kept walking. James would soon see Mary come out of the church and Eve was pleased for him that he was there on that day. What had happened without the knowledge of the guests however was Mary's baptism, conducted very hastily and very quietly a week before the wedding. Eve never had her daughter christened and she could not marry in the church because of that. George was not prepared to marry Mary unless she went through the ceremony, so she did. Eve attended and was at least now spared having to look at the insidious Ramsdon. Reverend Arnold was friendly and kindly towards her. Eve therefore only had to accept the fact that her daughter was being christened, which she managed to do.

After their marriage, George wanted Mary, for the time being at least, to move in with his family on West Way Farm, which the Wades had run for many years. He had laboured on the land since he was a child, but after returning from the war, George did not feel inclined to remain doing so. He had learned some mechanical skills whilst being in the army, and felt he wanted to use them to better himself and his new wife. But Eve was unhappy with her daughter moving in with the Wade family and put up some money for them to rent a small cottage on the edge of the village. James had sent extra income for her to give to his daughter, and Eve used that for the purchase of a year's rent. George hated the thought of accepting Eve's money, but Mary cried at having to live with so many people that she did not know. Again, he reluctantly had to relent.

With Mary gone from her home, Eve suffered another form of grieving. She tried to be fine with her daughter now married and off on her new life. But Eve missed Mary dreadfully, and felt uneasy about her new son-in-law, who was already showing signs of impatience towards his delicate wife. But Mary never complained to her mother about George, and in many respects, he was a good husband. He managed to get a job at one of the local cotton mills, maintaining their machines, which was a very respectable position. His income was reasonable and Mary quickly built up a comfortable home for the two of them. Materially, she wanted for little. George had however 'ordered' his wife to attend church every Sunday, which she intensely disliked doing. Mary had not been brought up as a Christian, nor had she been given much bible instruction. In the discussions she had with her mother since childhood about God and religion, Mary was always encouraged to think for herself and not to blindly believe anything either written or said without questioning it. Now she was expected to follow a faith that she felt nothing for. But after weeks of pressure, arguments and bullying from George, Mary capitulated and knuckled down to at least acting as if she was a devout Christian. George was not going to relent this time. When Eve asked her daughter if it was her own choice to go to church, Mary told her it was, so Eve could not interfere.

Then, later that year, Eve received four pieces of news; one very good, one she did not care much about, one she was vaguely interested in, and one which was very bad. Mary was with child; that was the very good news. Eve was happy to hear that she was going to be a grandmother. Margaret visited with the other three news reports. Squire Frederick Addington had died. That was the news Eve cared little about. James Addington-Barlow was now to take on his uncle's title and inheritance, which was the news that Eve had a passing interest in, him being James's son. The very bad news was that a flu pandemic, known as Spanish influenza, which had been raging across America and Europe, was now sweeping through Britain. The newspapers reported that the flu had already killed thousands of people abroad, although it was difficult to find out how many had succumbed to this virulent disease. But Margaret had heard rumours of villages down the south of England losing over half of their people in a few short weeks as the pandemic took hold.

This was confirmed when Nurse Ann came to see Eve two days after Margaret's reporting and expressed her fears about the flu reaching Elmsley. She and Doctor Finnan were trying to make some preparations for it coming to the village, but he was already seeing patients at his surgery suspected with having it and was visiting some very sick people. He asked Ann to ask Eve, if she would help look after those going down with the virus. Eve was surprised to hear Finnan request her involvement, but instantly agreed to assist them in any way she could. Within weeks, numerous folk in the community were becoming sick with the influenza. Some were dying, and they were not the old, frail and infirm, nor were they the very young; those who normally are taken with such an epidemic. These influenza victims were, prior to catching this flu, seemingly healthy and robust young individuals, and they were falling like flies. Eve was very concerned. She begged Mary to keep away from other people and try to isolate herself from the community. But that made little difference, as George brought the influenza home to her. He had reported not two days earlier to Mary that over half of the employees at his mill were suffering with the disease, and many had died from it.

The attack came on George very quickly and he was suddenly taken ill. Doctor Finnan was called, but with so many now sick, Mary had to nurse him herself at home, which of course made her vulnerable. Eve was unhappy with that prospect, knowing her daughter was at risk, and offered to see to George herself. But he refused, so Mary had no choice but to look after her husband, who was getting worse by the day. Mary was feeling ill herself with early pregnancy and after a few days passed, Eve refused to stand by and do nothing and insisted on helping her daughter. Whilst she had no direct contact with George, she supported Mary in the background. Eve also gave her daughter remedies to slip to her husband without him knowing. Ann had told Eve what symptoms to look for and explained what she had observed so far in her patients. This helped Eve to use certain remedies to hopefully lessen the most damaging of the symptoms.

George's fever eventually broke and the influenza began to recede. However, as he got over the worst of the disease, Mary went down with it. Being still very weak, George was in no position to refuse Eve nursing her daughter and therefore had to endure her presence in his home, which he was not happy about. His family made it worse with their comments when they visited George. But Eve had no intention of abandoning her daughter and told him and his family that in no uncertain terms.

Eve nursed Mary night and day. She was very ill, and within days of contracting the influenza, Mary lost her baby. George was devastated, as was Eve, but her focus had to remain on saving her daughter's life. Ann came to see to Mary after the miscarriage, on George's insistence, even though Eve could have managed without her help. Because Mary was so ill and had also miscarried, Ann suggested Doctor Finnan see her also, which he did do. After observing how Eve was already treating Mary, Finnan proclaimed that he had no more to add to her care, and told George to let Eve get on with her nursing, as she was doing a fine job.

Mary went to the very edge of life and losing her baby weakened her resistance greatly. As she had done successfully with George, Eve managed to prevent the worst of the influenza symptoms from damaging her daughter. She did not suffer any haemorrhaging from her nose, stomach, or intestine or any bleeding from her ears. The next worry for Eve however, was that as the disease progressed it could cause pneumonia, and Mary's chest was sounding very weak. Eve increased the steam baths and vapour treatments, whilst getting as much sustenance into her daughter that she could physically take.

Slowly but steadily, Mary began to recover. Eve maintained high treatment levels and insisted on nursing her daughter until she was definitely and completely over the influenza and out of danger. George could not fault his mother-in-law's care for his wife and genuinely thanked Eve for saving her life, and possibly his own. He was not a stupid man and realised that he must have been given some of her remedies as well. He had to recognise that Eve had possibly saved them both. Doctor Finnan visited a much-recovered Mary and even he admitted to Eve that she had performed 'something of a miracle here', although his statement was not meant to enhance her status as a medicine woman. Nevertheless, it did. When word got out that both George and Mary had gotten over the influenza by Eve nursing them, many folk who had lost loved ones wished they had called on her instead of Doctor

Finnan. Eve was not pleased to hear these reports however, as the doctor had been fair and kind with her. However, Finnan, although stern and rigid, was also an intelligent and even-handed man. He did not get upset when he heard the remarks about him, nor did he hold it against Eve that she was successful in treating her family members. Finnan was above such things.

His interest in Eve, like Pastor Ramsdon, had been one of curiosity, but unlike Ramsdon, he was not hostile towards her. Finnan had heard many stories about Eve Locke. Some made her sound like the devil's own, whilst others gave her saintly qualities. Having observed at close hand the way Eve treated George and then Mary when ill, Finnan was impressed with her knowledge and abilities. He was also intrigued about her remedies and wanted to know more. The doctor set in his mind that once the influenza passed away from the village, he would meet with Eve and talk about her traditional way of healing.

Mary was well on the way now to making a full recovery. However, early one morning, Dru came to George and Mary's cottage in a panic. Lillian was desperately ill. Eve went to her immediately and began the treatments. But, within two days, Lillian's condition grew much worse. She became gravely ill. Doctor Finnan visited urgently and did what he could to help her alongside of Eve. But Lillian haemorrhaged and then slipped away. Although her suffering was reduced by some of Eve's painkillers and sleeping drafts, Eve was devastated that she could not save poor Lillian. Dru was so shocked by his wife's sudden death he just walked out of his home in stunned silence and did not return for three days. Thomas, recovered from his war injuries, looked after his younger brother Edward. Eve offered to take them both home with her, but Thomas was capable and felt they should stay at their cottage and wait for their father to come back. When Dru finally returned, he looked like a shadow of himself. His eyes were dead. Now he had to face the funeral of his sweet Lillian and he dreaded it. Eve stepped in and made all of the arrangements, knowing that Dru was not able to do it. Before Lillian could be laid to rest however, Sarah's husband Ben went down with the virus also. Eve went immediately and nursed him. She moved Sarah and the children into her own cottage, away from the infection, and they thankfully did not catch it. Eve cared for Ben, who was not desperately ill with the disease, until he was out of danger, only leaving his bedside to stand by her brother at Lillian's funeral.

By the time the influenza pandemic was over, it had claimed almost a third of the population of Elmsley and a number of victims from the farms surrounding it. When Lillian was laid to rest, she had to be buried in an adjoining field to the church, because the churchyard was full. Saint Guthlac was given the land by a sympathetic farmer, whose own two young daughters had been taken with the virus. The ground was consecrated and the graves were dug. The toll of deaths alone of those that Eve knew well was horrific. Cuthbert Lamb lost a daughter, George Hopkinson, his wife and a grown up son. Henry Morely was also taken. It seemed as if most families had lost a loved one and that the entire village of Elmsley was in mourning. What was also pitiful was that some young men, returned after fighting for years in the war, fell as victims of the influenza. The disease was not selective. That was brought home to Eve by a letter she received from James. His middle son Harry had died of it, having not long returned from France, uninjured, after fighting in the war for three years. Harry had come home a hero with medals and had just become engaged to a young lady from Danberry, a nurse he met at the hospital there. She had been caring for his older brother, and they met on one of Harry's visits to him. James, his wife Jayne, and two other sons were overwhelmed with grief at this loss and James was finding it hard to accept that Harry, having survived the war, could be taken from him this way. Eve felt so sorry for him and his family.

She knew only too well the pain of losing a son and her letter back to James was full of her sorrow at his loss. There was little consolation she could give him. The war was unfair and unkind in taking her Seb, and it was a crying shame that Harry died of the influenza. None of it made any sense and she did not have the words to express her sympathy at this tragedy.

It was a dreadful time for everyone. A dark and sad cloud hung over the village, as funeral after funeral took place and the streets remained quiet and the losses were being counted. News came into Elmsley over the months that followed of how many the influenza had killed; not thousands of people across the world, but millions. The numbers were staggering. No village, town or. city in the whole of Britain was said to have escaped the ravages of the pandemic. It had been reported that up to a quarter of the country's entire population had died. These were dark days, even with the influenza no longer claiming any victims. Wives, husbands, mothers and fathers, sisters and brothers, were left grieving over such a senseless loss of life, and it would take years to recover from this devastation.

Dru was not coping at all with Lillian's death. He went through the motions of living, but his mind and soul were not truly connected to his body. Eve did her best for her brother, but she knew he had given up and she was helpless in the face of his grief. She also knew he felt that this was his punishment for the accident he had that killed his first wife Alice. His anger was that his poor, innocent Lillian had paid the price for his own terrible mistake. Now he was lonely and without the woman that he loved by his side. Dru was slowly dying, and nobody, not even his sons, could prevent it. Thomas increasingly took responsibility for his younger brother and for the running of the smithy and forge. Although he was very capable, Eve was concerned for her nephew. His life became very difficult. Coping with his father alone was hard, especially as Dru took to drinking too much again. Most of his time was spent at the Bull Inn, as well as much of his income. In so doing, he was destroying his business. Thomas had to go and bring his father home regularly from the Inn, so drunk, he could not walk. Eve constantly talked to Dru, begging him to stop drinking and ruining his sons' lives, but he just nodded agreeably, promised to stop, then continued on as he was doing. His business increasingly suffered and there was less work around as it was. Where his wealthier customers once had teams of horses and carts, which all needed his services, they were now purchasing the new motorised vehicles, or automobiles, as they were known. Dru had also become so unreliable that the customers he did have were losing patience with him, even though they felt very sorry for his loss of Lillian. But they too had farms and businesses to run and reluctant as they were, some eventually began to move their custom to other smithies in the area. Still this did not register with Dru. He seemed past caring anyway, and no amount of advice, badgering or pleading seemed to get through to him.

Thomas went to see Eve one evening to discuss something important. He felt that his father should sell up the business and their cottage and make a new start somewhere else. Thomas had met a number of soldiers from Australia during the war and heard stories of vast acres of land for sale at low prices, and of a living to be made that was free and healthy. He had enough knowledge of his trade to get work to begin with to keep them going, and then he would go into sheep farming. His Australian comrades told him how easy it was to become very wealthy in their country and Thomas had gone as far as applying for assisted passage. He thought they should all go to an area called New South Wales, and it was an opportunity that he felt they should take. If his father remained in Elmsley, he would surely kill himself with drink or die in a fight. Dru had taken to causing arguments at the Inn and been hurt a number of times. It was as if he was doing all he could to destroy himself.

Eve was far from pleased to hear Thomas's idea. She had lost her son, her daughter was married and had left their home, and now her nephew wanted to move himself, her brother and other nephew to the far side of the world. She could go with them, Thomas told Eve. She laughed and thanked him, but she would stay where she was, near to her daughter. Her roots were in Elmsley and that is where she belonged. Although she would hate for Dru and his sons to go so far away, Eve told Thomas that she understood his reasons for wanting to leave. The next task for him to do was to talk to his father.

Chapter 30

A year later, on the 19th September 1920, Dru and his two sons, Thomas and Edward, left Liverpool Docks and sailed to Australia. Eve, Mary, and Sarah made the journey to see them off. Eve and Dru promised to write to each other, and Eve said she would one day visit them once they were settled, but in their hearts they all knew that might never happen. Eve did not like travelling, and Liverpool was as far as she had ever ventured from Elmsley. But it helped everyone to believe that they would see each other again one day. And now that Mary was married, Eve had a son-in-law who would look after her, Dru surmised. Of course he will, she agreed with him. 'Yes, they would be fine in his absence, and he was not to worry about them.' The most important thing was that Thomas would look after his father and young brother Edward, and they all had the chance of a better life.

Dru made a good profit on selling his business and cottage, and was starting afresh with a respectable purse. All that remained were the final goodbyes. They hugged and kissed and hugged again before Dru and his lads walked up the long gangway and onto the ship. Eve, Mary and Sarah, waved to them until it and they were completely out of sight, then Eve cried her heart out. She had no idea how she was going to be without her brother. They had their differences in the past, but since childhood, he always looked out for her. Dru had always been there in her life.

Once back at Elmsley, when Sarah and Mary had both gone off to their respective homes, Eve returned to her empty cottage. She stood in the middle of her silent kitchen, exhausted and sad. She looked at the two chairs either side of the range, remembering Granny Anna sitting in hers, knitting and chatting away to her mother, who always sat in the other. Eve thought about the biscuit and bread-making days at the table when she was younger, and how her mother used to get flour all over her face, deliberately, Eve realised as she grew older, just so that she could tell her off and wipe it away. She heard her mother singing as she cooked supper and remembered how pleased she always was when she got home. Eve could see herself chopping up the herbs to make the remedies, and remembered how she would taste them sometimes without her mother knowing, thinking they might taste nice, and being horribly shocked when they did not. She thought about how her mother used to go over and over the list of the names and addresses with her of where the remedies needed to be delivered to, and how her mother would insist on wrapping her own special woollen scarf around her neck against the cold when she went out in the winter. The scarf still hung on the hook behind the front door. Eve remembered the summer evenings when she would take too long to do her rounds, because she was off somewhere chatting or exploring, and then return to find her mother waiting at the front door, holding a lantern in her hand, lighting the way home. She thought about Joseph coming to live in the cottage, and how he would walk in every afternoon with cakes and bread. Eve missed him so much. She remembered the night she invited Joseph to her bed and how shy and unsure he looked. He had been the most wonderful man she had ever known, and she wished that she had been more loving towards him, and that she had told Joseph she loved him sooner than she did. But that was then, and this was now. Eve could not control her desperate feeling of loneliness. She sat in her mother's old chair and cried again. She already missed Dru and her nephews and Australia to her might just as well have been on the other side of the moon.

The whole of that last year had been unsettled. Dru had agreed to emigrate as soon as his son spoke of it, and the months were filled with learning as much as they could about Australia, selling the smithy and forge, then the cottage and everything in it. Sarah and Ben were struggling. He lost the manager's job he had at the mill. The owner's son returned from the war and took back his old position. He saw Ben as some sort of threat and made sure his father let him go. It was months before he got another job. George helped out eventually, and found him a position in the cotton mill where he worked, but Ben had to go back on to the machines and take a severe cut in his wages, which was difficult with a wife and two children to support. He would often talk of going to Australia, just as Thomas had done. Ben repeatedly said that if they got the chance, they should go as well. Life sounded so much easier out there and working at the mill was hard work. Eve told Ben to keep in touch with Dru and Thomas, and if he really wanted to go, as much as she did not want to lose her sweet Sarah and their children, she would help his family with the cost of the passage. Eve could see how much the mill work was exhausting Ben. She had come to realise over the years that he was not as robust as he looked, and ever since he had suffered from the influenza, he remained below par. Of course, Eve tried to get Ben to take some of her tonic, but he was very old fashioned and did not believe in any medicine of any description, either from her or a doctor. Eve did not remind Ben that she had used her remedies on him when he was ill.

Then Margaret, Eve's old neighbour and provider of all the local gossip, passed away quite suddenly. At her funeral, many people expressed surprise at her age. Most thought she was in her mid-sixties, but Margaret was actually seventy-nine. It seemed that she had a heart attack, confirmed one day by Doctor Finnan, when Eve met him whilst shopping in Ashton. He had enjoyed several meetings with Eve over the last two years, and they had found some common ground. Finnan had even sent some of her remedies off to friends at his old medical school in Edinburgh, for them to try out on volunteer patients. According to his colleagues, they were having some success, but proper trials would cost money, and their budget, what with the war and then the influenza pandemic, could not go to that expense at this moment in time.

Eve saw Mary quite regularly and her daughter told her she was happy, but Eve thought that some of the light had left Mary's eyes. Her whole life seemed to have been consumed with taking care of her husband. She had even stopped making her beautiful pictures, as George did not think his wife should waste her time on such trivial doodling. That was not what God gave her hands for, according to him. Eve was very disturbed to find this out and tackled George one evening on this subject. She had called at their cottage to see Mary, who was out, and found him alone. When she asked George about her daughter and her painting, he became quickly angry and brusquely told her not to try and interfere with him and his wife.

"Tis nowt to do wi' you what Mary does or doesn't do," he rounded on Eve. "Don't ya think ya've done enough damage to her," he added nastily. Eve was stunned.

"An' what damage would that be?" she asked.

"Ya never brought her up to be a decent Christian woman, that's what!" George replied loudly. "Fillin' her head wi' all that nature nonsense; tis ungodly, that's what it is." Eve stared at him. He realised that he had just expressed some of his true feelings and waited for her to react. She did not, just turned to leave. As she walked out of the front door however, George, feeling he now had little to lose, shouted after her.

"'Mary will not be doin' any of those pictures again. Ah've destroyed all that paintin' stuff she had her mind in to," he stated arrogantly. "She's my wife an' she'll do what ah say. Tis her only chance of salvation. Now she's away from you an' yar ways ah'll make sure sh' repents." Eve was at first shaken and then horrified by what George had just said to her. She stopped at the door and turned to face her son-in-law.

"Ah allus thought ya wor a bigot George, but ah never took ya for a cruel man," she told him directly. "Ah've stopped myself from interferin' wi' yar marriage before now 'cus ya worn't harmin' my Mary. But stoppin' her from doin' her lovely pictures is cruel. Ah'll tell ya this now George. Ah'll not stand by an' watch ya hurt Mary. If ya have destroyed her paints, ya'll get her some new ones, or ah will. An' ya'll nay stop her paintin' ever again. Do ya hear me?" Eve was shaking with temper. "An' don't think that ya just dealin' wi' a woman that's gettin' on in years an' on her own. Ah can defend myself an' my daughter if need be, an' if ya think ah can't, ya'll be makin' a big mistake." Then she turned and left.

George was livid and wanted to run after Eve and shout at her some more but thought better of it. A short while after, Mary returned to find her husband in a very strange mood. She often felt apprehensive these days when she walked into her home. The atmosphere indoors depended entirely on what mood George was in, and that depended on whether or not she had upset him, which was becoming increasingly easy for her to do.

"Did ya tell yar mam that ah stopped yar paintin' yar pictures?" he asked Mary in his usual interrogation voice. She looked surprised. "Well, did ya?" he persisted, not getting his answer quickly enough.

"Nay," Mary replied. She was puzzled by her husband's sudden outburst.

"Then why did sh' come here an' accuse me of

treatin' ya cruelly?" George spat out.

"Ah have no idea," Mary said, slightly bemused.

"Do ya think this is amusin'?" he said irritably. Mary could sense her husband's temper mounting and tried to pacify him.

"Of course ah don't. All ah said to my mam wor that ah don't paint anymore, because ya don't like me to. Ah never told her ya wor cruel to me," Mary explained.

"Well don't go sayin' anythin' about us to yar mam," George told her indignantly. "Tis none of her business. An' ya can tell yar mam that ah don't want her to come here again." Mary became very upset at this.

"Ah can't tell my mam that," she argued. "An' tis my home as well as yours."

"Ya'll do as ah say," he shouted back at her and stormed out of the cottage. Mary wanted to rush straight to her mother but did not want Eve to see her as upset as she was. She knew that would only make things worse between her and George. Instead, when he had left for work the next morning, not having said two words to her since his return home late the night before, Mary went to see Eve. She told her what had happened, only in Mary's version, her and George had a 'talk'. She omitted to tell her mother about his aggressive questioning and shouting. However, it was what Eve expected her son-in-law would do, and she was also not surprised to hear that he did not want her to go to their home again.

"Ah'll come to see you mam," Mary told her. "'Tis probably best that ya stay away till George calms down." Eve looked at her daughter knowingly. She knew he was never going to 'calm down', as Mary put it. However, Eve did not want to cause Mary any more grief from her husband; she had not been fooled by her daughter's description of their 'little chat'. Eve now had the full measure of George Wade, and she was disappointed and concerned, not for herself, but for Mary, because she deserved someone better than him. Mary was a sweet and gentle soul and George was turning into a horrible bully. However, Mary would not have a bad word said about her husband and repeated time and time again that she loved him. Against that, Eve was powerless, and therefore agreed not to go to their cottage.

She was heartened to hear from Mary, some two weeks later however, that George had taken her in to Danberry and purchased a box of water colour paint blocks, some brushes and some special painting paper.

"George just said, come on, we'll go an' get ya some new paints an' things an' ya can start to paint again," Mary told her mother excitedly. "Ah couldn't believe it. Tis good of George to let me do it, seein' as what he feels about me paintin' pictures an' all." Eve was pleased to see her daughter happy, but not pleased to hear her praising George for his generosity in allowing to her paint again. But she smiled agreeably.

"Aye, tis good ya can do yar paintin'," she said. "An' is George still bullyin' ya to be a perfect Christian?" Eve could not help herself. She remained unhappy to have heard from George that he was going to help her daughter to repent, and wanted to hear Mary's account of it all. Eve was good at reading between the lines.

"Mam," Mary said. "George doesn't bully me. He just gets a bit impatient wi' me at times, that's all. Ah want to do things the right way now, not just fer George, but fer myself as well. It doesn't mean ah don't believe in the same things as you do, but ah believe in Jesus Christ too. Ah've told George that ah'll really try and learn about the bible...ah want to do that mam. Ah really do." Eve did not know whether to laugh or cry. She never thought she would hear her daughter say what she had just said, but judging by Mary's face, she was completely serious.

"So none of this is coming from George?" Eve asked.

"Aye, it did at first," Mary told her, "but then ah

understood what he wor sayin', an' ah want to be a good Christian now," Mary said convincingly. Eve had to accept her daughter's declaration and said no more to her on the subject. Whatever Mary had told her however, Eve knew the truth of the matter, and she determined in her own mind that she would keep a close eye on Mary and on George's behaviour towards her.

After the trauma of Dru and his sons leaving and her daughter getting married and leaving home, things did settle down for Eve over the months that followed, and she began to live her life without her brother and nephews. She also had to cope with living on her own, which she had never done in her life. She tended all of the family's graves, keeping her promise to Dru to care for both Lillian and Alice's resting places. She spent some time each week with her kin, talking, sometimes crying, and other times just sitting in silence. It gave her solace and peace, and helped with her loneliness. Eve often saw Nathan in the churchyard. Both his parents had passed on and there was only he and John, Sarah's first husband, living at the farm now, Henry Morely having been taken with the influenza. Eve and Nathan regularly spent time together chatting and something of a genuine friendship built up between them over the time.

Eve kept away from her daughter's home and did

not say anything to George when she happened upon him in the village or local towns. She greeted her son-in-law politely and with friendliness, but no conversation passed between them other than that. Mary came to see her often enough, so it did not matter, and by her accounts, George was being fairly pleasant. Eve's life settled into a simple routine and she was reasonably content. She still received a generous allowance from James Barlow, and with it was able to save some money and help others in a small way as well. She often bought clothes for Sarah and Ben's children, and provided small food parcels for them and a number of other very poor families in the village.

Eve spoke to Doctor Finnan from time to time and helped Nurse Ann when asked. She sometimes had visitors to her cottage seeking her knowledge and advice; Eve's reputation for having the second sight had spread far beyond Elmsley. She even had people calling on her from York, which was some forty miles away. Of course, Eve remained careful as to what she told her visitors, and was mindful of not openly predicting futures. It was against the law and she knew that there were still some in her community who would like to see her silenced. Eve spent much of her days gathering the ingredients for her remedies, and in the evenings she made them up and delivered them. Nothing much changed in Eve's life for the next year or so.

Then Mary visited her one afternoon with some upsetting news. She and George were moving away and probably going to live in London. Eve was mortified. She had not expected to hear such a thing. Why London, she asked? What about George's job? He was doing well at the mill, Eve thought. Mary sat with her mother and explained what had happened. She had not mentioned anything before because she did not want to worry her. However, she and George had problems which they could not simply resolve.

Three weeks earlier, George had an argument with Mr Blanchard, the owner of the mill where he worked. It was a fierce and terrible argument, according to Mary. A man, a young worker there, had died. He fell into one of the new machines that Blanchard had installed at his mill and was killed instantly. George was very upset, as he had warned the owner on a number of occasions that these latest machines he had purchased, although more efficient, were dangerous for the men that worked them. They had no adequate safety guards and the moving parts were very exposed. But his warnings were ignored. In a heated discussion, when talking about the dead man, who left a widow and three children behind, George rounded on Blanchard and accused him of neglect. As much as his work was valued, the owner sacked George on the spot. There was no rescinding. Blanchard told him to leave his employ and mill immediately, and not to expect any kind of reference from him either. Eve was most unhappy to hear this story.

"But surely George could get other work local?" she asked Mary.

"He's tried every mill in the area," Mary told her. "He's even been prepared to take a wages cut an' all, but some of the mills are closin' down. They reckon that tis now cheaper to get cotton from India, so they don't have to pay the wages here, and wool is not so much in demand anymore. So, they just don't need as many mechanics. George says that we either go to London or we emigrate, like Uncle Dru did." Eve felt sick. "Ah don't want to leave ya mam, but ah have to go wi' my husband, don't ah?" Eve could not disagree with that.

"But what will George do in London?" she asked.

"Well, he's allus kept in touch wi' a man he met in the war. Fred Black, his name is," Mary replied. "Fred lives in the east part of London an' he works on the docks there, by the Thames. He told George that if he can get down to London, he'll get him work; they need men there apparently, loadin' and unloadin' the big ships. Fred says that the pay is really good as well. Tis hard work mind. He told George that we can rent houses cheap down there too, right near the docks. George is real set on goin' mam. If ah don't say yes, he said he's goin' to go an' get us a bookin' on a ship to Australia. Ah don't want to go there mam. Ah couldn't be that far away from you." Eve hardly knew what to say. Of course she did not want Mary to go to Australia, but London..? The prospect of her daughter going anywhere away from her was daunting, but London was at least within reach.

Apart from missing her, there were other things that, if Mary moved any distance, Eve had to reconcile herself to. She would finally have to face the fact that Mary was not going to carry on the family duties or traditions. Marrying George was Mary's first step away from that life, and moving to London and far from her, would be the final and closing chapter of the Shetcliffe ancestral line of cunning folk. Mary had the inherited gift, but Eve always knew in her heart, ever since Mary was a very small child, that she would never use it. It was not within Eve's power to force her daughter to take up her inheritance; Mary had to want to do that herself. This was the only way it could, and should, be. Of course Eve was sad, but all she could do was write her own story and, when the time came, pass the family's books on to her daughter. Eve knew that once she died and Mary took charge of these treasures however, that George would undoubtedly have them destroyed. But if that was to be the fate of the ancestral books, then destiny could not be denied. After much thought about her daughter Mary, and once she let go of her disappointment, Eve was at peace with this eventuality. Now all she could do was wait to find out what was going to happen.

Three months later, Mary moved with George to Stepney, London. They rented a small house, and, as he said he would, Fred Black secured George employment on the docks, shifting cargo. Both Mary and Eve cried as they parted, with Mary promising to come back and see her mother as often as she could. Eve told her that she would pay her fares and that she must come to see her soon. She gave her daughter a substantial purse to keep for her own use, such as for travelling back to Elmsley. Of course they would write regularly, and Eve extracted from Mary a promise that she would tell her if she needed anything or if she wanted to come home. If she did, then all Mary had to do was to say, then she would make it happen. But Mary went off quite happy, apart from leaving Eve. She was looking forward to a new life in London. Things seemed to be so different there. People drove automobiles and travelled on trams and trains to go to many places. There were lots of schools for her future children, and shops, and parks, and all manner of things that she had never experienced.

With Mary finally gone, Eve was deeply sad. Her whole world had suddenly collapsed. Apart from knowing that she would miss her daughter, Eve was also concerned, because she could protect Mary if she stayed close, but London was far away. Distance would weaken any protection she could give her and she feared for Mary. With her leaving Elmsley, Eve had to release her daughter into the hands of fate, and she knew that fate was not always kind. She wrote to James and told him that Mary and George had gone to live in London. Eve felt he should know.

However, determined to put on a brave face for Mary's sake, Eve set about writing to her every week with the news of the village and the people in it. She also wrote with the latest news from Australia. Dru and his sons were doing well and were very happy with their new home. Thomas had fulfilled his ambition and purchased a sheep farm and it was making them a good living. He married an Australian lady called Beth Anderson and they were expecting their first child. Edward was travelling around the country. He had not made up his mind yet about being a sheep farmer, but Thomas expected him to return and settle down one day. Dru heard from Edward regularly, so was not worried about him. Thomas had also heard from Ben, who wrote asking him if he could give him any work, or help him find work if he brought his family over to New South

Wales. So Eve wrote to Mary that Sarah, Ben and their children might soon join her uncle and nephews in Australia.

Mary wrote back to Eve about her house, the people she was meeting, Londoners, who she could barely understand, nor they her. She sent Eve pictures from newspapers, postcards and all sorts of things she thought her mother might find interesting. Mary was still painting, when she had time. To make ends meet, she told her mother that she had taken in some homeworking, sewing cuffs on dresses. Between George's wages and the extra income Mary was earning, they had a fair living.

And so the next year passed. Mary had visited Eve three times and stayed with her for a few days on each occasion. It was wonderful to see her daughter and she treasured those visits. And Eve, as hard as it was for her, went down on the train to London once. She booked into a small, local hotel and visited Mary's house when George was at work. He knew Eve had come to London, but they did not meet. Eve was content that her daughter's life was reasonably comfortable and that she remained well and seemed happy. James had written to Eve not long after Mary had moved, expressing his disappointment that she had left the village. He was surprised that they had gone to live in London and was concerned for his daughter's well-being. James asked for Mary's address, which, after some consideration, Eve gave him. He told her that he would still honour his allowance and asked if she would forward some extra money to Mary, to help her in her new life in London. In his letter, James confessed to Eve how often he used to pass through Elmsley just in the hope of seeing his daughter, which he did do on several occasions. He told Eve that he had also seen her in the village and in Ashton, and thought that she was still as beautiful as the first day they met, all those years ago. Eve secretly enjoyed reading this, even though she dismissed it as nonsense.

Then Eve received a letter from George. He wrote, telling her that he did not want his wife travelling all the way up to Elmsley again. She was carrying his child and he did not want her to go so far away from home. What should have been good news for Eve, finding out that her daughter was going to give her a grandchild, was tinged with sadness, as she knew that she would only see Mary if she went to London herself. That meant that Mary, for the time being at least, would not be able to stay with her and they could not enjoy those special few days together in the cottage again. Eve wrote back to George telling him that she understood and would be coming down to London soon to see Mary. She wrote to her daughter and said the same. Two weeks later Eve visited Mary, staying in the local hotel again. As she was still not allowed to go to her home, Mary met her mother there. She looked very pale, Eve noticed straight away. She was carrying a child, but still Eve was not comfortable seeing Mary look so white and so listless in the way she moved about.

"What's wrong sweet?" she asked her. They were sitting in the tea room at the hotel.

"Oh, ah just feel tired," Mary replied.

"Are ya eatin' the right things an' restin' like ya should?" Eve asked.

"Aye," Mary said. "Ah'm fine. Just get tired quickly."

"Tis the first three months that's the worst," Eve told her. "Ya'll pick up. Ya know what ya have to do Mary, so make sure ya do it fer the baby's sake." Mary nodded. She had been given enough knowledge about pregnancy and birthing from Eve to be able to manage her own. "An' how are ya getting' on wi' George these days?" Eve asked. She was not convinced that Mary was just tired. She sensed that there was something wrong.

"George is workin' really hard mam," Mary told her. "He has to be at the docks very early in the mornin', and don't get home till late. He's tired most of the time. Ah'm not sure that we did the right thing in comin' to London, but George is so stubborn, he won't admit that."

"So do ya think he might eventually give up an'

come back to Elmsley?" Eve said.

"Ah don't think so," Mary said. "Ah can't see us comin' back to Yorkshire at any rate. There's nay work up there fer George. Now we've got the baby on the way, ah don't think he'll risk changin' jobs again. At least not till the baby's born."

Eve would have liked to have heard that her pregnant daughter and her husband were coming home, but even she knew there was little work in the area. A number of mills had recently closed down and many of the youngsters in Elmsley had also left the village and gone down south, just like George and Mary had done. The work would be just as hard, but at least there was work to be found. Times were very difficult, especially up in the north of England. The country had still not recovered from the war, and even though there was a shortage of men, the farms needed fewer labourers, as machines were now taking over where once the land needed more hands to work it. Businesses were struggling and local factories employed fewer people. Even the big houses were not retaining as many staff as they used to before the war. With things as bad as they were, Eve had to agree that George stood a better chance of earning a living wage down south than up in Yorkshire. And with a child now on the way, he needed steady and reasonably well-paid employment.

Before that year was out, Ben, Sarah and their children left for Australia. Thomas had offered Ben work on his sheep farm and help with accommodation until they could set themselves up over there. They had been granted assisted passage and sailed off late November. Eve was very sad to see Sarah and the children leave, but knew it was the right thing for them to do. Ben could not have survived many more years working in the mills and she was pleased that Thomas would help them settle in the new country. Again, Eve said she would visit there one day and they promised to write. Her world was slowly disappearing as each beloved person left her life.

Chapter 31

Elizabeth Florence Wade was born on the 26th July 1927. She was a beautiful, healthy baby with a mass of dark hair and deep purple eyes, destined to turn chocolate brown. Eve had been travelling to and from London during Mary's pregnancy, more frequently towards the end of her daughter's confinement, in the hope that she would be near her when the birth came. George had made it perfectly clear that he did not want Eve at his wife's birthing however, and Mary had to agree to that, even though she wanted her mother there. George had put so much pressure on his wife that she eventually capitulated, and Mary told Eve, for her sake, to accept that she could not be present when the baby was being born. Eve was very upset. She had always expected to help deliver her own grandchildren, as her mother and her grandmothers had done for generations. However, seeing the stress that this was causing Mary and how torn she was, Eve did not show her daughter how wounded she felt. That helped ease Mary's own disappointment and fear of hurting her mother.

Eve got the news, in a very short letter from Mary, that the baby had arrived, a week after she was born. She immediately wrote back and said she would be travelling to London in a few days. Before

Eve could even post her reply however, she received another letter from Mary telling her not to come, as George had forbidden her to see the baby. Mary begged her mother in the letter to please understand, just for the time being, that George was afraid for the baby and did not want her to have anything to do with his daughter. She would talk to him, Mary reassured her. She would make him see how unkind and unchristian he was being towards her, Mary wrote. She must be patient, and let her work on her husband. He was a good man really, but he was concerned that she would somehow taint his baby girl. Mary then told her mother how George disliked everything that she stood for. He had become more devout and more obsessed with his religion since they moved to London. Eve must be assured that he was not unkind or cruel to her however and that in every other way, George was a decent husband. He was just consumed with the belief that she, Eve, was sinful and did ungodly acts. Mary told her mother that she had tried many times to tell George that this was far from the truth, but that only resulted in her having to pray on her knees for hours, denying her mother and her grandmothers pasts to God. Please understand, she pleaded again with Eve. Please wait and she will come and see her. Mary told her mother that she would visit Elmsley as soon as she felt strong enough to travel. The baby was fine and well and beautiful. She would have some photographs taken of her and send them as soon as they were ready. Mary again asked Eve not to worry for her or little Elizabeth. She ended her letter imploring Eve to forgive her husband.

Eve was heartbroken. She read Mary's letter again and again. The more times she read it, the more the dislike of George built up in her heart. She had to be careful not to allow this to turn to hatred, but that was difficult. George had taken her daughter away and now he was denying her even seeing her only grandchild. But Eve was helpless. If she took revenge on her son-in-law, she hurt her daughter, who was still professing in her letter that she loved George dearly. She would also damage her granddaughter. No, there was nothing she could do. She would wait and speak to Mary when she came to visit.

In the meantime, she wrote to James. Eve had to confide in someone, and he seemed the right person to do that to. In her letter she told him of the birth of Elizabeth and that she and Mary were well. She then told him of her distress at being denied seeing her granddaughter and how she knew that George would not ever allow his mind to be changed by Mary. James wrote back to Eve telling her that he was sorry that George was acting in such a manner. He was also concerned for Mary. He had been to London on business and whilst there, had passed through the road that she and George lived in. He was not happy with the area and thought it was run down and grubby. He could not understand why they went to live there and asked if there was anything he could do to help bring Mary and her husband back to Elmsley. Perhaps find employment for George? At least then, they could both see something of their grandchild; it could not be avoided. Eve replied that even if he could help George, she did not believe that he would return with Mary and the child to Elmsley, but she would certainly put this proposition to Mary when she visited her. Eve also thanked James for his continued support and concern.

It was seven months later when Mary finally came to see her mother. She visited, but without the baby. Eve had half-hoped that she would have Elizabeth with her, and her heart sank when she saw Mary get off of the train in Danberry Station without her. Nathan Morely had taken Eve in by horse and carriage that morning to collect Mary and bring her back to Elmsley. Upset and disappointed not to see the baby, Eve was none the less overjoyed to hold Mary in her arms again. They hugged and cried and then Nathan took them back to Eve's cottage. Mary explained that she could not leave the baby before now, but as she was reducing her breast feeding, she could leave her overnight with some of her milk. Mary then told Eve that she was sorry, but she would have to make the long journey back to London early the next day. Eve was devastated. She had barely twenty four hours to spend with Mary, after not having seen her for months. Things would improve Mary told her. As Elizabeth got older, she would be able to spend two days with her when she visited. George had told her that he would let her come up often and he would look after the child at those times.

It was very hard for Eve. She looked at her daughter in some amazement. She had not complained to Mary or told her how desperately unhappy she was at being denied her granddaughter, but could Mary not see how dreadful that was for her? Could she not make some kind of stand with George and insist he was fair with her mother? In a quiet moment, once Mary had returned home, Eve sat and thought about the whole situation. She had mentioned to her daughter that George could possibly get work near Elmsley, if he wanted to leave the docks. But Mary's response to that was that he would never return to live there. She said that they were now quite happy where they were and they liked London and George enjoyed his job. Mary also told Eve how George had become very involved with his local church and was being trained as a lay preacher. Apart from looking after the baby, she herself was doing a lot of work for the church and had been baptised again to reaffirm her commitment to the Christian faith. She also revealed to her mother that she had stopped painting for ever. It was only for idle hands, just as George said. Eve thought back on this conversation, remembering Mary's expression as she said these things, and now came to the horrible realisation that her daughter was rapidly slipping away from her. Mary had become everything that George wanted her to be and had buried her natural self, her character, and even her inheritance. Her daughter had denied who she was and where she came from. Eve cried, because she now knew she had to give up trying to keep some kind of hold on Mary or have any influence in her life. She had only tried to do this for her daughter's sake, not out of maternal selfishness. Eve also believed she would probably never see her granddaughter; George had made such a good a job of separating her from Mary and Elizabeth.

When she thought back to her daughter as a child, Eve remembered how she always gave in to Seb whenever he bullied her. Mary always let her little brother have his own way and that is exactly what she was now doing with George. But Mary was a willing partner in this, and so Eve was powerless. As long as her daughter partook in George's plans, Eve could do nothing. As she sat in her front room staring into the flames from the fire, she understood that she must accept what was now before her. She would see Mary when George allowed her to visit and her granddaughter would probably never know her; she could not think that George would let Mary even talk about her to Elizabeth. Eve had sent Mary off home with some gifts for the baby and some money for her purse, should she need it for herself. But she knew Mary would possibly not give the baby her presents, not if George knew she had sent them down, and would no doubt give him the money as well, her not keeping anything for herself...that would be wicked!

And so the time passed. Eve's life changed very little, except she felt the years catching up with her. Mary visited every few months and told Eve all about her life, her and George's work at the church and about Elizabeth. Eve had been given a photograph of her granddaughter, and saw her own mother in her dark eyes and dark brown locks that she had grown. Elizabeth was now five years old. On her last visit, Mary told Eve that she had recently lost a baby. She had only been two months pregnant when she suffered a miscarriage. It would seem that as hard as she and George were trying, Mary could not fall for another child and keep the baby. She confessed to Eve that this was her third failed pregnancy since the move to London. She had not told her of the others because she did not want to worry her.

However, Mary was upset at the loss of this last baby, as she felt that she was getting too old to have any more children now. Eve did not say a great deal to Mary when she told her of the miscarriages, except to give her sympathy and a loving hug. Mary would not be allowed to take any of Eve's remedies, so it was pointless her even suggesting she did. Eve looked closely at her daughter however, and was satisfied that physically she was fine, and told her that if she was meant to have more babies, then she would. That was what the Reverend at her Church had told her, Mary said to Eve. He also said that it was God's will. Mary believed that, but was still disappointed, as she would have liked to give Elizabeth a brother or sister. Eve was more interested in Mary's health and told her that when a woman is older, it was not kind on the body to be pregnant. Then Mary admitted to her mother that George was very unhappy with her for not producing more babies. He took it as some kind of punishment from God, 'divine retribution' he called it, and said that she needed to purify herself further from her past and then she might have another child successfully.

Eve was furious at hearing this and finally exploded. All of her pent up feelings flooded out and she told her daughter exactly what she thought of her husband and his ridiculous religious nonsense.

Eve also told Mary that she thought George was a bigot, a bully and a cruel man. She said he should actually be ashamed to call himself a Christian, because a true person of that faith would not do some of the things he did. Mary was shocked and very upset to hear Eve speak so of her husband. But Eve was in full flow now and added that she, as her daughter, should have stood up to George and not let him be so cruel in not allowing Elizabeth to know her. She, as her daughter, should also be ashamed of herself.

They did not part harmoniously. Eve had said what she thought and how she felt but she knew that Mary was deeply upset and after she had left, Eve felt sorry that she had distressed her. Of course Eve wrote soon after and apologised, hoping that Mary would forgive her outburst, but she did not reply. Eve wrote many times, but it was a full year before Mary sent her a response. Her letter, when it came, was very harsh and in it she accused her mother of interfering with her life and trying to come between her and her husband. Eve was very hurt by Mary, but she knew she was reading George's words, not her daughters. Eve wanted to write back and defend herself and her actions, but decided that it would be a waste of time. Instead, she ignored Mary's accusations, and wrote back in her reply about the news in the village and what was happening with their family in Australia.

It was another year before she heard from her daughter again. This letter was not so angry and just gave her mother news of herself and Elizabeth and how she was growing up fast and getting on in school. Eve replied and asked for a photograph of the girl, which some months later, Mary did send. Eve had written to James during this time and told him of her estrangement from Mary. He was upset for her and said that he would try and find out about their daughter and granddaughter when he visited London himself on business. James reported back to Eve some months later that he had actually seen Mary in the street one day and that she was with a young girl, presumably Elizabeth. He told Eve that Mary and the child looked well. They wore nice clothes and seemed fairly prosperous, in comparison with many of those living around that area of London. He said that the child was a pretty little thing with long dark brown, curly hair, which tumbled out from her blue hat that matched her smart blue dress. Eve was immediately transported back in time as she read this, to when she stood staring at Jayne Addington that day in Ashton, in her blue hat and beautiful blue dress. James said to Eve that he trusted that his sighting of Mary and Elizabeth had at least calmed her concerns for their health, and that he hoped their falling-out would be of a short duration. Eve was gladdened and reassured to know that James had seen her daughter and granddaughter. She lived in the hope that after some pleasantries had passed between her and Mary by letter, then she might go to London and at least meet up with her daughter, even if only for a few hours.

Apart from her unhappiness over the situation with Mary, things remained fairly settled in Eve's life. She was getting older and had gained a modicum of respectability in the community. Some of those now growing up in Elmsley did not see her in quite the same way as their parents and particularly their grandparents did, or had done so. However, Eve would still often be referred to as the 'witch', but this was said in a less denigrating manner than it had been in the past, although the pious amongst the villagers still viewed her with suspicion and mistrust. Few people would sit where she had sat or would say too much in her presence. When Eve walked down the street, wherever that was, she knew she was looked at and whispered about. To some extent, she quite enjoyed the attention and certainly did nothing to allay the fearsome reputation she had acquired over the years. Eve wore her hair, as she had always done; lose about her shoulders, only now it was pure white. Her milky complexion was aged, but still held a youthful glow.

Her eyes were as blue as ever, made more pronounced by the colour of her hair. She was slightly fuller in her figure, but still retained her straight posture and slim waist from years of walking the hills and fields and dales near Elmsley. She was fit and strong for her seventy years and still striking to look at. Those men who had yearned for her in younger years, even now, found her pleasant on the eye. She was also as vibrant and as tough as ever. Eve knew how to look after herself and her body.

Some old acquaintances of hers passed on during this time. Pastor Bell died quite suddenly. He had become something of a friend to Eve over the years. She attended his funeral, much to the dismay of a number of people in the village, but then they did not know of their friendship. Samuel Jowett also passed away. Eve had been called to him by Mrs Jowett and stayed at their home and nursed Samuel in his final days, with the knowledge and blessing of Doctor Finnan. Samuel was to be the doctor's last patient, as he was retiring from his practice, passing it on to a young doctor by the name of Doctor Aldred. Aldred's wife, Rachel, a trained nurse, took over from Nurse Ann, who retired herself when Finnan did. Ann moved near to some of her family in Liverpool. Eve had tried to persuade her to stay local, as she and Ann had become close over her time there, but Ann was looking to her old age and a cousin had offered some rooms in her boarding house and she took them. And so, yet more people in Eve's life were gone.

In her letters to Mary, Eve kept the conversations light and friendly. When she felt that her daughter had forgiven her for her outburst, she wrote asking if they could meet in London. Mary sent her a reply, some two months later, agreeing to meet. So Eve made the journey down to London again. Mary was altogether well, as James had reported on his last sight of her, but she was much changed. Mary had a certain air about her. Eve thought that she looked like her daughter, but she had lost her smile, her light heartedness and her joy for life. Eve was pleased to see Mary, but deeply saddened at how much she had altered. It was Mary, who was speaking to her, but Eve could hear George in much of what she said; she sounded just like him now. Eve pushed this away however, and just enjoyed her daughter's company for as long as she would sit with her. Eve had booked into the local hotel for two days and thankfully saw Mary on both of them. It was just as Eve was leaving to make her way to the station to catch the train back to York, when she caught sight of her daughter standing across the busy main road from the hotel. Mary was holding the hand of a young girl. Eve was looking at her granddaughter for the first time. It was the last thing that she thought could ever happen and she paused for some moments, not knowing whether to cross the road to them or not. But before she could decide, Mary smiled at her kindly, and then turned and walked away with Elizabeth. Eve went to shout after her, but with the noise of the traffic, with trams passing and people walking busily about everywhere, she did not. Instead, she stood in silence and watched as Mary and the girl walked along the main road for two hundred yards or so then turned down one of the streets leading off of it. Eve was both disappointed and happy at the same time. She wished she could have spoken to Elizabeth or hugged her, but this was the closest she had been to her granddaughter and it filled her with hope for future meetings. Then she recalled Mary's smile. For a few fleeting moments, Eve had got her daughter back.

All the way home, on the long journey back up to Yorkshire, Eve felt more content than she had done for years. This was at least progress and she could not wait to write to James and tell him what had happened. But her happiness was short-lived. The letter she received from London just days after was from George. Mary had told him that she took Elizabeth to the hotel where her mother was staying, just to show her the child, Mary explained to him.

George told Eve that he was furious that she had encouraged his wife to disobey him. He had given Mary strict orders that his daughter should have nothing to do with her. Now Mary was not allowed to visit or see her either. Eve was sickened by this letter and immediately wrote back to George and to Mary, separately. She told them both that she was coming down to London the following week to speak about the whole affair. A week later, Eve made the journey down south and went directly to Mary's house. She stood at the front door for some time, but there was no answer. Eve made her way to the local hotel and waited there for a few hours, then went back to the house. She still received no answer, but a neighbour, who had seen Eve call there earlier, came over.

"If yer lookin' for Mary an' George, they've moved," the lady said. Eve stared at the woman.

"Moved?" she asked.

"Yeh, they moved last week," the woman repeated. "It was a bit sudden. But they went...oh, er, Tuesday last."

"Do ya know where they moved to?" Eve questioned her.

"Ain't got a clue luv," the woman replied. "They was 'ere on the Monday, then early Tuesday mornin' the van came an' took all their furniture and stuff, an' they was gone. Never said a bye or leave to anyone." Eve was stunned. She did not know what to say.

"Are yer family?" the woman asked. Eve nodded a yes. "Oh," she sighed, sympathetically. "Oh, I am sorry luv," she said. "P'raps they just forgot to tell yer." Eve nodded again. She stood not knowing what to do. Eventually, the neighbour turned to go back into her house, but Eve called after her.

"Please," Eve said, "if ah give ya my address, will ya let me know if ya find out where they've moved to? Mary is my daughter."

"Yeh, course I will dearie," the woman said cheerfully. "My name's Doris, Doris Green," she added. "If I see that daughter of yours I'll tell 'er to get in touch with yer straight away. I didn't 'ave much to say to 'er husband mind, but I always used to speak to Mrs Wade and that lovely little girl of 'ers."

"Aye, that's Elizabeth, my granddaughter," Eve told her. She then thought of something. "Would anybody else livin' down this road know where they moved to?" she asked. The woman shook her head.

"I doubt it," she replied. "I think I was the only person round 'ere they spoke to. They kept themselves to themselves pretty much." Eve thanked the woman, wrote her address on a piece of paper and handed it to her. When the woman went indoors to her house and Eve was alone in the road, she became very upset. After a few minutes, she left and returned to her hotel. There were only three places she knew of where she might find some information about Mary or George. She could go to the docks, where he worked, although how she might find him, Eve could not begin to think. There was the church they belonged to and then there was the school Elizabeth attended. The first place Eve went to was the school. She walked to Burley Road Junior School, a few streets away. After calling in to see the Headmistress, Eve was told that Elizabeth had been taken out of school the week before, because the family had moved. She did not have a forwarding address for the Wade family to give her. Eve then walked to a number of churches in the area, finally finding the one to which George and Mary had belonged. The vicar welcomed Eve, but told her that he knew her daughter and husband had moved away, but he did not know where to. He expressed his surprise at their departure, as he thought it rather sudden. But he had discussed their move briefly with George beforehand, who told him that he had been promoted and they were moving to a better house in a nicer district. The vicar reassured Eve that the family were all well and the move was deemed to be a good one. She left the church feeling more anxious however, as she thought that George would of at least have told his vicar where he was going.

The following day, and for the two days after that,

Eve roamed around the docks at Stepney, in the areas accessible to her. It was a forbidding place for anyone, let alone an elderly lady who was a stranger to London. She had no idea where to look, but she spoke to as many people as she could in the hope of finding somebody who knew either George or Fred Black, his colleague. At the end of the third day, Eve had found no one. Distraught, she left London and returned home. With nowhere else to turn, she wrote to James. Eve had limited resources and therefore could not afford to travel backwards and forwards to London very often. Perhaps he could search for their daughter, she thought, when he went down south on his business trips? At any rate, Eve wrote and told him of Mary and George moving. James replied that he was concerned to hear they had simply moved without telling her where. He advised Eve to wait and hopefully she would be written to by Mary. Meanwhile, of course, he would do what he could to find out their whereabouts. However, Eve did not receive any letters from Mary, and even James, as hard as he tried, could not find the couple.

Chapter 32

By the fifth month of not hearing from her daughter or being able to locate her, Eve did the unthinkable. She visited the Wade family's home, intending to appeal to the fair-mindedness of Martha Wade, George's mother and Elizabeth's other grandmother. Eve believed that Martha would have some way of contacting her son and perhaps she would understand the pain that she was going through, not knowing where her daughter and granddaughter were. Nathan Morely took Eve one evening to the Wade's farm, which was some three miles outside of the village. He waited for her by the farm entrance, but within sight, and Eve walked the fifty yards up a muddy track to the farmhouse. It was Allen, one of George's brothers, who opened the door to her. For a few moments, he did not recognise Eve, but whist he was puzzling over her identity, she asked to speak with his mother.

"What do ya want wi' mi mam?" Allen asked her brusquely.

"Ah would like to speak to Martha please, if ya don't mind," Eve insisted. He stared at her and hesitated for some moments before calling out at the top of his voice to his mother.

"Mam, tis Eve Locke," he yelled. Silence followed. Allen stood glaring at Eve, a slight smirk on his face as he recalled who she was. She looked back at him in disregard. Minutes later, Martha Wade shuffled to her front door. She looked totally astonished to see Eve standing on her doorstep.

"What are you doin' 'ere?" she asked rudely.

"Ah've come to ask ya if ya know where my daughter has moved to," Eve replied humbly.

"Aye, ah do," Martha said.

"Can ya tell me where so ah can contact Mary?" Eve asked.

"Nay, ah can't," Martha snapped at her. "An' ah'll ask ya ti leave mi farm," she added nastily.

"Please," Eve pleaded. "Ah just need to know that Mary an' Elizabeth are well. Ya're a mother and grandmother. Surely ya must know how ah feel?"

"They're well," Martha said coldly. "But my George doesn't want anythin' ti do wi' you."

"That's maybe," Eve tried to argue, "but Mary is my daughter. Ah just need to know where sh' is. Tis cruel o' yar son to deny me even seein' my daughter an' the child. Tis cruel." Martha was not moved. She stood officiously glaring at Eve, her arms folded in front of her.

"Tis yar own fault Eve Jennus, or Locke, or whatever ya call yarself now," Martha rounded on her. "Ya've been doin' bad things all o' yar life, an' now tis comin' back ti ya. God is punishin' ya fer all the evil things ya've done."

"What are ya talkin' about woman?" Eve replied angrily. "Whatever ah've done is nowt to do wi' God. What yar son is doin' to me is wicked, an' he calls himself a Christian?"

"Get yarself away from mi door," Martha shouted at her. Then Allen, a large man, stepped forward from behind his mother and, with some force, lunged forward and pushed Eve to the ground. Martha gasped in horror; she did not expect her son to do such a thing and grabbed his jacket, pulling him back into the doorway. Nathan saw what Allen had done and rushed as fast as he could to Eve's assistance. He was furious.

"What do ya think ya're doin' man?" he yelled at him as he helped Eve up from the ground. "Ya've got nay right to treat Mrs Locke that way."

"Then get 'er away from our door," he shouted back. "An' how ya can defend that witch, ah can't understand. Sh' killed yar brother William!"

"That's nonsense," Nathan said loudly. "That's just superstitious nonsense."

"She's evil," Martha said. "An' my George's protectin' 'is family. 'E'll nay let ya see Mary again or Elizabeth. Tis God's will," she shrieked. Nathan, who was still holding Eve, looked on in astonishment and disgust at Martha Wade and her son.

"Let's leave here," he put to Eve. "Let's go. These people are not worth speakin' to. They call you evil.

Tis them that's evil." He ushered Eve away from the Wade's front door and walked her back to his cart. She was very upset. They left the farm and rode back to the village in silence, save for Eve's quiet sobs. When they reached her cottage, Nathan climbed down and walked around to help Eve from his cart. He gently pulled her to him and held her there for some moments.

"Is that how ya've allus been treated? He asked her.

"By some, aye," Eve replied. He shook his head in sadness and pity. She looked up at Nathan and touched his face. "Thank ya fer yar kindness Nathan," she said, wiping her eyes. He nodded an acknowledgement. "Ah must look a pretty sight?" she added shyly.

"Ya look fine to me," Nathan told her. "But then ya allus did." Eve smiled at him and studied his face for a few seconds. He was still handsome, she thought. His hair was white, just as was hers, his face lined and weather-beaten. But still his eyes shone with care for her.

"Oh Nathan," Eve sighed, touching his face again, "if only things had been different."

"Aye," he replied. "If only my stupid brother hadn't have thrown that stone at ya all those years ago. The ridiculous thing is, as a lad, William wor sweet on ya Eve, just as ah wor. He used to go to t' village just so

478

he could see ya...he told me that years after."

"Oh Nathan," Eve said. "Ah never knew. Ah didn't hurt William," she insisted again.

"Ah know ya didn't Eve," Nathan reassured her.

"An' you wor sweet on me?" Eve asked, smiling.

"Aye," Nathan said simply. "Allus wor, allus will be." Eve was almost embarrassed by this declaration and grinned like a young girl. She then kissed Nathan on his cheek.

"Another time, another life," she told him. He smiled one of his rare smiles.

"Aye, another life," he replied.

Eve was deeply upset that the Wades would not let her know where Mary and her granddaughter were. Their attitude towards her had been no surprise, but she was taken aback by the venomous nature of their attacks. She had no option now but to accept that she would get no help from them. Eve was running out of ideas as to what to do next. She did not give up however, and spent the next year travelling to London whenever she could afford to, looking for Mary. This became the main focus of her life. She regularly heard from James, his letters always telling her that he also had no success in finding their daughter and granddaughter either. Eve often had letters from her nephew Thomas and from Sarah also. Thomas gave her all the latest news about his little family and of Dru, and also of

Edward, who himself was now married with two children, both boys. Edward had settled down and eventually bought his own farm, some thirty miles from his father and brother. They were all well. Sarah wrote telling Eve of her life, her family news and what was going on in Australia. She had not liked it there at first and missed England and her Mother Eve dreadfully. But she could see how Ben was much better living there, and they had recently opened a store in Sydney and were selling hardware. Eve smiled when she read this; she could not imagine Ben as a storekeeper, but the more she thought about it, the more she agreed it probably suited him. They were making a good living and Sarah had another child, who she named Eve. Sarah sent her photographs of the family, the store and a special one of her new baby. Eve was content that her brother and his family and Sarah and hers were all fine and happy in their new lives.

The first year of Mary being missing was the worst for Eve. She was heartbroken at not knowing where she and Elizabeth were, and during that same year, she lost her dear brother Dru. Thomas had only recently written telling Eve that his father was unwell, but it was not considered to be serious. However, the next letter told her that Dru had slipped away in his sleep. He did not suffer and died peacefully, according to Thomas. He wanted Eve to know that Dru spoke a lot about her that final month of his life, and said how much he loved and missed her. They were all sorry that he could not have seen her one more time before he died. Thomas assured Eve that his father enjoyed life to the full, right up until his final days. He had been very happy living on the farm and pottering around looking after the chickens and geese, and Thomas told her it had been the best thing for her brother to have gone to Australia. Again, Eve cried her heart out. She had always told herself that she would visit Dru one day. Of course, that was never going to be very likely, but now it was too late.

By the fourth year of not knowing where her daughter was, the stress of it was taking its toll on Eve. It had aged her and damaged her spirit. She was becoming something of a recluse. She did not go out very much, even locally, and her trips to London had ceased; she could not cope physically or emotionally with the endless and fruitless searching. Eve had almost given up hope of ever seeing her daughter and granddaughter again.

She made fewer remedies and pastes these days. Those she did make were only from the herbs and plants she grew in her own garden. She no longer walked the fields and woods and dales around Elmsley searching for flowers, fungi, wild herbs and plants, and those who wanted Eve's mixtures collected them from her cottage. She still had visits from folk wanting to be told things, and she no longer cared about the consequences of using her gifts. If she saw it, she told it. Two exceptionally severe winters in the area had been forecast by her, and also an outbreak of cattle disease as well. Local farmers always listened if Mother Eve gave out one of her warnings. People living some distance away, as well as local people, often sought Eve's advice, as she called it, and listened to her thoughts about future events, as she called them. She still had 'unnatural' powers, according to the local rumours and there were still plenty of people alive in the village who could recount every time she was found to be correct in her prophecies over the years. The religious in the community, in their unremitting attempts to discredit Mother Eve, still declared her as being ungodly, but this largely fell on deaf ears. Eve's thoughts were too useful and too accurate to be forsaken.

Then one day, Eve happened to mention to someone she met in the street that she had recently been having frightening thoughts. In them, everything appeared black and there was death all around. She had no idea what these visions meant, and hoped it was not another pandemic coming to the village. Mother Eve's thoughts circulated rapidly around the village and local area, and were of some concern to those who believed in her gifts. Of course, to those that did not, she was accused of scaremongering. However, what was to transpire two months later made clear to her and others, exactly what she had seen. It was the 4th of September 1939, and news came into Elmsley that the Germans had invaded Poland. This had happened on the1st day of the month, and two days later, on the 3rd, Britain and France subsequently declared war on Germany. Everyone in the village and local farms were in a state of total disbelief and shock. Some said the news was utter nonsense, others argued it was true, but as the newspaper reports began to flow in, so the reality of the situation hit home. Many people in the community had not recovered from the previous war and its devastating effect on families in and around Elmsley. Now, just twenty years later, it was all happening again. Mothers and fathers, wives, sisters, aunts and girlfriends, began to fret at the prospect of their loved ones being called upon to fight, yet again. It was a dreadful time for the whole country and disastrous news for Eve's community.

Public meetings were held in the village hall to discuss the issues and men from the Government Ministry visited with war instructions and new laws. One of those was that there was to be enforced full-conscription on all males between the ages of 18 and 41 in Britain. Once again, the men and boys of the village and local farms were to be taken to fight for their country. Some of those working on the land and in the local factories were exempt, because they could not be replaced, but mostly, they were all called up. With the outbreak of yet another war, Eve became even more anxious at not knowing where Mary and Elizabeth were. She felt afraid and alone. Thankfully, James was still in contact with her and continued with his financial support, much of which Eve saved.

Over the past few years, he too had still been searching for Mary. James was too old to travel backwards and forwards to London himself, but he had employed agents to look for her. It seemed incredible, but she could not be found. Eve began to wonder if they had left the city altogether, but in her heart, she did not think so. Her only consolation was that George would be too old now to be called up to fight, so at least Mary and the girl would not be left to cope on their own. Another year passed and there was still no contact from Mary. Then, on the morning of the 8th September, some dreadful news came over the wireless. London had been bombed the day before; the dock areas having been particularly badly hit. Eve was sick with fear, but tried to convince herself that Mary and her granddaughter were safe. Perhaps they had moved away from Stepney after all, she told herself?

Perhaps they were not even in London?

Then, the following day, news came in a telegram to Eve. George and Mary were dead. Eve was so shocked she could not speak or move from her chair for some hours. She felt as if her whole life had ended. Her daughter's house had taken a direct hit by a bomb. The family were sheltering under the stairs, but that was not much protection from the blast. Elizabeth was not killed though; rescued by a policeman, who pulled her out alive, and fairly uninjured, from the rubble. Mary had left Eve's address with the vicar of their local church and instructions that, in the event of anything happening to both her and George, then her mother, Mrs Eve Locke, was to take their daughter Elizabeth and look after her. The vicar, Reverend Petty, had notified the police in Stepney of this letter immediately after he heard the tragic news of the deaths of his parishioners. It was the following day when John Smithy, the new constable in Elmsley, came to Eve's cottage with the contents of this letter, and asked if she would travel to London to collect her granddaughter. Eve immediately prepared herself to go there. Before she left home, she telephoned the Reverend from the police house, telling him that she intended to bring her daughter and her husband back to Elmsley for burial and could he please tell her where their bodies were.

Every horror went through Eve's heart and mind that night before she left for London. Somehow James had heard the news of the deaths of George and his daughter Mary, on a visit to his son at Addington House and he called immediately at Eve's cottage. After her complete shock at seeing him standing on her doorstep, she invited James into her home. He was distraught at his daughter's death and openly wept. In the many long distressing hours that followed, James and Eve held each other, cried, talked, cried again and consoled one another. Eve was glad he was there and glad she could share that night in James's company. Their history was set aside as they discussed the arrangements for bringing Mary and George's coffins, and the young Elizabeth, who did not even know her grandmother, home. James told Eve that he would pay for everything and have his agent organise the entire proceedings for her.

He was as good as his word. Eve was to travel to London and collect her granddaughter from the hospital, where she was being cared for. They would stay at a hotel whilst an agent of James made all of the arrangements at the funeral parlour in Stepney, where the Reverend Petty told Eve that Mary and George's bodies were being held. The agent arranged for them to deliver the coffins to the station and have them loaded on to the train to take them back to

Yorkshire. Another agent in Danberry would make further arrangements to collect the coffins from the station and have them taken, by hearse, to Saint Guthlac Church. He would also make the preparations with the Reverend Arnold for the funeral and burials. Eve would give her approval to everything upon her return to Elmsley. And so it was set in motion.

Eve was taken to Elizabeth on her arrival at the hospital. The girl sat, obviously traumatised, staring silently out of the window. Eve carefully approached her and spoke.

"Elizabeth?" she said softly. "Ah'm yar grandmother. Ah've come to take ya home wi' me." Elizabeth turned to look at her. Eve could see some cuts and bruises about her face; superficial the doctor had told Eve, before she entered Elizabeth's room.

"Where's my mummy and my dad?" Elizabeth asked Eve.

"Have ya not been told?" Eve asked her calmly. Elizabeth stared blankly at her. She looked confused and tearful. Eve went over and sat near her. "Yar mammy an' daddy, they wor killed my sweet."

"I don't know who you are," Elizabeth said.

"Ah know," Eve replied. "Ah'm yar grandmother. Ah'm yar mammy's mother. My name is Eve." Elizabeth continued to stare at her.

"I want to go home," she said and began to sob. "I want my mummy."

"Elizabeth," Eve said. "Yar mammy's gone my sweet child. Sh' wor killed in the bombin' of yar house. Yar mammy and yar daddy wor killed. Ah'm sorry lass. Ah can't believe it myself. My poor Mary's been taken. There's just you an' me now." Eve was trying hard not to get upset for the child's sake. Elizabeth did not respond to what she had just told her, but just continued to cry. Eve sat in silence whilst her granddaughter sobbed for the next hour, screamed into her pillow, and walked the floor in anguish. Eve knew exactly how she felt. Later that evening, Elizabeth left the hospital with Eve and they went back to the hotel. It would be a long, gruelling and desperately sad journey home the next day.

The train was held over at London and Blackwell Station, whilst Mary and George's coffins were taken aboard the end carriage, and then Eve and her granddaughter took their seats in the coach next to it. The following few days happened in a blur for Eve. As arranged, the funerals were held at Saint Guthlac Church and Mary and George were interred next to one another in the churchyard. James had ordered Reverend Arnold to have them laid to rest in his private part of the cemetery. James went to the funeral, much to the interest of some folk in Elmsley. The Wades also attended of course. They were content to know that George was being given a decent Christian funeral and took James's gift of the burial plot for their son as a goodwill gesture, given that George had been a hero in the First World War.

Elizabeth had barely said two words to Eve or anyone else since she had been brought from the hospital in London. She remained traumatised by the loss of her parents. Added to this was that she did not know what to make of the village, the language and her grandmother. It was all very strange and foreign to her and she hated every minute of being there.

The child was almost thirteen. Even at this tender age, she was beautiful. Her dark brown eyes matched the colour of her long dark hair. Her complexion was peachy with slight rosy cheeks. Her figure was developing and showed the promise of a slender and curvy body. Eve was stunned at how lovely her granddaughter was. She certainly took after Mary in many ways, except her eyes, which held a glint of determination and strength that her daughter did not have. James had found it difficult to take his eyes from his granddaughter at Mary and George's funeral. He was also astonished at the girl's looks and was proud to know she was his flesh and blood. In a quiet moment after the service, he reassured Eve that he would look after both of them and promised her financial help towards Elizabeth's future. He told Eve that he had made his will and that he would make sure they were secure when he dies.

Now Eve had to try and help her granddaughter settle into a new life, one that was very different from the one she left behind in London. This was going to be very difficult. Elizabeth was distressed, angry, confused, hurt and deeply sad. It was going to take Eve some time to calm her down and mend her broken heart. Eve also had to deal with her own loss, which brought back all the pain of losing her only other child, Seb, her husband Joseph, and her mother and father and of her dear Anna. Eve's heart needed mending as well.

A further problem arose, just days after the funerals. Martha Wade wanted her and her family, quite naturally, to be able to see Elizabeth. It transpired that she had seen her granddaughter over the years periodically, so Elizabeth knew her vaguely. Eve was not against this happening, in spite of the way the Wades had treated her in the past, but she wanted to set some conditions in place before agreeing to let the Wades spend time with her granddaughter. Eve insisted on them not vilifying her to Elizabeth or trying to impose any of their beliefs on to her. When Martha Wade heard this, she was furious and refused to 'obey' anything that Eve ordered. This placed Eve in a very difficult position.

She discussed the situation with Nathan when he visited her one evening. He thought she was mad to even contemplate letting the Wades near Elizabeth, but Eve wanted to be fair. She knew the pain of separation and would not want to inflict that on anyone. At the same time, she was not prepared to have them turn her granddaughter against her either. In the end, Eve decided to hold firm to her conditions. Martha would not agree to control her views and opinions of Eve and wanted Elizabeth to be brought up a Christian. Eve was not prepared to let herself be denigrated and told them that Elizabeth would be allowed to choose her own path, not have it determined by others. And so, for the time being at least, the Wades were refused access to the girl. Allen Wade was not about to accept this however.

Chapter 33

Allen, of all the three of George's brothers, was the most unpleasant. He was an oaf. He lumbered along and had the manners of a pig. Eve had always disliked the fellow intensely. He was rude and ignorant, not just to her, but to many others in the village. Eve thought that perhaps he had suffered a trauma at birth, or had an accident. But whatever the cause, he was mentally slow and often aggressive. Allen was the youngest of the seven Wade children, George being the eldest, and, along with two of his sisters, remained at home with his mother. Old Mr Wade had died just after the First World War, not long after George returned from the front.

Allen took one look at Elizabeth and was instantly besotted with her. Eve did not realise this until she saw him pass her granddaughter in the street one afternoon. He was fawning all over her in a very sexual and completely unacceptable manner. Poor Elizabeth was totally embarrassed and frightened by the man. He was tall and very broad and stood over her young frame quite menacingly.

When Martha told Allen that Eve would not let them have Elizabeth visit their farm, he threw a tantrum and smashed some things in the kitchen. This was not unusual behaviour from him, but

Martha was worried all the same. She had been complaining to her son about Eve, but Allen became very angry and as he destroyed things, dashing them to the floor, he stated that this was what he intended to do to Eve, if she did not let them have Elizabeth. He wanted her to come and live with them at the farm. He fantasised what he would do with Elizabeth if she were living under the same roof as him.

No, the situation had back-fired on Martha, and now she regretted firing up her son's temper. His sisters tried to talk to Allen and tell him that it was never intended that Elizabeth live with them, just perhaps visit, but he would not hear any of it. In Allen's mind, he wanted Elizabeth in the house with him and that was it. After listening for weeks to her son demanding she go and fetch her granddaughter and bring her to the farm, Martha sent one of her daughters to warn Eve. The sister turned up on Eve's doorstep one evening and told her that Martha had sent a message that she should to be mindful of Allen. The sister explained his growing obsession with Elizabeth and that he wanted her to live with them. Martha did not think he would do anything silly, but she reported that her son was not easily controlled by her these days and she could not keep him on the farm and away from Elmsley. Eve thanked the sister and asked her to take back her gratitude to Martha as well. She then set about protecting Elizabeth from her uncle.

One evening however, just as Eve was cooking supper, Allen knocked on the door of her cottage. She called out to see who was visiting so late in the day. He answered and asked, quite nicely, to be invited in. Eve was reluctant, but all the same, she opened her door to him. Allen walked in friendly enough and greeted her and Elizabeth, who was drawing some pictures at the table; she took after her mother in artistic skill. Eve and Elizabeth returned his greeting and Eve offered him some tea. He accepted and was served with tea and a slice of fruit cake. The conversation was polite and simple, for a while. Then Allen addressed Elizabeth directly, asking her if she would like to go and live with him and his family at their farm. The girl was unable to reply and looked to Eve for help.

"Ya don't 'ave ti get 'er say so," Allen told Elizabeth. She rose from her chair and moved across the room to Eve, fearful and confused. "Ya can make up yar own mind," he persisted.

"Ah think ya'd better go now," Eve told Allen calmly. He stood up, having to stoop as his head touched the low beams across the ceiling.

"Ah just come ti ask little Elizabeth if sh' wanted ti come an' live wi' us," he replied aggressively. "Ya don't 'ave any more right ti 'ave 'er than us."

Eve held steady. "Ah'll ask ya to leave now Allen,"

she repeated calmly. "Elizabeth is stayin' here. Sh's not goin' to go an' live wi' you. Sh's livin' wi' me."

"Ah don't 'ear 'er sayin' that," Allen said loudly, moving slightly towards Eve. She told Elizabeth to go upstairs to her room and lock the door, which she did. Eve then took a deep breath.

"Ah'll only say it once more Allen. Ah want ya to go," she stared the man in the face. He tried to glare back at her, but was shifting his eyes, finding it difficult to focus on hers. He shuffled his feet about for a few seconds, looked at the floor then made his way to the front door. He turned as if to say something, but Eve put her fingers to her lips in a 'silence' gesture and Allen could not, and did not, speak his intended words. Soon after, he had gone. Eve locked her door behind him. Minutes later, Elizabeth came back downstairs.

"I don't like him Nanna," she said to Eve. Eve smiled. That was the first time her granddaughter had ever called her Nanna.

"Don't you worry about him," she told Elizabeth. "Ah'll make sure he don't come near ya again. But ah need ya to tell me if any boy or man around here ever tries to talk to ya or touch ya. Ah need to know straight away. Remember that my sweet, won't ya?" Elizabeth nodded.

Allen Wade, it was hoped, would not trouble Elizabeth again. He tried to speak to her one day in

Elmsley however, but his throat closed up, instantly. He thought he was going to choke and found himself gasping for air. Eve believed that after such an experience, he would not attempt it again. But Allen Wade had a low level of intelligence and clearly did not understand what was happening. Frustrated, he turned on his mother and accused her of not wanting to take in her granddaughter and of not trying to get her away from Eve Locke. On one occasion, he struck her about the face in temper at not getting his own way. Eve heard about this incident through village gossip and felt some pity for Martha. But she could not help the woman. Firstly, she was not asked to interfere, and secondly, if she did, the only way to stop Allen would be to immobilise or remove him and Martha would not really want that. She needed her son to help work the farm. Whilst Eve thought perhaps Martha was actually reaping what she had sown, her concerns about Allen remained. She was not wrong.

Eve was out in the village buying some food when she came across Wade in the street. He began by shouting at her, then he threatened to hurt her, then he attacked, throwing her to the ground. Eve struggled to get up; it was not easy at her age. But Wade pushed her again and she fell back on her knee, which hurt her badly. Fortunately, the butcher, Mr Harper, who saw what was happening out of his shop window, came to Eve's rescue and ordered Wade to stop his attack. Harper helped her from the ground and stood with her until Allen had moved off down the road. Eve was shaken and in pain. After she gathered herself together, she limped home, where Elizabeth attended her grandmother's badly cut knee.

"What 'ave ya done ti our Allen?" his sister Agnes shouted at Eve when she opened the door to her three days later. "What 'ave ya done ti 'im?"

"Ah've done nothin' to yar brother," Eve responded. "Ya have nay right to come to my home. What are ya thinkin' woman?"

"'E's not come 'ome," Agnes shouted again. "We know ya've done somethin' ti 'im." Eve stared at the woman. She did not know what to say to her, as she was not really interested in what had happened to her brother. But Agnes was going to tell her anyway.

The Wades were expecting Allen home from the village after he had delivered some chickens to the butcher shop. They had spoken to Mr Harper the following morning, when Allen had not returned the evening before. He told them about him attacking Eve in the street, just after he left his shop. Harper added that he intervened before Allen really hurt Eve, but by the look of her, he had already caused her some pain. Fearing Eve, the Wades had assumed that she would have made Allen pay for what he did to her. They had searched for him in the whole area, as did some friends from neighbouring farms, but to no avail. There was no sign of Allen. He did not drink, so excessive alcohol was not a factor, and his horse and cart were found tied up in the village, where he had left them, so he must have been on foot.

"If ya never 'ad anythin' ti do wi' Allen's disappearin', then can ya not tell us if yar can 'see' what's 'appened ti 'im?" Agnes asked Eve, who was stunned at such a request. For as long as she could remember the Wade family had always castigated her, calling her evil for having the second sight. Now, when they want help, they thought they could simply ask for her assistance and she would give it.

"If he's walkin', then he can't be far," Eve said. "Ya just have to keep lookin'. Tis not cold out, so that won't have killed 'im. An' he's strong. Just keep lookin'." Agnes left and returned to her mother's farm, reporting back on what Eve had said. But Martha was not convinced that she did not cause some harm to her son.

Two days later, they found Allen. He was sitting upright, leaning against a tree, just outside of the village. He was obviously missed during the first search, as he was facing away from the road. A more thorough search of the area however, had located his body. The police were called and enquiries began. Of course, Martha Wade and her family accused Eve, but there were no obvious injuries on his body and the police, quite sensibly, could not see how a seventy-six-year-old woman could have killed Allen Wade and then sat his very large, heavy body up against a tree. It was deemed to be simply ridiculous. A later post mortem found that he had died of a massive heart attack and the following inquest decided that he must have sat down and simply died; no other logical explanation could be found. Why he was walking along that particular road leading out of the village, having left behind his horse and cart in Elmsley, nobody could explain, but there was no reason to think that Allen Wade had died in suspicious circumstances. The Wades remained unconvinced that Eve was not to blame for his death, and made their beliefs known in the community, even though there was certainly no legal case for Eve, or anyone else to answer either.

After the unfortunate death of Allen Wade had slightly faded in most people's minds, Eve and Elizabeth settled down to something like a peaceful life. Eve taught her granddaughter at home. Elizabeth tried going to a local school, but found it very hard to fit in. She spoke differently, and acted differently from the other youngsters her own age. Elizabeth was also singled out for being the granddaughter of Mother Eve, and was constantly bullied for being a witch, just like her. Some parents of other children at the school did not want their sons and daughters mixing with her because she was a descendant of the Shetcliffes; a name that echoed down the centuries and was still tainted in the eyes of a number of Elmsley folk.

Soon after Elizabeth reached the age of thirteen, Eve introduced her remedy book to her granddaughter and Elizabeth was very enthusiastic about studying the traditional healing ways. She soon learned about the flowers, plants and fungi and wild herbs that were used to make up the remedies and curing pastes, and where to find them. Like the females in her family line before her, Elizabeth became a regular sight in the fields and hills and woodlands around Elmsley, gathering ingredients for her grandmother's cures. Eve also began to pass on to Elizabeth the old knowledge and she was a willing, eager and very promising student. Mary and George had brought their daughter up in the Christian faith and Eve did not prevent Elizabeth from continuing in those beliefs if she wanted to. But the girl chose to follow the path that Eve showed her and was happy to take on her inheritance. Over the next year or so, a great love built up between the ageing Eve and the young vivacious Elizabeth. Eve told her granddaughter all about her mother and how she grew up with her loving brother Seb, and how they lost him in the Great War. She told Elizabeth, now known as Lizzy to Eve, stories about their ancestors, of her own mother Mary and grandmother, Elisa, and what had happened to them in their lives. Eve spoke of her Granny Anna and of her dear husband Joseph, and of her brother Dru and his sons, who went to live in Australia. She showed her photographs of their families and also pictures of Sarah and Ben and their children. Elizabeth would sit leaning against her grandmother's knees, listening to these tales. She gradually began to feel at home with Eve and living in Elmsley, although it was difficult to get on with youngsters her own age. Many girls would not befriend her and were a little jealous of the beauty that had arrived from London to occupy the fantasies of the local lads. She always had young admirers chasing after her wherever she went. Elizabeth found this attention hard to cope with. She was mostly alone, save for one or two friendships she did manage to make occasionally, but these did not last long. Her education and intelligence were superior to her peers and her city ways, too progressive and foreign for their parents.

The terrible tragedy of losing both her mother and father, and the memories of the bombing raids faded slightly as time passed. Eve made sure that her granddaughter did not hear much of the radio, which talked nightly of the horrors of what were happening around the country's cities. Stories were constantly coming in of the bombing of nearby Hull, which was said to have been attacked almost as badly as London, and the villagers did occasionally see German planes flying overhead, either on their way to or from their bombing campaigns. Of course, Eve could not make Elizabeth immune from it all. The war, although their village was never bombed itself, was all around them. News regularly came in of men from the community losing their lives, and at these terrible times, the atmosphere in the whole area was one of loss and grief. Eve tried to help by talking to the bereaved; it was the least she could do.

Elizabeth was growing up fast. Her childlike figure was blossoming into a curvaceous and sensual figure. However, her mind was not maturing as quickly as her body and she was naive and innocent in her actions. Eve grew concerned, as she became aware of the growing attention being paid to her granddaughter, not just by the young lads in the village but from some of the older men as well. She needed to watch Elizabeth very carefully and try to instil in her an understanding of the dangers of showing too much of her body in public and also how some of her movements could be deemed provocative to a man. This is a difficult task when a young teenage girl does not know about the sexual act, or have the slightest idea of how a man is aroused. But Eve managed to help Elizabeth gain some awareness of her effect on the opposite sex. Eve also had to accept that Elizabeth would soon start to be interested in boys as well.

She was now almost sixteen and had been seeing her period for almost two years. Eve explained very clearly and candidly to her about sex, pregnancy and birthing and all the issues surrounding them. Elizabeth was bright, and grasped very quickly what being a woman was all about. Eve encouraged her granddaughter to talk freely about her fears and confusion regarding boys and sex. But what she could not do, was help Elizabeth go through the trauma of growing up and all the hormonal changes that accompanied that.

As she entered her sixteenth year, it was almost as if a light had been switched on in her head. Elizabeth became sullen, argumentative, miserable and sometimes impossible to speak to. She disappeared for long spells in her room and Eve was struggling to keep control of her. Elizabeth would begrudgingly help mix up the remedies for her grandmother, before going out, sometimes for hours on end. Eve would ask her where she was going, but her questions were met with an angry response from Elizabeth for her to be left alone, before the girl would run out and slam the front door behind her. A neighbour once told Eve that she had seen her granddaughter some miles away, walking alone on the moors. This terrified Eve and she tried to speak to her about it, but just got the same response. All Eve could do was give Elizabeth as much protection as she could and hope that her granddaughter would eventually get through these testing years and settle down.

That year was a great strain on Eve. She was no longer a young woman and was finding the emotional outbursts of Elizabeth hard to deal with at times. And then, early the following year, in the space of two months, Eve had two items of dreadful news to deal with. Firstly, Nathan Morley died. It had been a very cold and damp winter, and now, going into spring, the rains persisted. He went down with what appeared to be influenza, Eve eventually heard, which rapidly turned to pneumonia. His brother, John, got him into the cottage hospital at Ashton quite quickly, but Nathan passed away suddenly that night. Eve was beside herself with grief. She was also angry that John did not call on her for help. She would have gone to Nathan if she had known. As it was, he had been dead two days before she even found out he had been taken ill.

There were very few people at the funeral. Many in the village were sick of death and few of Nathan's relatives attended, save John, a sister and her husband, and a couple of friends. Both parents had passed, so it was a quiet affair. The family owned plots in the churchyard, so Nathan was able to be buried next to his parents and his two brothers, William and Henry. John said very little to Eve that day, but he did thank her for going to Nathan's funeral. He understood that a friendship had developed between them over the years, even if he did not know how deep it was. John had kept away from Eve for decades and was still very much afraid of her. He also feared that with Nathan gone, he was somehow less safe. What actually happened to John was unfortunate. The day after laying his brother to rest, he became ill with the same symptoms as Nathan had. Now it was confirmed to be a particular strain of influenza that was the cause of both Nathan's death and John's illness and rumours abounded that they could have caught it from some of their animals. Within two days, John was also admitted to Ashton Hospital with pneumonia and after a short time, subsequently died. Eve did not attend his funeral.

She was barely coming to terms with the loss of Nathan however, when she heard further bad news. James had been taken ill. Eve found this out because his son, James Addington-Barlow called at her home early one evening to tell her. Elizabeth was out walking, fortunately. Eve nearly passed out when she opened her front door to the man; he looked so much like his father, just a generation younger. She had seen the young James before, but always at a distance. He was handsome, with much the same build as his father. He was not quite as friendly however. Eve invited him into her home but he looked around the room in some discomfort at being there.

"I've come to talk to you about matters concerning my father, James Barlow," James said to her. Eve offered him to sit down, but he declined. The young James was tall and looked awkward standing in her low-ceilinged cottage. Eventually, unable to sustain a bent neck, and because of his war-injured leg, he reluctantly sat down. "My father has asked me to come and speak to you on his behalf, as he is sick."

"What's the matter wi' him?" Eve asked.

"I'm not at liberty to say," he replied curtly. Eve looked hard at him.

"Please tell me what's the matter wi' yar father," she insisted. "He's my friend," she added calmly.

"I know what you are to my father," James said bluntly and stared at Eve. She gathered from that remark and from the man's countenance that his father had told him something of their relationship.

"An' what is that?" she asked.

"My father has explained your association with him," James told her. "I understand that you had an affair that resulted in your having a child between you. Your daughter's name was Mary, recently deceased." He fidgeted uncomfortably in his chair. Eve offered him a drink, which was refused. "I understand that my father has always acknowledged his daughter and has given you and her an allowance over the years and still does. My father informs me that there is now a granddaughter living with you, Mary's daughter, by the name of Elizabeth Wade." Eve had sat silently listening to the young James making this pronouncement. She was very surprised to hear him say what he was saying. As she listened however, it struck her that this was beginning to sound like a death-bed confession.

"How ill is James?" she · asked, now more concerned.

"Very ill," the young James replied matter-of-factly. Eve became distressed.

"Is he in hospital?" she asked.

"He was, but he wanted to die at home," James said.

"Can ah go to him?" she asked.

"No," James told her. "My mother does not know anything of you and she must never know either."

"Please," Eve pleaded. "There must be a way fer me to see James. Has he not asked fer me?"

"He has asked to see you," James admitted, "but my mother is by his bedside most of the time. She will not leave my father. I really don't see how you can visit him. It's impossible." Eve sat down upset. James was dying and she wanted to be with him, touch him, kiss him, look at him, one last time.

"Please," she said again. "Ya must find a way."

"I can't make you any promises, but I will try," James told her. "But this is not for your sake," he rounded on Eve. "You had no right to have an affair with my father. He was married. You had no right to do this to my family." Eve looked at him.

"Do what?" she asked. "Have ah ever interfered wi' yar family? 'Ave ah ever caused yar father any trouble? It wor James, bless him, who wanted to do right by me. Ah've never asked him fer nowt, not fer me or Mary, ever." She could understand James's disdain of her for loving his father, but she was not about to be castigated by the man as being some kind of parasite. What did he know, really, of what passed between her and James?

"No, you haven't," he replied. "And that's the only reason I'm here. My father asked me to speak to you and tell you that he does not have long to live. He asked me to pass this letter directly into your hands. I have no idea of its contents, but he told me to assure you that he has set aside some allowance for you and your granddaughter upon his death." Eve took the letter from James and placed it on her table, unread. "Well, I have delivered my father's message and letter to you, so now I will leave," he said, getting up. Eve would have liked to spend a short time speaking to James, but it was clear that he did not want to talk to her.

"Ah've allus loved James," she told him as he made his way to her front door.

"I am not interested in anything you have to say about my father," he replied. "I will honour his commitment to you, as he has directed me, but only if you stay completely away from our family and keep your word never to reveal our connections. We want nothing to do with you or your granddaughter. My father said that we could rely on your integrity and your discretion. I hope that's true."

"Ah don't care about the money. Ah just want to see yar father." Eve said. James did not reply, just turned sharply and left. Eve then tried to gather her thoughts. She felt desperate again, just as she had done all those years ago when she saw Jayne Addington take the arm of James in Ashton and then they both walked away from her. Later that night, when Lizzy was home and fast asleep in her bed, Eve worked to make it possible for her to see James. She spent some hours in silence, holding the one item she had that belonged to him. It was a button from his jacket that she found on the floor of Joseph's bakery, after they had made love that evening. She had kept it in her special box. All those years past, all those memories saved, all those moments lost. As she sat holding her small treasure, a cold realisation flowed through Eve's heart. She suddenly knew it was too late; James had passed away. She could not begin to grieve though. Eve half hoped that her feelings were wrong, but she had a knowing that she could eventually not ignore. By the morning light, Eve had said goodbye to the greatest love of her life. Now she would read his letter.

My dearest Eve,

I wanted you to know that I have loved you with all of my heart, ever since that first day when I saw you walking towards me along the lane. There has never been a moment when I have not regretted what I did to you. I made a terrible mistake and I have paid for that. I am only sorry if I have caused you pain. I have never forgiven myself for turning away from you.

We had a beautiful daughter, our Mary, and it broke my heart when she was so cruelly taken from us. I am so very pleased and grateful that I lived to see our granddaughter, Elizabeth, who will grow up into a beautiful woman.

I have left my son, James, in charge of the allowance for you and the child. He will have spoken to you by now, so you will know that I told him about us and our love. It is up to him whether or not he can forgive me, but I have charged him with showing you respect. There is a matter however, that I have not discussed with James or any other person alive, but I am now about to tell you. This story should not die with me; it belongs to you.

Before my father-in-law, the old Squire Edmond Addington died, he confided in me a secret that only a very few people ever knew about. He told me this in confidence, but instructed me to use this information if need be to protect your mother and you and your brother Dru, from any member of his family, especially Frederick. This is what Edmond told me.

When they were both very young, your grandmother, Elisa Shetcliffe and he, were lovers. Edmond said that he adored and loved her passionately, and had it not been for their coming from completely different worlds, he would have married her. Elisa fell pregnant. Edmond's father, the then Squire, when he found out about your grandmother and the baby, ordered his son to cut all ties with her. It would have been scandalous and ruinous for his family for them to have any association with the Shetcliffes, who were not only from a low class, but had a bad reputation in the area. The Squire also offered Jabez, Elisa's father, who worked for him, to pay for his daughter to be sent away to have the child, and then to give it away. But Jabez and Maria, Elisa's mother, refused, as did Elisa. She had no intention of giving up her baby.

What then transpired was that your grandmother stayed in the village and gave birth to a little girl, who

511

she called Mary. Edmond's father set over to Jabez and his family a cottage and some land, that which you now own, in exchange for absolute secrecy as to who the father of Elisa's child was. Both parties kept their word. So, Eve, your grandfather was Squire Edmond Addington. He was your mother's father. The Addington blood runs through your veins.

It is up to you what you do with this information. I think it is only right that you know your grandmother's secret. I have instructed my solicitor to deliver to you all of the signed documents from Edmond Addington, proclaiming this account to be the absolute truth.

All that is left is for me to do is to say goodbye to you my love. I fear that we shall not see each other again, as my time is approaching fast.

Please forgive me.

James.

Eve read the letter many times. She was heartbroken and dismayed. For the first time, she believed that James had truly loved her. He had been kind and generous towards her over the years, but that could have been guilt, or honour and decency, all of which James had. Now she felt his love. Regarding the old Squire Edmond, Eve was astonished to know he was her grandfather, and yet, when she thought back to the time she stood before him when she was a young girl, younger than

Elizabeth was now, she remembered a few seconds, a very few moments, when he looked at her in a particular way. Yes of course she now realised, the Squire looked at her with certain recognition. Eve had always been told that she looked like her grandmother, Elisa. Perhaps he saw his beloved in her face? Perhaps that was why he showed leniency towards her that day in the court room? And to think, Frederick Addington was her and Dru's cousin. More inconceivable to Eve was that Jayne Addington, James's wife, was also. She, Eve Locke, was the cousin of the woman who took away the love of her life. That was very difficult for her to digest.

From Eve's mother's life story, it would appear that Mary never knew who her father was. But Eve was not so sure that her Granny Anna did not know. Her mother Mary once told her that Elisa, her mother, had very few secrets from her little adopted sister. But what would she, Eve, now do with this knowledge? She herself had not told Elizabeth who her real grandfather was. She had not lied to her granddaughter, but the girl assumed that Joseph had been her mother's father, and Eve had not encouraged her to think differently. Any further complication of the family line might be just too confusing for Elizabeth. So Eve decided to keep it from her, at least until her death, after which her granddaughter would find out from her story. Then it would be there for Elizabeth to do with what she will.

Chapter 34

Eve could not, of course, attend James's funeral. It was decided by his family that he should be buried in Swithindale, in the churchyard of Saint Olave's, an old parish church near his estate. Instead, she took a slow walk out of the village to the wooden gate at Britchet Lane, where she placed a simple bunch of flowers and stood for some time, thinking about James and the times they used to sit on the gate and chat and laugh, before running off across the field. He was now physically gone to Eve, but not to her heart. He would be part of the precious memories she stored and often, in quiet moments, recall.

The year that followed James's death saw another hard winter, and as the spring approached, news came into the village that the German army was retreating. The end of the war seemed in sight. Elizabeth was now a young woman of seventeen and she spent as little time as possible at home in the cottage. Eve understood that her granddaughter wanted to spread her wings, but she feared that Elizabeth was still too young to be sensible. Then, one afternoon, the girl ran indoors screaming and crying hysterically. Eve tried to find out what had happened to her, but Elizabeth would not speak. She just ran to her room and locked herself in, not coming out for hours. Eve was concerned and pressed Elizabeth very hard to find out what had gone on, once she eventually emerged later that night. After much coaxing, she told Eve that she had not been harmed in any way, she was just very upset. Elizabeth, according to her story, had been seeing a young man for some time, but his brother had found them together and now she feared that his family would separate them. Eve tried to find out who the boy was, but all her granddaughter would tell her was that he was the son of a very rich family and, knowing they would not let them see each other, they met in secret. This was not good news for Eve. She demanded to know who the boy was, but Elizabeth flatly refused to tell her.

She would soon find out however. James Addington-Barlow called at Eve's home a few days later. Eve sent Elizabeth to her room after inviting the man in. The young James stood before her, looking even more unfriendly than at their previous meeting. He was clearly very angry and came straight to the point.

"Your granddaughter has been having a relationship with my brother's son, Toby," he told her. "I need hardly tell you that this has to be stopped immediately." Eve nodded an acknowledgement of what she had just heard. She hardly knew what to say; the entire picture emerged before her eyes. "My brother, Charles Addington-

516

Barlow, has been told about our father's indiscretion with you. I had no choice, once I realised who his son was secretly meeting. I have to tell you now Mrs Locke, there will be no further allowance given to you or your granddaughter from the Addington-Barlow estate. You have broken our trust and our arrangement." Eve went to say something in her defence, in her granddaughter's defence, but, looking at the superior expression on the young James's face, she could not bother herself too much.

"Elizabeth does not know who Toby is to her," she did say however.

"Your granddaughter was trying to seduce my nephew," James turned on Eve. "Toby is just a young man, barely seventeen, and knows no better. Clearly, your granddaughter has done this sort of thing before." James looked at Eve scornfully. "The boy has been sent away and will never see her again. Do you understand what I am telling you?" James mouthed slowly and loudly, as if Eve were deaf and stupid. She did not reply immediately, just studied him quietly for some moments before speaking very deliberately and in the same manner as James had spoken to her.

"Please leave my home," she told him. "Ah'll ask ya to go now. Ya've done what ya came here to do, an' ya've said what ya came here to say. An' Squire Addington-Barlow," she added, "never speak that way about my granddaughter again. Sh's just an innocent child. And, Sir, make sure that ya never come to my door again either." He glared at Eve, then turned and left. When James was gone, Elizabeth crept down the stairs.

"What did he say to you Nanna?" she asked nervously.

"He said ya wor seein' his nephew, an' that they've sent him away," Eve told her. It was no good lying to the girl. "Ya have to let this lad go Lizzy. He's not fer you." Elizabeth did not take this news well and screamed her way back upstairs and slammed the door. Eve heard her crying well into the night. It could not be helped. Elizabeth could not be told the truth, not at this time. If she was in love with this lad Toby, then it would be too traumatic for her to hear that she was related to him, that they were cousins. Eve did not know how far their relationship had gone, but if they had performed sexual intercourse, then Elizabeth must not find out they shared the same bloodline, in more than one sense. She was far too immature to be given this information therefore Eve had to remain silent, at least for now.

She tried to find out what had gone on between her granddaughter and Toby, but Elizabeth went silent about the whole affair and refused to talk about it or even hear the boy's name mentioned. Eve could see how desperately upset she was and understood her pain only too well, but she was unable to help. This was something that Eve had little control over and her granddaughter would have to find her own way through it.

Elizabeth had just barely started to recover from Toby being sent away, when she heard that he had been married off to a girl from another wealthy family. This news almost totally broke her spirit as well as her heart. It took months for Elizabeth to come out of the deep depression she went into over this whole affair. But, little by little, she came through it.

Once Eve was able to speak to her about what had happened, she told her granddaughter all about losing the love of her life as well and how she understood her heartache. From this experience, Eve and her granddaughter seemed to grow closer, and as time went on Elizabeth calmed down and became more settled with her life. She stayed at home more and the only time the pair ever argued was when Elizabeth brought up London, and how much she missed the city and wanted to go back there. She put it to Eve that she should go to a college or find work in London; there was little in the village that she could do, and transport to any of the local towns was limited. But Eve would make a great fuss about her going to the city. She was afraid for Elizabeth and wanted to keep her as close as possible for as long as she could.

But as the years passed, Eve knew her time was approaching. There were things she needed to settle and get in order. To this aim, she saw a solicitor in Ashton and had made over to Elizabeth all of her worldly goods. Throughout the years, with the generous allowance from James, she had managed to save some money. This she would pass to her granddaughter, along with the cottage and the small plot of land behind it. Apart from the contents of her home and some few pieces of jewellery, there were the family books. Elizabeth knew and understood what was in the books and also what their value was. She had been allowed to see the contents of the remedy book and had been learning over the years from the second book. The third, containing her family's stories going back many generations, remained a mystery until she would claim her inheritance.

Eve arranged her funeral with the Reverend Arnold. She was to be laid to rest next to her daughter Mary. James had signed over one of his plots to her when Mary died, so that Eve could be assured a resting place near her dear child for eternity. She knew this would cause a commotion in the village, as many folk would find it hard to accept that she would be buried in that part of the churchyard. It was in the 'good' Christian part, not over on the north side, which was the only place a descendant of a Shetcliffe should ever be allowed to be interred, according to some folk in the community. But Eve did not care about that. She owned the burial plot, courtesy of James Barlow, so there was nothing they could do.

Again, as with the three previous years, winter came in early. It had already snowed twice and it was still only November. The evening before, heavy snow had fallen on Elmsley. Eve felt chilled and had not ventured far from the fireside all of that day. She sat in her mother's comfy chair, sipping some hot tea. Elizabeth went out early to do some shopping in the village, and then she planned to collect some holly from the old tree that bordered the end of the garden. She was going to make the winter wreaths.

It was very quiet in the cottage. Eve leaned over to switch the wireless on, but thought better of it, and was content to sit back in her chair and watch what was left of the day's cold, winter sun stream through the window, brighter than usual as it reflected off of the white snow. She was at peace. Her mind drifted back to her childhood with Dru and she thought about her Raggy Polly, which she still had, and she recalled sitting on the front step of her father's cottage, playing with her dolly. She remembered the smiling face of her grandmother Elisa, and how she used to kiss her forehead gently. She thought of her dear father, Thomas, and when he used to tease her and pretend he was asleep and then suddenly sit up, making her scream. She remembered her lovely mother Mary. How kind and gentle she was. How sweet her temper was. She thought of Granny Anna and recalled how upset she got when nobody would eat her fruit pie that day because it was not sweet enough, and then, when she tasted it, she realised she had not sugared it. How they all laughed. Eve then saw Joseph coming in and out of the cottage with his bread and cakes. She remembered their wedding day and how happy he looked. She thought about the days she birthed her daughter Mary and her son Seb. Joseph was a good father to both of them. How could she have lost them all? Eve began to weep, softly. In amongst her tears, she saw James. He was young and handsome, with his curly hair and long eyelashes. She remembered their love-making, when he pulled her to his warm body and they joined for the first and only time. She could still feel the sensation of absolute love and surrender. She thought about Dru's boys, Thomas and Edward, and Sarah and Ben and their three children. How grown they were all now. She remembered old friends; Margaret and her gossipy ways, and the quiet Nathan, such a gentle soul. All her loved ones...all gone to her. Eve was tired. She would just have a little sleep she told herself.

A shadow fell across the room as the sun disappeared behind yet another snow-laden cloud. The room became dim, save for the light of the fire, but it was warm and cosy and comfortable. Eve pulled her shawl around her more tightly, rested her head back and began to drift off. Elizabeth would not be long, she had told her grandmother, and when she returned, she would cook some supper for the pair of them. Eve closed her eyes, but thought she heard a noise that she was not used to and opened them again. Standing in the doorway, was her mother, Mary. Eve smiled. Mary held out her arms to her daughter and then spoke, telling her that it was time for her to leave. She had come to take her home.

Eve called to Elizabeth; she had just heard her granddaughter come in. Elizabeth immediately rushed into the room and over to her grandmother. She knelt down next to her and held her hand. Eve needed to say goodbye and to give Elizabeth, daughter of Mary Elizabeth Wade, granddaughter of Eve Maria Locke, great granddaughter of Mary Elizabeth Jennus, great, great granddaughter of Elisa Mary Shetcliffe, and descendant of Esobel Mary Shetcliffe, her last and final breath.

Chapter 35

The day after Eve had passed away, and whilst her body still lay in its coffin in the darkened front room of her home, there were some strange rumours rapidly spreading through the village. A neighbour, who had called early that morning to pay her respects to Elizabeth and her farewell to Eve, noticed some strange footprints in the snow. They belonged to something that had entered the village and then circled around Eve's cottage. In some frenzied state, she spoke of her find to others. Elmsley appeared to have had a visitor during the night, the night that Eve Maria Locke died. The visitor left behind what some believed was unnatural footmarks. These footprints were large and deep, and seemed to have been made by an upright-walking creature with two legs. However, the creature, it was said, had a horny covering of foot. In other words, it had cloven hooves. Where the tracks were deeper and wider, around Eve's home, the creature must have stood for a time, its weight widening the print and melting the snow about its hooves. From the small crowd that gathered outside the cottage later that morning to examine the footprints, a woman's voice quietly spoke out.

"They're the Devil's footmarks," she said "He must of come to take care of one of his own."

* * *

Elizabeth

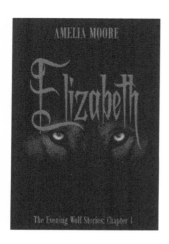

When the young, beautiful Elizabeth Wade goes to live and work in an isolated, rural North Yorkshire village as their school teacher, little did she know that she was to be accused of witchcraft and become the focus of suspicion, sexual desire and revenge, when a series of unexplained and terrible events befall the community.

It's the early 1950s and the people of Bridgeford are still steeped in superstition and fear of evil goings on in their midst. It is no surprise therefore that they turn on Elizabeth, a vulnerable and defenceless woman...or so she appeared to be.

Made in the USA
Charleston, SC
23 March 2013